THOMAS EAKINS

THOMAS EAKINS

Art, Medicine, and Sexuality in Nineteenth-Century Philadelphia

Amy Werbel

YALE UNIVERSITY PRESS

New Haven and London

Designed by Matthew Monk
Set in Janson by Matthew Monk
Printed in Singapore by CS Graphics

Library of Congress Cataloging-in-Publication Data
Werbel, Amy Beth.
Thomas Eakins : art, medicine, and sexuality in nineteenth-century Philadelphia / Amy Werbel.
p. cm.
Includes bibliographical references and index.
ISBN 978-0-300-11655-7 (alk. paper)
1. Eakins, Thomas, 1844–1916—Psychology. 2. Eakins, Thomas, 1844–1916—Sexual behavior. 3. Artists—Pennsylvania—Philadelphia—Attitudes. 4. Physicians—Pennsylvania—Philadelphia—Attitudes. 5. Philadelphia (Pa.)—Social life and customs—History—19th century. I. Title.
N6537.E3W47 2007
759.13—dc22
[B] 2006032500

A catalogue record for this book is available from the British Library.

The paper in this book meets the guidelines for permanence and durability of the Committee on Production Guidelines for Book Longevity of the Council on Library Resources.

10 9 8 7 6 5 4 3 2 1

For Fred, my Tom

CONTENTS

PREFACE

In 1985, I had the good fortune to sit in Lloyd Goodrich's living room on the Upper East Side of Manhattan. We drank tea, and for most of the interview his dry lips inhaled deeply on a cigarette that looked as though it had been planted there for several decades. He was an old man then, and I was a senior in college, working on an honors thesis about some drawings attributed to Thomas Eakins. He helped me with my project, and toward the end of the hour he looked into my eyes and advised me not to listen to all the rumors about Eakins. At that point, I hadn't come into contact with too many rumors, but years later I read them all—many in the files he had collected during years spent interviewing the surviving relatives, portrait subjects, and students who knew the artist.

Goodrich was old school. His world was John F. Kennedy, not Bill Clinton. He dutifully recorded all those stories about Eakins, flattering and not so flattering, but he didn't believe the unpleasant ones, or maybe he just didn't believe that they should be written about in detail. Many historians who love Eakins' paintings still wish for an era in which his accomplishments could be discussed without having to drag along the baggage of the scandals that dogged his life and followed him after death.

There is no doubt that Eakins was, and still is, a lightning rod for critical interpretation. He was smart enough to intuit many of the cultural land mines in his beloved hometown of Philadelphia—but then subversive enough to find ways to step on each one. The land mines were composed of assumptions and expectations about art, education, anatomy, gender, and sexuality. Mostly they consisted of conventions regarding the body—who could be looked at, studied, dissected, photographed, and depicted, by whom, and how. The problem of nudity, established in the colonial era, was never more difficult for American artists than it was in the late nineteenth century.

Eakins' response to the problems that faced American figure painters in this era often amounted to straightforward confrontation. He refused to limit his probing of humanity, or his teaching of art, using categories of class, race, sex, or age. Eakins instead intensely studied all the bodies around him with the eyes of a trained anatomist, and depicted them without hyperbole or garnish. At the core of the artist's accomplishment is a profound engagement with the body—not aestheticized and contextualized as many of his colleagues liked to see it, but as it is a feat of biology and engineering. For Goodrich, that vision and skill made Eakins a worthy subject for elevation to an emerging pantheon of American artists he helped to invent.

Today, historians are less interested than Goodrich was in nationalistic elevation. We live in a time of fallen heroes, and Eakins is a good one because he still manages to step on those land mines—even the ones he couldn't possibly have foreseen. In recent years, he has been cast by scholars as victim of a paranoid Oedipal complex, sexual harasser, pervert, philanderer, abusive uncle, misogynist, repressed homosexual, and slandered innocent. One of the great benefits of studying Eakins' art and life is that by looking at all these claims about a single man, some stretching back one hundred and twenty years, we can find the boundaries of propriety and perversion assumed by their authors, and see how those boundaries have changed. Few artists create works that probe and critique, and even fewer live their lives in a way that *forces* those around them to do so—Thomas Eakins managed to do both.

This book is largely about digging; it starts with Charles Willson Peale and his *Exhumation of the Mastodon*, uncovers the bones presented to male and female students of medicine and art in nineteenth-century Philadelphia, explores the grave-robbing scandals that rocked the city in 1882 and 1883, and concludes by unearthing the underlying values that guided Eakins through the difficult choices and moments he faced during his life. Digging, in a sense, is always what historians do; we dig up historical facts in order to shed light on them and bring attention to those moments that should not be forgotten as we move forward and contribute to the history of our own time.

The question of what Eakins actually did in the intimate moments of his life, and with whom, is of course fundamentally unanswerable. What we can determine is what such actions would have meant, and how scandal—and the art that provoked it—served to instruct and shape public culture in nineteenth-century America. We will never know if Eakins, as a man, committed acts that deserve our censure. It is undeniable that Eakins, as an artist, is still a force to be reckoned with.

ACKNOWLEDGMENTS

Historians of American art, and those writing on Eakins in particular, are blessed by an exceptionally generous group of colleagues. Various friends and mentors including Elizabeth Milroy, W. Douglass Paschall, Darrel Sewell, Alexander Nemerov, and H. Barbara Weinberg all have provided me with a great example and sound advice through years of research. I am grateful for more specific assistance with this project from Jonathan Weinberg, whose wisdom and brilliant insights make him easily a historian's best friend; Kathleen Adair Foster, the most generous and supportive scholar with whom I have ever worked; Marc Simpson, a diligent Eakins scholar and aid to those who write about the artist; Jules Prown, a most devoted adviser; Marta Braun, who reviewed my chapter on photography at a critical moment; and William Innes Homer, who graciously gave me a copy of Eakins' letters that he curated over many years.

No historian accomplishes anything without the help of reference librarians, and I am extremely grateful to Kristen Hindes, Naomi King, and Michelle McCaffrey at St. Michael's College, Jack Eckert at the Countway Library of Medicine at Harvard Medical School, F. Michael Angelo at the Thomas Jefferson University archives, Barbara Williams at the Drexel University College of Medicine archives, Angie Chapple-Sokol at the Dana Medical Library of the University of Vermont, and various staff over the years at the library of the College of Physicians of Philadelphia and other Philadelphia archives.

In researching this book, I spent a great deal of time buried in the stacks of the Harvard libraries that continue to inform and inspire me as they have for twenty-three years. I extend thanks to the enormous staff that maintains that collection, and also to the much smaller staff of the Irving House, my home away from home in Cambridge. Thanks also are due to Katherine Lane for her gracious hospitality and the opportunity to relive my student days in Somerville.

This project would not have been possible without the professional, collegial, and financial support of various administrators and colleagues at St. Michael's College through the course of many years. Marc and Dana vanderHeyden, John Kenney, Susan Summerfield, Jan Sheeran, Elizabeth Inness Brown, William Wilson, and members of the faculty development council all have aided me enormously through their devotion to the support of scholarship. Gregg Blasdel and Will Mentor, understanding department members, have picked up my slack at times when this project overwhelmed other responsibilities. I am especially grateful to Lance Richbourg, who demonstrates the ideal of perfect loyalty as a friend and co-worker on a daily basis. Kelly McDonald, Madeleine Rabideau, and Jim Millard provided indispensable administrative support.

I have felt honored this past year to work with Patricia Fidler, a consummate professional in the field of art historical publishing, as well as others at Yale University Press, including my editor Phillip King, Michelle Komie, and Kristin Swan. Thanks also are due to Professor Ned Cooke of the History of Art department at Yale University, and to the Yale Publications in the History of Art series, which helped offset reproduction costs. No graduate could enjoy a more supportive alma mater.

Finally, the largest measure of my gratitude is due to my sons, Graham and Emmett, who truly are the wild things that make my heart sing, to my parents, Harvey and Glenda Werbel, and to my dear partner Fred Lane, who edited this text with love and care, and taught me how to be a real writer.

CHAPTER ONE

From Benjamin Franklin to Thomas Eakins
A Century of Philadelphia Scientists, Artists, and Provocateurs

Sometime between 1883 and 1885, a colleague photographed Thomas Eakins unclothed and holding aloft a naked female student at the Pennsylvania Academy of the Fine Arts (fig. 1). In recent decades, this image has been tendered as the most tangible proof of the artist's indiscretions. Although the scene undoubtedly is worthy of critique, it also is worth noting that Eakins hardly was the first indiscreet Philadelphian. More than a century before that shutter snapped, Charles Willson Peale sketched an attractive teenager, probably Polly Stevenson, seated on Benjamin Franklin's lap in a London townhouse, her lips planted on his cheek and her hand suggestively placed on his groin (fig. 2).[1] The teenager, of course, was not Franklin's wife.

Perhaps surprised at the scene he encountered, Peale nevertheless saw fit to record it in a pencil sketch that his principal subject seems not to have minded. Although he already had fathered an illegitimate son, Franklin could afford to be secure in his flirtations and liaisons in the late eighteenth century—they never arrested his progress in politics, business, or social engagements. Nor did the impropriety of the moment lessen Peale's admiration for Franklin. Charles Willson Peale went on to work collegially with his passionate friend in the Pennsylvania legislature and the American Philosophical Society, and to paint him in a more formal and celebratory manner. In fact, Franklin was the first subject Peale chose for a series of portraits that documented America's "illustrious personages."[2]

Franklin's proven and infamous moral infractions did not impede his rise, but a century later Eakins suffered dramatic professional and personal consequences for challenges to convention that are much more difficult to assess. Although the woman in Eakins' arms is nude, for example, and also clearly not his wife, there is little in the photograph that suggests a sexual liaison. In Peale's sketch, Franklin has been interrupted by an intruder while enjoying an amorous moment; Eakins and his student, in contrast, are not in a private residence where we might assume they should not be together, but rather at the center of an academy classroom surrounded by easels and a modeling podium. The audience here is not intruding, but rather stands in the place of an art student drawing or painting the models at the center of the room. In this case, the record provided by the photograph is especially helpful: this is not a pose that models could hold long enough for artists to complete a thorough study.[3]

The nudity of both participants in the photograph is undeniably startling, but perhaps even more surprising is the fact that the students who participated in classes with Eakins at the Pennsylvania Academy mostly understood and agreed with his insistence that serious students of art undress and model, and never complained that their professor's relationship with them was anything more than purely professional. Franklin would have been bemused: the idea that a naked woman in a man's arms could be a sexless affair would have been more shocking to him than the pose itself.

If Eakins had been graced with Franklin's social skills, particularly in the art of self-promotion, the course of his life might have gone more smoothly—he ended up on far fewer lists of "illustrious personages" by the time of his death in 1916 than he probably deserved. On the other hand, the two men lived in different times, and it is hard to imagine Franklin's free spirit thriving so vibrantly in Eakins' time. Philadelphians held vastly different attitudes toward social provocateurs in the second half of the nineteenth century than they did in the second half of the eighteenth. Henry Adams complained succinctly of his own (later) era that "American art, like the American language and American education, was as far as possible sexless. Society regarded this victory over sex as its greatest triumph."[4]

Indeed, Philadelphia was a very different city in 1880 than it was in 1770. Franklin and Eakins nonetheless define two ends of the same historical and cultural thread, with Charles Willson Peale and his son Rembrandt between as densely interwoven strands. The juxtapositions and continuities evident in the lives of all these men make it clear that Eakins, despite all his nonconformity, fit squarely into a tradition of artisan-artist-scientists who negotiated issues of class, gender, and sexuality while making their unique contributions to the cultural history of Philadelphia. Comparison of the experiences of these men illuminates both important continuities—and disruptions—in the warp and weft of American cultural life in the nineteenth century.

In canvassing the lives of Franklin, the Peales, and Eakins, many similarities emerge. All four men arose from what Franklin liked to call "middling" circumstances, counted themselves as Philadelphians (although only Eakins was born in the city), and involved themselves in a catholic mix of scientific study and invention.[5] For Franklin, these intellectual passions were pursued along with a diverse career in publishing and statesmanship; the Peales and Eakins combined their love for science, medicine, and engineering with ambitious careers as artists and art teachers. All four men viewed themselves as furthering the goals of an increasingly cultured and progressive young nation: the "cradle of democracy" that served as home provided them with fertile soil in which to nurture this ambition.

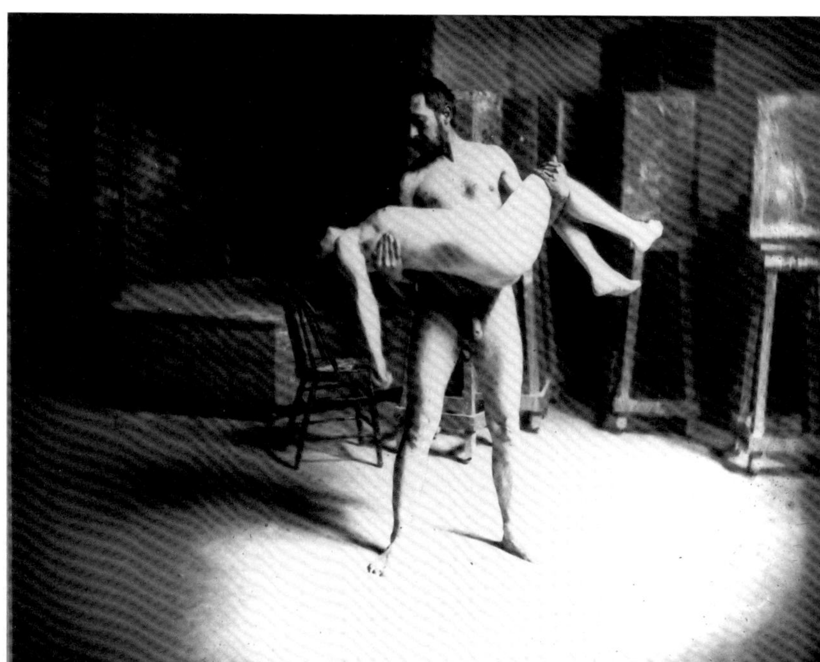

Fig. 1. Circle of Thomas Eakins, *Thomas Eakins nude, holding nude female in his arms, looking down*, c. 1885. Dry-plate negative, 4 × 5 in. Courtesy of the Pennsylvania Academy of the Fine Arts, Philadelphia, Charles Bregler's Thomas Eakins Collection. Purchased with the partial support of the Pew Memorial Trust.

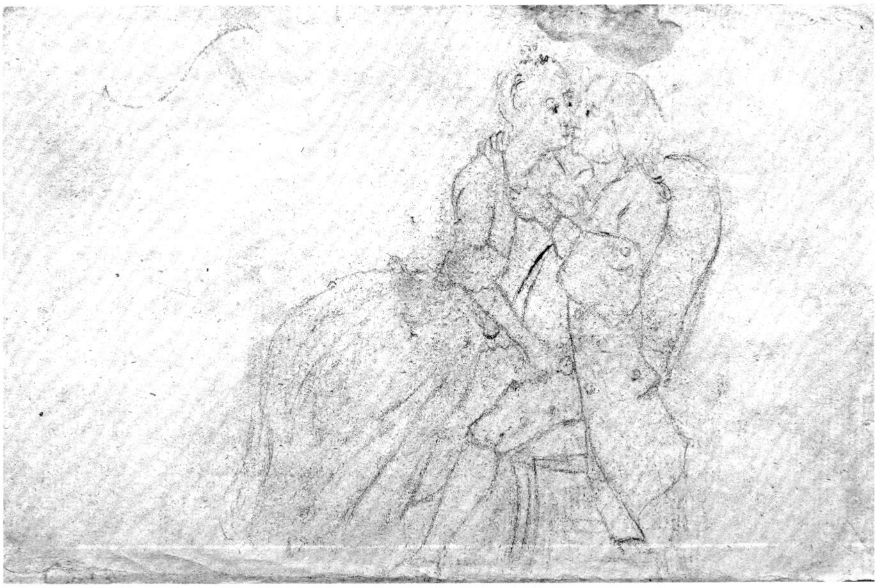

Fig. 2. Charles Willson Peale, *Scandalous Sketch of B. Franklin and Young Woman*, c. 1768. American Philosophical Society, Philadelphia.

The accomplishments of Franklin, the Peales, and Eakins are unimaginable set against the backdrop of any city other than Philadelphia. Historians have termed Philadelphia our "first city" because it gave birth to the Declaration of Independence and the U.S. Constitution, the city of "brotherly love" due to its Quaker roots, and the "private city" due to the quiet nature of its aristocratic associations and clubs. In the nineteenth century, Philadelphia also was renowned for its manufacturing, medical education and hospitals, and relatively cosmopolitan atmosphere as the nation's second largest and most diverse city.

The prospect of financial success in this relatively promising market, along with patriotic fervor, drew Charles Willson Peale from Baltimore in 1776 and encouraged him during the next decades of his life. In Philadelphia, Peale plotted a course followed by succeeding generations of artists and museum curators. Just as Franklin led a generative life as an inventor, politician, postmaster, and newspaperman, so Peale in the artistic realm laid the groundwork for the development of an American—and particularly Philadelphian—art scene. The longevity of Peale's example is evident in the similar course of Thomas Eakins' life, which played out almost exactly a century after Peale's—the men were born 103 years apart, in 1741 and 1844, respectively.

Peale's experiences as a child no doubt were much more frustrating than those of Thomas Eakins. Charles Willson Peale was the son of a Maryland schoolteacher who had been convicted of participation in a forgery scandal when he was clerk in a London post office as a young man. The criminal court that tried Peale's father condemned him to exile in the colonies, and the colonial branch of the family never inherited its family estate in England.

Due to the scandal and conviction, young Charles Willson was raised in quite modest circumstances. In the eighteenth century, it was standard practice for boys and young men without means to be apprenticed to a tradesman—public schools were still decades in the future. And so, at the age of thirteen, young master Peale was apprenticed to a saddle maker. Finally released from service at the age of twenty-one, when he already was married, Peale began his own more self-directed career as a portrait painter at a relatively mature age. The enterprise was not entirely successful, and among the traumas of his early life, Peale spent some time on the run from debtor's prison.[6]

Eakins enjoyed a rather pleasant childhood, in contrast—he was the son of Benjamin and Caroline Cowperthwaite Eakins, a couple whose subsistence derived from Benjamin's highly regarded labors as a calligrapher and writing master, and his investments in real estate and railroads.[7] Unlike Peale, Eakins was born far enough into the nineteenth century to enjoy the benefits of the public school system Benjamin Franklin and his descendants had helped to create—he attended neighborhood grammar school until 1857, and then Philadelphia's prestigious and selective Central High School from 1857 to 1861. From 1861 to 1866, Eakins' activities are largely undocumented; the artist's early lack of clear focus paralleled Peale's—he waited until the similar age of twenty-two to commit himself to a career in art. The disparate childhoods of these artists contributed to a central difference: Peale had little formal schooling (his grammar and spelling throughout his life exhibit scant awareness of the niceties of these subjects), whereas Eakins benefited from intensive training in general, medical, and art academies and, of course, fine handwriting at home.

Although education in America clearly had come a long way in the period between Peale's childhood and Eakins', both men recognized early in their careers that they could not achieve success as artists without European training. For Peale, display of some talent in portrait painting led a group of Maryland gentlemen to sponsor his study in London from 1767 to 1769, where he was befriended by Benjamin West and taught the mannerisms of a proper British portrait artist. The trip was momentous for Peale in several ways. It was at this time that he learned he would not inherit his father's estate. Charles Coleman Sellers credits this discovery with provoking Peale's adoption of the meritocratic (and strongly Whig) sentiment that "the true nobility was that of virtue and talent, open to all." When Peale returned to Maryland, he combined his fervent revolutionary patriotism with his new career as a portrait painter, "adding battle flags, replete with rebel device and sentiment, to his repertoire."[8] The time Eakins spent in Paris a century later, from 1866 to 1869 as one of the first Americans to study in the ateliers of the Ecole des Beaux-Arts, also provoked strong nationalist sensibilities.

The professional lives that Peale and Eakins shaped upon their return from Europe included a similar combination of painting, invention, and teaching consciously devoted to the furtherance of American meritocracy. Their personal lives hardly could have been less similar. Peale's historians never have had any occasion to debate his sexual proclivities—the artist fathered seventeen children (many of them named after famous artists) with three wives. While Franklin scholars differ in their tabulations of how many of his widely documented flirtations were actually consummated, for Peale no such speculation seems necessary. David C. Ward's concise summary of this aspect of Peale's life is typical: "His family was the literal and figurative expression of his potency."[9] Heterosexual lust and consummation are clear in the biographies of Franklin and Peale, with nothing to suggest any other, or lack of, desire.

Eakins, on the other hand, presents a smorgasbord of titillating sexual non sequiturs that have nourished a cottage industry of speculative historians.[10] He is known to have participated in witty and somewhat flirtatious correspondence with Emily Sartain for many years, and then is reputed to have been engaged for five years to Kathrin Crowell before her unfortunate death from meningitis in 1879.[11] Five years later, at the age of forty, he married a promising Pennsylvania Academy art student, Susan Macdowell, and the couple resided together until Thomas' death in 1916, although the marriage produced no children. Eakins frequently appears with nude young women and men in photographs by his circle, and with nude men in his own painting *Swimming*, and he often shared bunks with his friend and traveling companion Samuel Murray. None of these men are known to have suggested a sexual relationship with the artist.

Of the many women Eakins photographed, painted, and taught, several did complain about his unconventional approach to nudity, and many of the artist's acquaintances recall that he badgered them to pose in the nude. Of these many women, only two specifically accused him of misconduct. Lillian Hammitt, a student, and Ella Crowell, the artist's niece, exhibited unstable behavior before and after their dealings with the artist, and later were diagnosed with "mania," a popular catch-all phrase of the time signifying a variety of largely emotional difficulties. Their complaints against Eakins, though known only through secondhand sources in their own day and even more difficult to assess today, undoubtedly lend a tragic sadness to the artist's story. Lillian Hammitt claimed that Eakins had promised to leave Susan and marry her, and newspapers later recorded the sight of her wandering the streets of Philadelphia in a "bathing costume" before her institutionalization.[12]

Ella Crowell committed suicide in 1897, which led to the

artist's permanent estrangement from his beloved sister and her family, who blamed him for their daughter's death. Writers in recent decades have used these events in the artist's life to claim that he was adulterous, incestuous, or a slandered monogamous heterosexual innocent. Others have discussed his images of naked men and close male friendships and assumed homosexuality. In short, Eakins' biography offers a bevy of speculative possibilities, but no demonstration of sexual proclivities and relations as clear and unequivocal as Peale's seventeen children.

Another central difference between the two men is evident in their contributions to patriotic causes. At the time of the Revolutionary War, Peale's efforts on behalf of the young nation were substantial. As Charles Coleman Sellers recounts, Peale "captained a company of [Philadelphia] militia, joined Washington before Trenton, fought at Princeton, and was on active service through the next year's campaign."[13] A few years later, Peale served as a delegate in the 1779–80 term of the Pennsylvania state legislature, a session notable for its passage of the nation's first law banning the practice of slavery. In contrast, Eakins passed up the opportunity to serve as either politician or soldier. At twenty-one, he bought his way out of the draft lottery that might have sent him to the front lines of the Civil War. Eakins' decision not to serve, presumably made jointly with his Quaker-descended family, is indicative of a change in the nature of the times, as well as the differences between the men.

In the mid-1770s, at a time when the British quite literally were at the gates of Philadelphia and then inside them as an occupying force, few men avoided service. In the 1860s, however, home ground was uncontested and any Philadelphian who produced the twenty-four-dollar fee could avoid the draft. Whatever his thoughts about the uncertain future of the nation may have been during these ill-documented years, it is clear that Eakins' patriotism was of a far less passionate and self-sacrificing strain than Peale's.

Although Eakins never took up arms for his country, he did follow Peale's example of patriotism by using art to preserve the images of national heroes, including America's most prominent physicians and scientists.[14] Beyond their nationalistic purposes, such commissions also were simply good business. Organizations including the American Philosophical Society, Jefferson Medical College, the University of Pennsylvania, and the College of Physicians of Philadelphia all served as sources of work for Philadelphia's nineteenth-century portrait artists.

For both Peale and Eakins, painting portraits of scientists was more than just a sideline. Peale spent substantial time repeatedly painting the first three presidents of the American Philosophical Society alone—Benjamin Franklin, David Rittenhouse, and Thomas Jefferson. Eakins too enjoyed relatively good sales of his paintings in the scientific community throughout his career, despite the controversies that later constrained sales of his other works. The artist's medical portrait subjects include, most notably, Benjamin Howard Rand (1874), Samuel D. Gross (1875), John H. Brinton (1878), David Hayes Agnew (1889), Jacob Mendez DaCosta (1892 and 1894), William S. Forbes (1905), William S. Thomson (1907), and Edward Spitzka (1913) among many others. At Jefferson Medical College and the University of Pennsylvania, painted tributes to their historic faculties by the Peales and Eakins reside collegially together.

Portraits of scientists were popular in America in the late eighteenth and nineteenth centuries, not only because they depicted venerable citizens but also because they celebrated the particularly democratic triumphs of men who had risen in society by virtue of their hard work and intellect rather than any birthright.[15] Benjamin Franklin was the best example of a "middling" man whose scientific achievements had brought him into the royal courts of Europe as a distinguished guest.[16]

Peale and Eakins both pictorially displayed their appreciation for the implications of a portrait practice that elevated and commemorated individuals on the basis of their achievements. Although each artist painted men of both the middle and upper classes, the format and effort in their portraits seldom depended on the subject's financial means—in the gallery Peale devoted to "illustrious personages," each man occupied the same square feet of canvas. Eakins likewise chose to paint enormous canvases when the project suited him, as opposed to more traditional financial considerations. Both artists drew on a rich historical tradition in constructing such portraits, but they also broke some new ground of their own, including the democratizing scale of their works.

The traditional iconography included in the portrait of a "man of science" was established in the Renaissance, and included attributes associated with scientific pursuits—instruments, books, and writing implements, and sometimes bust-length sculptures of scientific predecessors. The poses were in the tradition of somber thinker-as-melancholic portraits, typically capturing the subject engaged in reading, writing, or actually using scientific apparatus. These were men of action—or at least deep thought.[17] Charles Willson Peale followed these conventions, as we can see in his portrait of David Rittenhouse, by portraying the self-taught astronomer pointing to a diagram of a comet he had observed in 1770 (fig. 3). Although Peale followed British precedent fairly well in composing his tribute to Rittenhouse, he did refrain from costuming his subject in the turban and banyan in which British painters often depicted their subjects. Science in England was frequently the province of wealthy dilettantes, and painting them in expensive loungewear helped denote that high status.

An interesting exception to Peale's more typical avoidance of this custom was his portrait of the celebrated Philadelphia physician and medical professor Dr. Benjamin Rush. The unusual choice of turban and banyan in this portrait reflects the preference of the portrait subject for rather different purposes than his British counterparts. In a quote that foreshadows complaints about Eakins a century later, Rush wrote for a medical lecture: "Loose dress contributes to the easy and vigorous exercise of the faculties of the mind. This remark is so obvious, and so generally known, that we find studious men are always painted in gowns, when they are seated in their libraries. Sometimes an open collar and loose shoes and stockings, form a part of their picture. It is from the habits of mental ease and vigor which this careless form of dress creates, that learned men have often become contemptible for their slovenly appearance, when they mix with the world."[18]

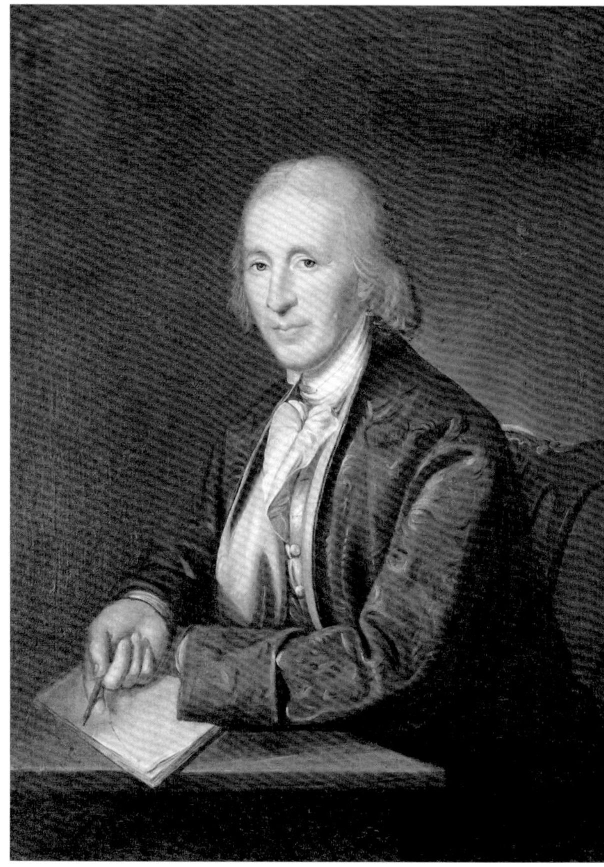

Fig. 3. Charles Willson Peale, *Portrait of David Rittenhouse*, 1791. Oil on canvas, 37 × 27 in. American Philosophical Society, Philadelphia.

Eakins never painted his sitters in turbans and banyans, but he did follow Rush in adopting a casual manner of dress that was frequently described in terms similar to "slovenly." Eakins also typically asked his portrait subjects to choose informal clothes that demonstrated patterns of frequent wear.[19]

Eakins' desire to capture his scientific and medical portrait subjects at work rather than posturing was sometimes taken to an extreme. Indeed, in many cases the artist seemed more interested in the science than the man behind it. Benjamin Howard Rand, for example, almost disappears behind the chemistry equipment shown beside him in his large portrait (fig. 4), and Henry Rowland's spectrograph is the brilliant focal point of his scene (fig. 5), with the formulas he developed an unusual distraction as carvings into the frame the artist constructed himself. Rand's desk is a good example of the "slovenly" mess that frequently results from the intense mental exertions of a pioneering scientist.

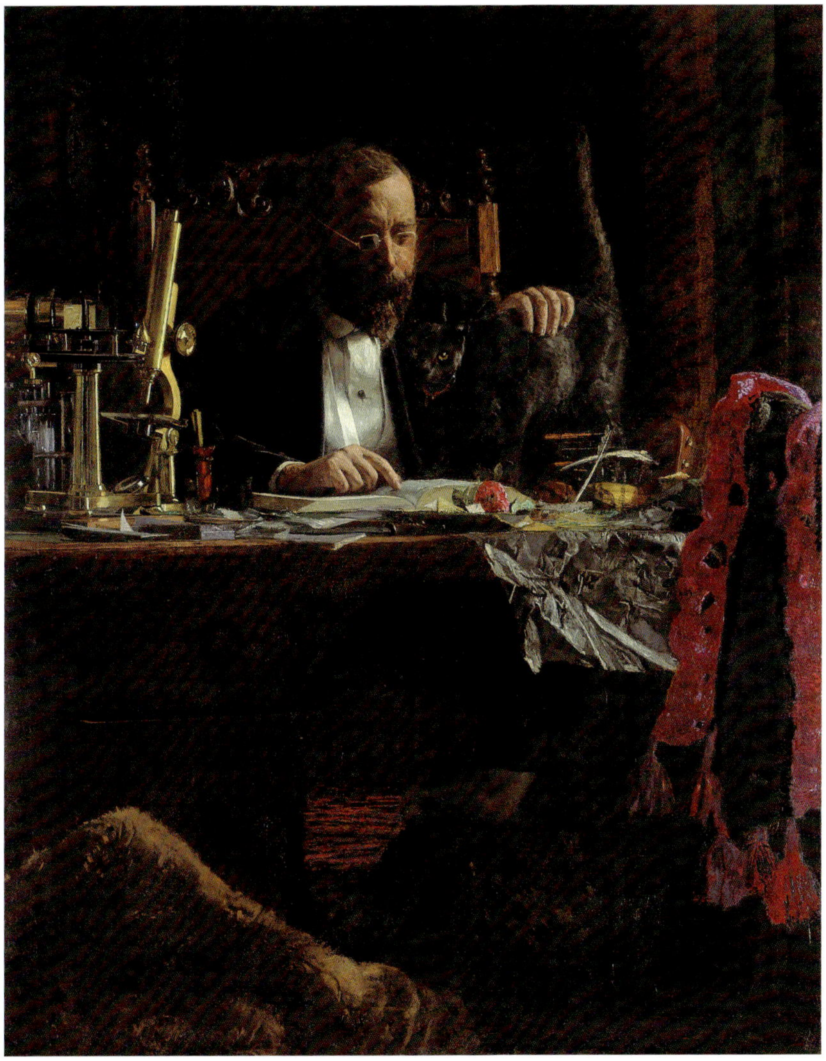

Fig. 4. Thomas Eakins, *Portrait of Benjamin Howard Rand, M.D.*, 1874. Oil on canvas, 60 × 48 in.

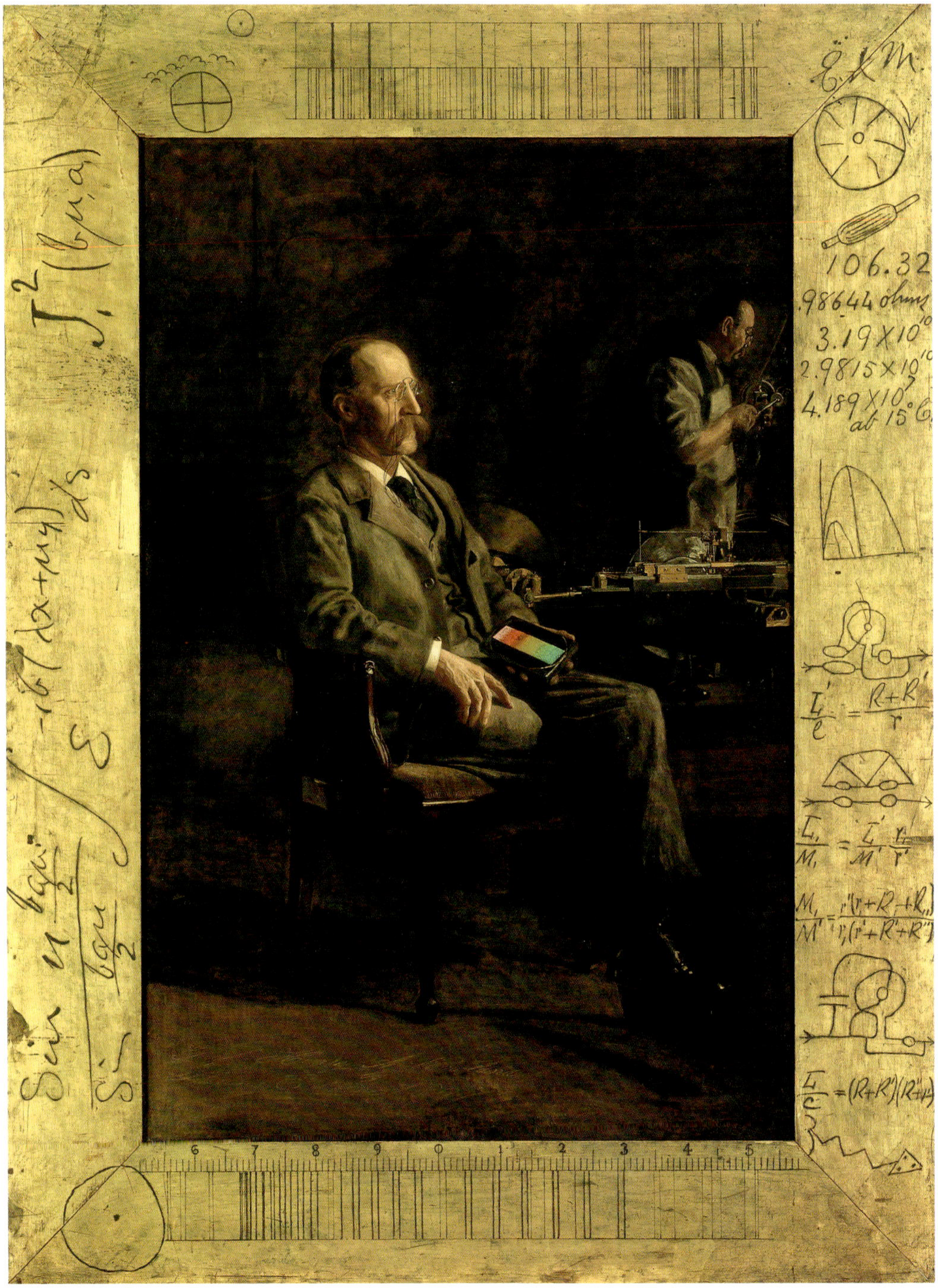

Fig. 5. Thomas Eakins, *Portrait of Professor Henry A. Rowland*, 1897. Oil on canvas, 80¼ × 54 in. Addison Gallery of American Art, Phillips Academy, Andover, Massachusetts. All rights reserved. Gift of Stephen C. Clark, Esq.

Both Eakins' emphasis on the *work* of making scientific progress, and on the content of the sitter's research programs, is not surprising. Eakins himself was an unrelenting laborer, famous for his elaborate studies for finished works, which sometimes included large perspective drawings, oil sketches, wax models, and photographs. Franklin and Peale were equally tireless workers before him. Franklin's "retirement" at forty-two gave him, as he put it, "leisure to read, study, make experiments, and converse at large with such ingenious and worthy men as are pleased to honor me with their friendship."[20] In his supposed leisure time, Franklin pursued scientific investigations so famous as to hardly need recitation. Franklin, of course, was the progenitor of a multitude of inventions from the battery to bifocals, and his love of invention extended beyond the practical to such amusing efforts as the use of "electricity jolts to cook turkeys." Franklin also took pleasure in mathematics and wrote to a friend that he enjoyed "whil[ing] away his time as Assembly clerk by constructing complex 'magic squares' of numbers where the rows, columns and diagonals all added up to the same sum."[21] Eakins' friend Samuel Murray likewise recorded that the artist "worked out problems of painting by trigonometry and algebra, and worked mathematical problems for fun with some of the greatest mathematicians, for example with Dr. Johnson of Anapolis and with the English Professor Glasier, astronomer physicist."[22] Eakins used his mathematical skills famously in perspective studies for paintings, but also in his experiments with camera shutters and lenses.

Charles Willson Peale also experimented—with telescopic sights for rifles, porcelain teeth, arsenic-based preservatives for taxidermy, gas lighting, fireplaces, bridge design, and the use of illuminated transparencies as "moving picture" exhibitions.[23] Most famously, in 1776 Peale constructed an elaborate "Triumphal Arch" in Philadelphia to celebrate the end of the Revolutionary War. The wooden arch was filled with illuminated transparencies and paintings, and topped by statues of Peace and other goddesses. The most striking element of the work was also its downfall. To heighten the spectacle, Peale arranged for his sculptural figures to hold torches that were rigged to descend at a critical moment in the festivities, thereby lighting fireworks rockets.

Unfortunately, a stray torch struck one of the paintings, resulting in a chain reaction that destroyed the four-story arch, killed one bystander, and badly burned Peale and others.[24] In later years, Peale decided to forgo the fireworks for less explosive but still dramatic illusionistic efforts. One of those was an "Exhibition of Perspective Views with Changeable Effects," later called "Moving Pictures."

In this indoor show, Peale's arrangement of screens, transparencies, movable scenery, and Argand lamps foreshadowed Eakins' photography experiments with Eadweard Muybridge exactly one hundred years later; the copy on Peale's advertising brochure could just as well have been used to advertise Eakins' rapid-shutter studies of animals and athletes in motion: "MR. PEALE respectfully informs the public, that with great labour and expence, he has prepared a number of *perspective views*, with *changeable* effects, imitating nature in various *movements*. He flatters himself they will please: But how far he has succeeded in his imitations, is submitted to the judgment of the candid public. This manner of exhibiting pictures, imitations of choice parts of natural objects, in which *motion* and *change* is given, is entirely new, at least in this part of the world; and cannot be performed without much complicated and costly machinery."[25] True to form, Peale went on to justify the expense of the show to paying customers with lengthy descriptions of its excitements. Eakins was never such a practiced salesman.

Although neither Peale nor Eakins enjoyed Franklin's great fame and success as a result of their engineering efforts, all three can be credited with profound educational and institutional tinkering that still resonates to the present day. Following in Franklin's footprint as founder of the first public library (the Library Company of Philadelphia) and public college (the University of Pennsylvania) in the colonies, Peale contributed the Philadelphia Museum in 1791 as the nation's first museum, and the first *public* museum in the world.

Peale's efforts to educate the American public using the greatest achievements of science and art in his Philadelphia Museum set a course for his son Rembrandt's curricular reforms as an art educator, and also for Thomas Eakins. Although Peale's museum closed before Eakins could have profitably visited it, the younger artist nonetheless was imbued with the Franklin and Peale philosophy of institution-building as an educational reformer in his own right as director of schools at the Pennsylvania Academy of the Fine Arts from 1879 to 1886. Peale's museum is a good example of the types of problems all three men faced in promoting institutional growth and progress in Philadelphia.

When Peale established his museum in 1791, its home was in the quarters of the American Philosophical Hall. In those early years, exhibits were limited to a small collection of such nationalistic attractions as pheasants given by Lafayette to George Washington, and Peale was responsible for everything from taxidermy to advertising. Over the course of the next twenty years, the collections of the museum expanded at a furious pace, as admirers of the project contributed specimens to bolster Peale's displays of the diverse creations of man and nature. Museum records reveal that "during the second decade of the nineteenth century, the museum contained (among other things) 269 paintings, 1,824 birds, 250 quadrupeds, 650 fishes, over 1,000 shells, and 313 books in the library."[26]

Although Thomas Jefferson turned down Peale's request for federal aid to procure a larger building, Pennsylvania legislators did agree in 1802 to turn over the second floor of Independence Hall, which was empty following the relocation of the capital to Lancaster. At first, Peale was respon-

Fig. 6. Charles Willson Peale, *The Long Room, Interior of Front Room in Peale's Museum*, 1822. Ink and watercolor sketch on paper, 14 × 20¾ in. The Detroit Institute of Arts. Founders Society Purchase, Director's Discretionary Fund.

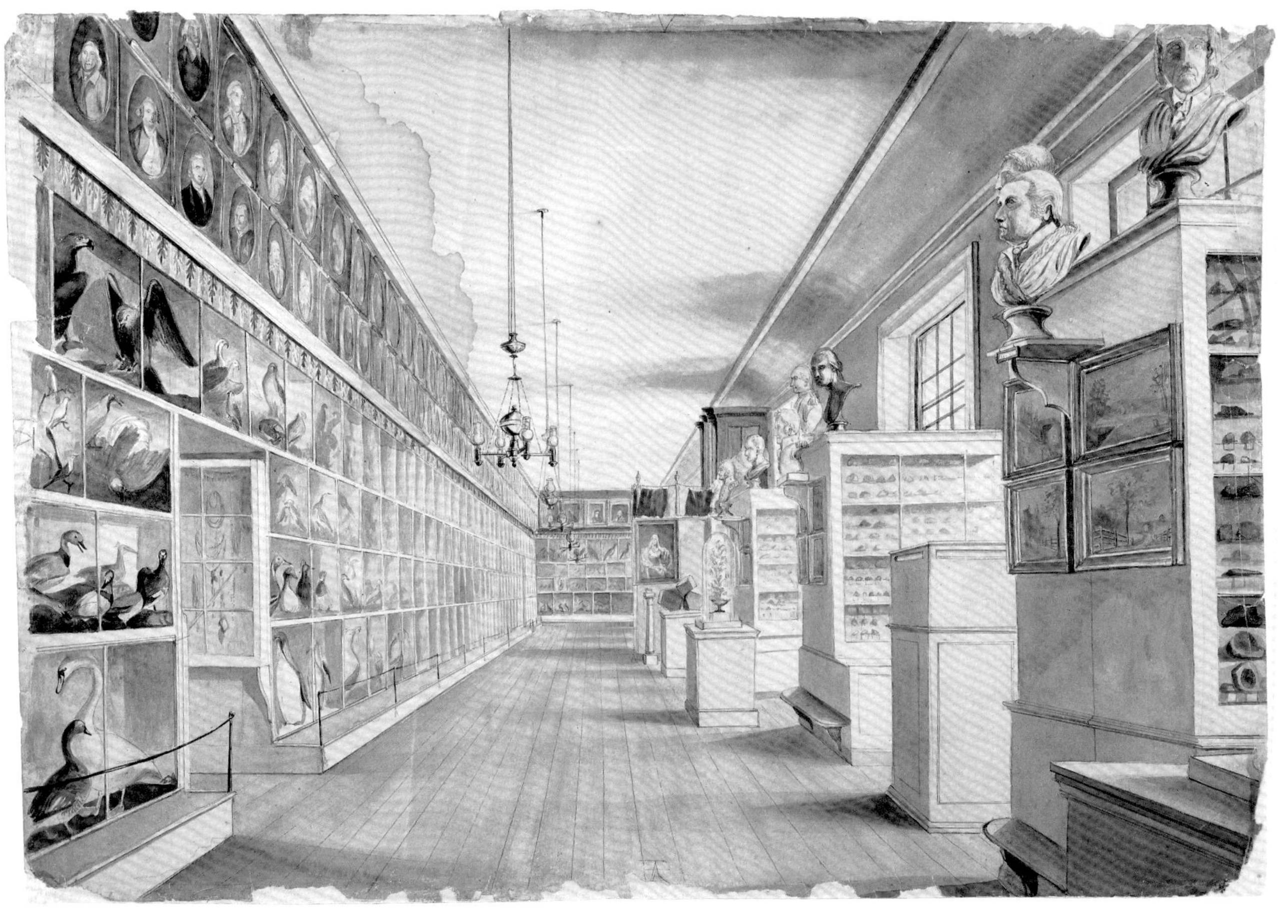

sible only for "maintaining order in the State House yard, a popular gathering place for drunks and prostitutes," but later he also was required to pay rent.[27]

In the first decades of the nineteenth century, above the din in the courtyard, Peale's museum evolved to include a living zoo, whose residents were "stuffed and mounted" upon their deaths, and also a wide assortment of preserved foreign and domestic animals and birds, bones, minerals, and fossils. The Philadelphia Museum was the obvious resting place for many of the famous acquisitions of such explorers as Lewis and Clark, and thus made a distinctively patriotic display.

In 1822, Charles Willson Peale depicted the famous Long Room of the museum in a watercolor that shows the arrangement of the collections (fig. 6). At the top of the hall were the visages of "illustrious personages" (including Franklin), preserved in an artistic version of taxidermy—as portrait subjects on the wall and as bust-length sculptures on top of the display cases. These heroes preserved in paint are in some ways close cousins to the dead birds and animals preening on stands beneath them. Rembrandt Peale's portrait of the famed anatomist Georges Cuvier is a good example of the stylistic results of the museum's emphasis on quantity over quality (fig. 7). Certainly, the younger Peale spent far less time researching Cuvier's tools and laboratory environment than Eakins would have done.

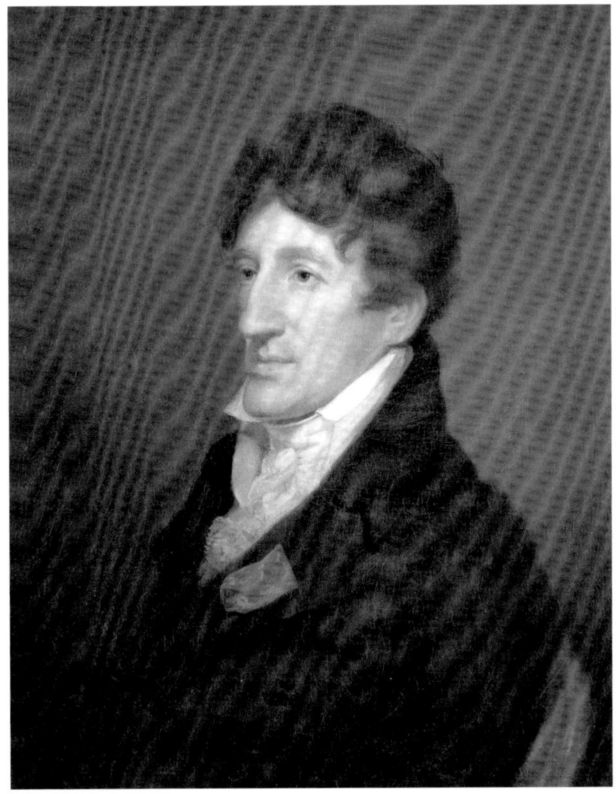

Fig. 7. Rembrandt Peale, *George Cuvier*, 1808. Oil on canvas, 27½ × 22¼ in. Courtesy, The College of Physicians of Philadelphia.

The most famous inhabitant of Peale's Museum was a fossilized prehistoric mastodon unearthed in Newburgh, New York, in 1801. Charles Willson Peale celebrated the find five years later in his canvas *The Exhumation of the Mastodon* (fig. 8). In proto-Romantic fashion, Peale chose to depict a most dramatic moment, rather than the occasion of the find itself. When we encounter the scene, all is nearly lost, as a violent thunderstorm threatens to flood the excavation site and literally sink the project. Busy workers fill buckets, pull bones from the water, and turn a great waterwheel. At the edge of the dig, Peale lectures to an assortment of family and friends, including the ornithologist Alexander Wilson and the entire Peale clan (although several of them never actually were on the scene).

The grand design of the canvas and Peale's intensive labor on it have raised questions about why the artist devoted so much attention to painting this archaeological excavation on an upstate New York farm. Lillian Miller writes: "In his mind, it was an heroic drama, full of struggle and travail, replete with both human and cosmic significance and containing within it those elements of awesomeness and fear that defined the sublime—an essential ingredient of eighteenth-century history painting.... To Peale, this was a theme that equaled the great themes of classical history and also seemed especially appropriate to American republicanism, for the courage it honored was called forth by civilian rather than military goals."[28] The same might be said of the effort Thomas Eakins exerted years later in painting his exuberant (and sublime) *Gross Clinic* (fig. 9).

In that painting, showing a surgical amphitheater at Jefferson Medical College in 1875, the excavator was instead a surgeon, searching for a bone tumor inside the open hole of a patient's leg. The waterwheel at the center of Peale's masterpiece is replaced by the more delicate digging tools of

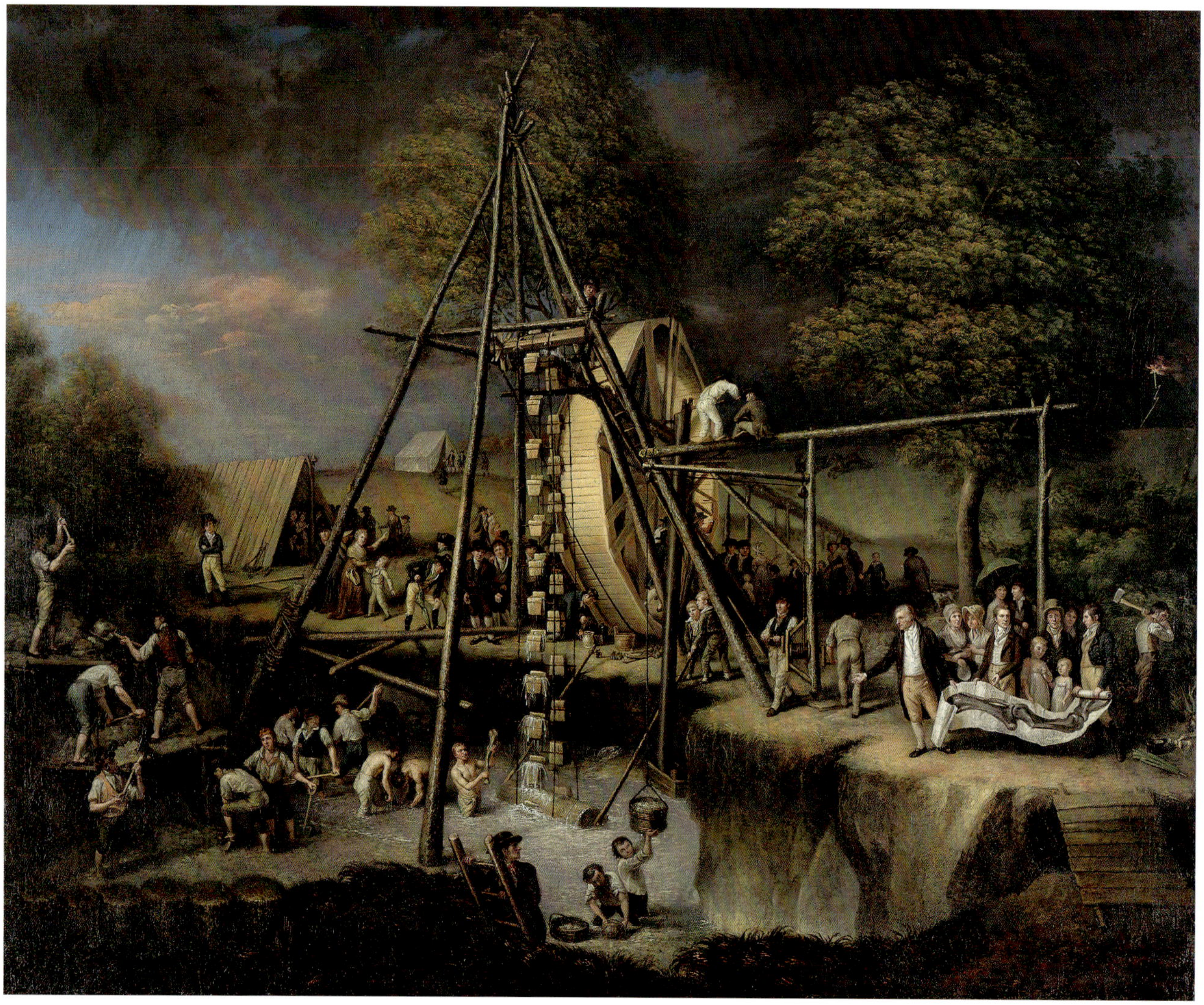

Fig. 8. Charles Willson Peale, *The Exhumation of the Mastodon*, c. 1806–8. Oil on canvas, 50 × 62 ½ in. The Maryland Historical Society.

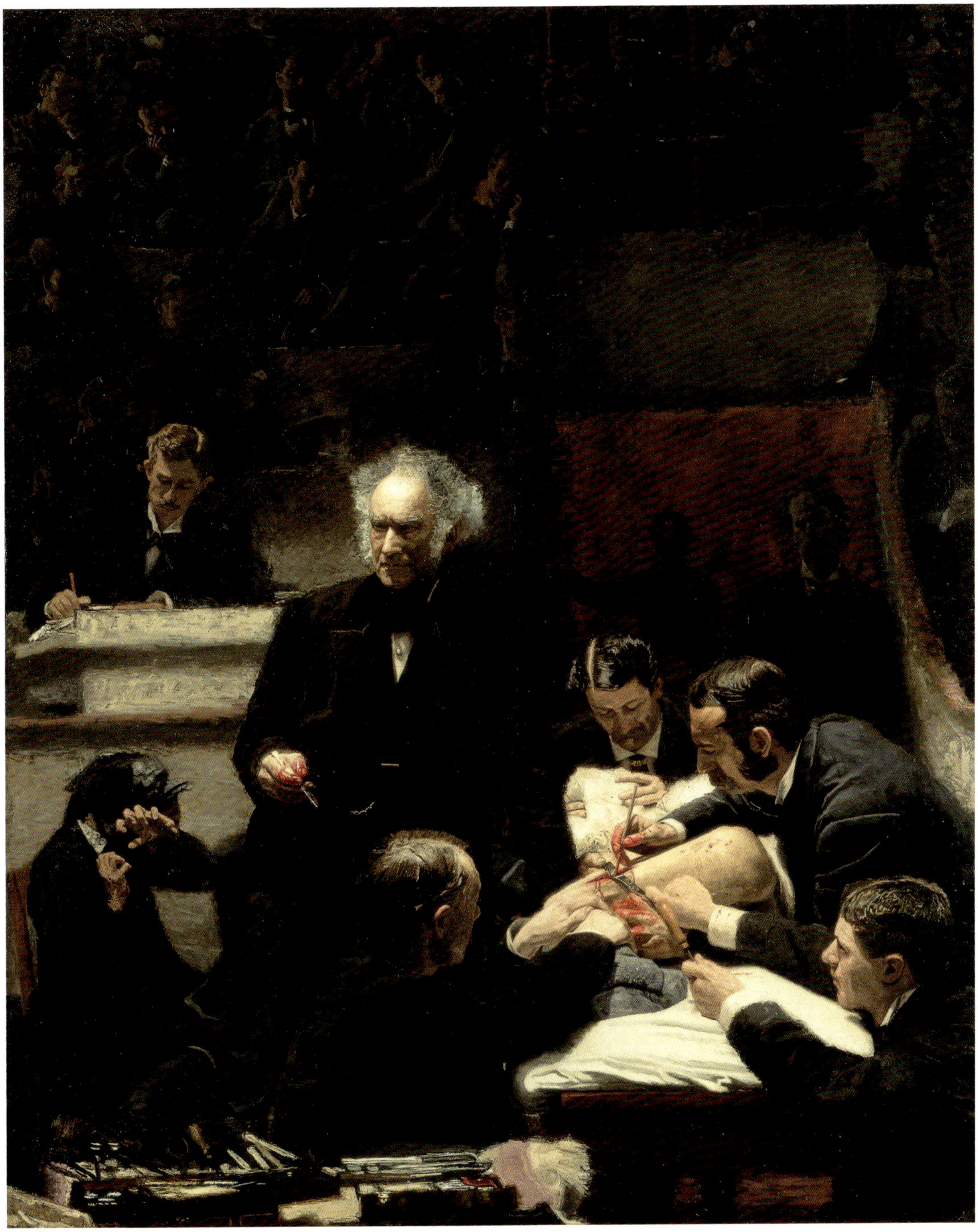

Fig. 9. Thomas Eakins, *The Gross Clinic*, 1875. Oil on canvas, 96 × 78½ in. © Courtesy Thomas Jefferson University, Philadelphia.

scalpel and knife, the fluids drained by sponges and rags rather than buckets. Despite these differences, both paintings use art to celebrate dynamic moments when an American community gathered on the threshold of new scientific uncovering and "civilian" triumph. The mastodon was the first accepted example of extinction, and therefore Peale's exhumation, according to Edgar Richardson, "helped add to man's understanding of geologic time, whose realization was one of the great intellectual events of the nineteenth century."[29] Eakins' grand portrait, painted for the Centennial Exhibition of 1876, captured a similar American contribution to science, exemplified by one of the most famous surgeons of the day performing his signature operation.

Beyond their celebration of American scientific achievements, both portraits also underscore teaching as an important element in the heroism of the scene. Peale lectures on the importance of the mastodon to the friends and family around him while the work of excavation proceeds; in *The Gross Clinic*, the surgeon is shown both healing the patient and lecturing to the students behind him. The art of teaching

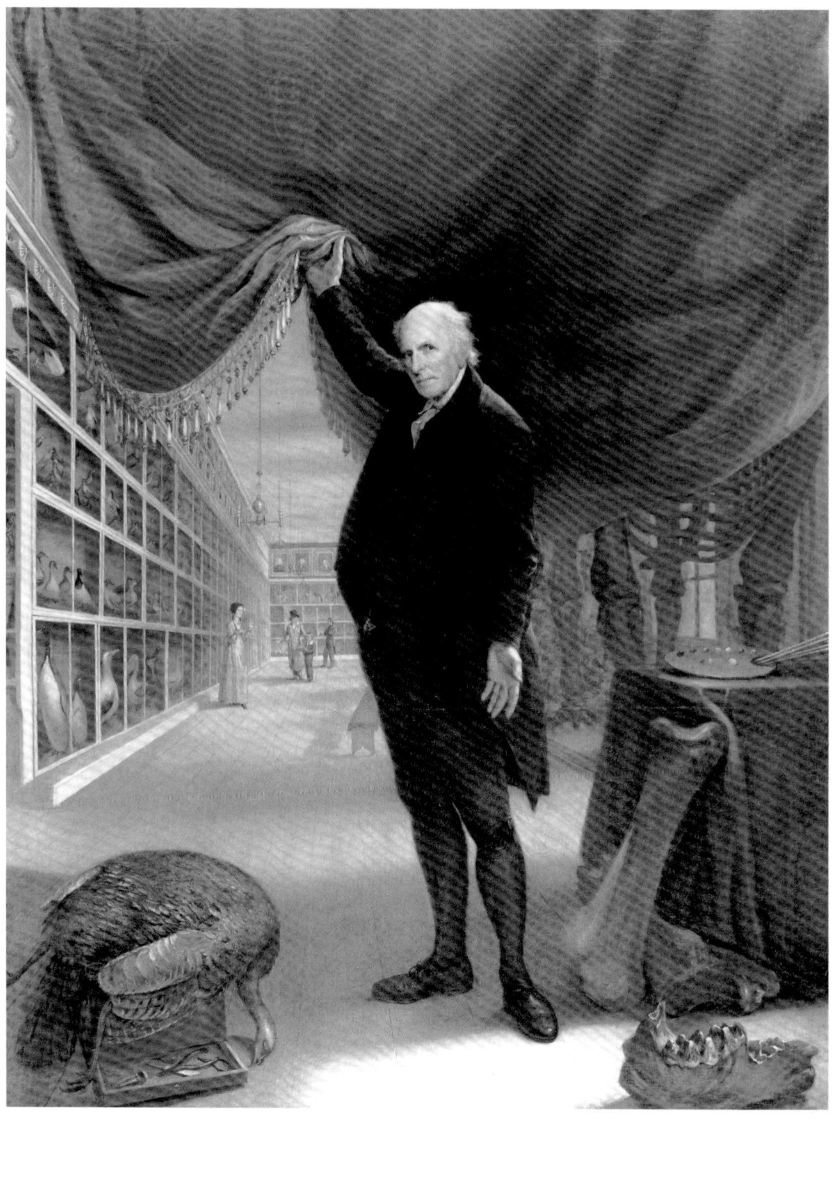

Fig. 10. Charles Willson Peale. *The Artist in His Museum*, 1822. Oil on canvas, 103 ¾ × 79 ⅞ in. The Pennsylvania Academy of the Fine Arts, Philadelphia. Gift of Mrs. Sarah Harrison (The Joseph Harrison, Jr., Collection).

is even more famously celebrated in Peale's *Artist in His Museum* (fig. 10), in which, as Miller writes, Peale "is at once the artist exhibiting the sources of his inspiration and the teacher raising the veil of ignorance from a dimly lit foreground to an illuminated background of knowledge."[30] For both Peale, presenting his collections to a fee-paying public, and Eakins, bringing the clinical lessons of Dr. Gross to the public at the Centennial Exhibition, the act of teaching was equally as patriotic as the act of scientific progress.

Although Gross, Peale, and Eakins all were prominent educators in the nineteenth century, the audiences they addressed varied widely. Peale's public was the most general of the three. In 1816, he declared his ambition as museum director "to form a school of useful knowledge, to diffuse its usefulness to every class in our country, to amuse and in the same moment to instruct the adult of each sex and age—with a zeal far surpassing the bounds of fatigue." As Sellers notes, this was an entirely new agenda. "European museums in the eighteenth-century had no concern for 'usefulness' to 'every class' and 'each age or sex.' Peale in contrast declared that the 'Fair Sex' and children possessed 'equal rights to every advantage.'"[31]

Peale's museum also was egalitarian in its goal of possessing, as he declared, "specimens of every genus; that there should be no c[h]asms, if possible to be avoided: and as the diffusing of knowledge is the greater object of such an institution, it ought to display the common as well as the uncommon."[32] One hundred years after the opening of Peale's museum, Eakins brought a similarly egalitarian impulse to his tenure as professor and director of the Pennsylvania Academy schools, by developing a curriculum open equally to male and female art students, and by offering study of a diverse range of artistic (and anatomical) subjects, from cats to humans.

An interesting note here is that, although Peale displayed humans in his encyclopedic museum only by means of art—in the form of painted and sculpted portraits, he had wanted to treat them in similar fashion as other species. Sidney Hart and David Ward write that he "seriously considered exhibiting the embalmed corpses of eminent men to show the highest level of the natural world. When this proved unworkable a substitute was found in [the] portraits."[33] Eakins displayed a similarly pragmatic approach to the body in both art studios and dissecting laboratories a century later. The principal difference between the two men on this point is that Eakins rarely retreated from an idea on grounds of practicality, or to appease public sentiment.

Although both artists shared a progressive approach to education, the qualities of each age suggested quite different agendas. Peale began painting when there were no arts institutions in the colonies, and their establishment was the first order of business. Shortly after Peale founded his museum, he also helped form the Columbianum (1794), an artist's society promoting education. The Columbianum was short-lived, but Peale persevered and soon helped found the Pennsylvania Academy of the Fine Arts in 1805; Eakins served as the academy's first director of schools in a major reorganization nearly three-quarters of a century later. Although Eakins' academy was many steps removed from the fledgling institution's earliest incarnation under Peale, nevertheless, the problems each man faced in the effort to build or improve artistic education in Philadelphia were similar.

Disgruntlement at the academy was a fixture in Peale's time as well as in Eakins', and in many ways the core set of problems did not change much in intervening decades. Both Peale and Eakins battled with trustees who oversaw and technically owned the academy. Tensions were perhaps inevitable: academy students and teachers were practicing artists, as opposed to aficionados and collectors, and most were relatively middling in class background and means compared with the much wealthier board members. It was the trustees who bore financial responsibility if the academy were to default on its loans; the question of who should control and determine the exhibitions and educational programs at the academy was therefore inevitably contentious.[34]

One of the most difficult issues debated by artists and trustees in these early years, both in Philadelphia and at the American Academy of Fine Arts (founded in New York City in 1802), was nudity. At the Pennsylvania Academy, nudity caused disgruntlement as early as 1807, when Rembrandt Peale and other Philadelphia artists launched a series of complaints at their overseers who, according to Lillian Miller, viewed even the exhibition of nude sculptures as "'extremely indecorous, and altogether inconsistent with the purity of republican morals'—this despite the fact that women enjoyed a separate attendance at the antique statue gallery on Mondays so that they could view the casts 'without blushing in the presence of their escorts.'"[35] The Pennsylvania Academy continued to provide segregated viewing opportunities through much of the century, a custom that was more acceptable to the Peales than it was to Eakins decades later.

Eakins' dismissal from his post at the academy in 1886 resonates with difficulties reminiscent of earlier times. Technically, Eakins was fired because he removed the loincloth from a male model in a class including female students. The trustees also undoubtedly (though not as publicly) were disturbed at reports and evidence that Eakins had been modeling in the nude both for and with coeducational classes. It is an amusing side note to the larger and serious issues in this painful episode that even here Eakins had some precedent in the example of Charles Willson Peale, who was pressed into service as one of the first "Academical" models in America. Nineteenth-century biographers commonly recounted the tale. In need of a model, Peale hired a muscular young baker he had seen stripped to the waist on the street in Philadelphia. The baker, however, was poorly informed about what he had been hired to do, and "becoming aware as he stripped of the staring eyes of the artists, made a hasty retreat." In response, Peale removed his shirt and the class began. The real story may not have been so dramatic, but nevertheless it is clear that both Peale and Eakins struggled to find suitable models for life study as compared with their European counterparts—and both ultimately disrobed themselves.[36]

Although Eakins was more strident and provocative in his solution to the problem, institutionally the outcome of these struggles between trustees and artists was remarkably similar. In 1810, students in Philadelphia formed their own Society of Artists of the United States, intent on studying nude models and viewing sculptures and paintings of the nude. Rembrandt Peale was named the second vice president and professor of painting at the society in 1811.[37] Three-quarters of a century later, many of Eakins' students followed suit after their teacher's forced resignation; in 1886 they created the Art Students' League of Philadelphia with Eakins as professor. In both cases, artists asserted their rights to study from the nude more freely than fiduciary trustees would allow. For artists of Peale's generation, however, this step solved only one of the problems related to nudity.

Much of the conflict between early-nineteenth-century artists and trustees in New York and Philadelphia concerned the exhibition, rather than just the production, of sculptures and paintings depicting the nude. If artists had no opportunity to sell the salon-style works they had been inspired to paint during years spent training abroad, there could be no hope of securing livelihood as *au courant* artists in America. The fear that the fledgling nation's best artists would stay in Europe was pressing. Both in New York and in Philadelphia, however, trustees were unwilling to risk censure.[38] In Europe, by contrast, Royal Academy exhibitions of ambitious paintings of human flesh were the means by which artists came to the attention of patrons. With little hope of such advantageous support, American artists had to find a different way to earn their keep: they needed a new business model.

Evidence of efforts to sell paintings of nudes in America is sparse in the nation's earliest years. One notable exception is an entry in the diary of Colonel Edward Lloyd in 1774 recording a payment to Charles Willson Peale of thirty-five pounds for a painting titled *Venus Rising from the Sea*.[39] The canvas presumably followed convention in displaying Venus in her birthday attire, although the work itself has not survived. Despite this tantalizing allusion to a lost painting, there is little other documentation of colonial and revolutionary nudes.

The situation is quite the reverse after 1806, when Adolf Wertmüller, Rembrandt Peale, and John Vanderlyn all embarked on exceedingly well publicized efforts to earn their livings at least in part as painters of "nudities." If one were to seek an original culprit for the centuries of shocking paintings (including Eakins') that have followed, Adolf Ulrik Wertmüller would be the best choice.

Wertmüller was unusually distinguished for an artist painting in America in the first decade of the nineteenth century. Born in Sweden, Wertmüller went on to train in Paris and to become a member of the French Royal Academy, the Swedish Art Academy, and first painter to the King of Sweden, Gustaf III, before his arrival in Philadelphia in 1795.[40]

Although Wertmüller had not planned to stay in America, soon after his disembarkation he fell in love, and after a brief trip back to Sweden he returned to Philadelphia and married the granddaughter of painter Gustavus Hesselius. Once resettled in his new home, Wertmüller investigated the possibilities for exhibiting paintings in America and decided on the promising example he found in the independent gallery of John Smibert. Smibert sold paintings from a room that was part of his house in Boston, and thus never shared a commission with a dealer.

Following Smibert's example, Wertmüller rented a room in a house on Filbert Street in 1806 and, according to William T. Oedel, "arranged the first public exhibition of a nude female" painting on this side of the Atlantic. Over the next four years, a substantial number of visitors paid twenty-five cents to see Wertmüller's *Danaë and the Shower of Gold* (fig. 11); the aging Swede had found the secret to successful exhibition of nude paintings in early America. Although prudish patrons were unlikely to hang such a subject in their parlors, they were more than willing to pay to see such works—if only to condemn them. When Charles Willson Peale saw the *Danaë*, he commented that "I like no art which can raise a blush on a lady's cheek."[41] The subject had been popular with veritable old masters like Titian and Rubens, but most visitors like Peale saw a naked woman on a bed looking perhaps a bit too happy about being impregnated by Zeus, who had taken the form of a shower of gold.

Wertmüller's gambit was so financially successful, however, that when he died in 1812 and *Danaë* was put up for sale, the painting was documented as having an "annual earning power of eight hundred dollars or more." In the second decade of the nineteenth century, the tawdry painting was still the top earner in Philadelphia.[42]

Rembrandt Peale was in Paris with John Vanderlyn in 1810 when rumors of Wertmüller's earnings filled letters from home. Optimistic about their prospects of matching the

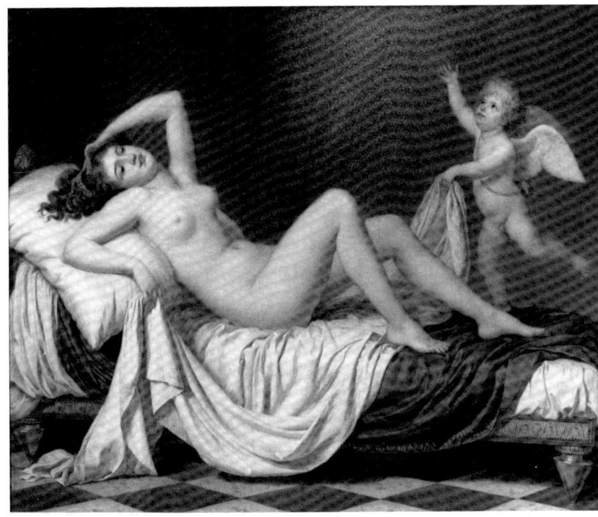

Fig. 11. Adolf Ulrik Wertmüller, *Danaë and the Shower of Gold*, 1787. Oil on canvas, 59 1/8 × 74 7/8 in. National Swedish Art Museum, Stockholm.

Swedish artist's success, both prepared for their return to America by painting large-scale nudes that might attract the same paying customers. Vanderlyn copied three famous nudes by Correggio and Titian in the Louvre, and finished his own composition, *Ariadne Asleep on the Island of Naxos*.[43] Peale followed Vanderlyn back to America in October 1810 and soon began construction of an addition to his house especially designed for the display of paintings, complete with skylights. For the price of twenty-five cents, visitors to "Rembrandt's Apollodorian Gallery" could see works in a variety of genres, including several copies of European paintings. Most of the paintings on view were large-scale works that demonstrated Rembrandt's French training—no selling point for an American artist in Philadelphia was more valuable. Eakins tried to bank on this same distinction a half century later.

Rembrandt Peale of course did not invent Francophilia when he returned from Paris in 1810. France was the great hero of the Revolutionary War. The French had come to the aid of the colonies at a critical juncture and had been first to recognize the independent nation. In celebrating the conclusion of the war, Charles Willson Peale filled his transparencies in the streets of Philadelphia with pro-French symbolism. As Sellers writes, "the success of American arms was vaunted, the vileness of the enemy exposed, and always, France glorified in a blaze of poetic allegory."[44]

Francophilia was still strong thirty-five years later, but it was complicated by a more entrenched set of concerns. Americans admired the skills artists brought back with them after spending time in Paris, but many of them also considered the importation of French attitudes toward nudity and sexuality as unwelcome immigrants (a concern that helped spur the first federal obscenity law in 1842, aimed at foreign, mostly French, imports). Nevertheless, market forces and the taste for forbidden fruit overruled espoused morality as they still do today.

In a display of thoughtful and cunning capitalism and perhaps in deference to his father, Rembrandt Peale modified Wertmüller's example by attempting to paint nudes containing moralizing examples of virtue that could be marketed along with the promise of naked female flesh. It took a few tries before Peale got the formula correct.

Rembrandt Peale's first effort at a profitable and acceptable nude was his monumental *Roman Daughter* of 1811, which he described as a "novelty" specifically crafted to entice paying visitors—the painting was not for sale (fig. 12).[45] Unlike the *Danaë*, here there was at least a moralizing narrative of filial piety and feminine sacrifice, which in Rembrandt's mind undoubtedly justified the awkward display of a large naked breast. How else could the story be told?

The Roman Daughter illustrates the story of a young woman who saved her father's life by secretly sustaining him with her own breast milk after he had been condemned to starve in prison. Charles Willson himself sat as model for the persecuted father, although it is unclear that he appreciated the end result. The titillating and somewhat embarrassing fact that the breast is being nuzzled by an old man's mouth definitely was not appreciated by critics—one reviewer also complained that the positioning of the father's hand at his daughter's pelvis was unfortunate.[46]

Peale's next large-scale work, *Jupiter and Io* (destroyed by fire in 1823), was even more controversial, prompting "A

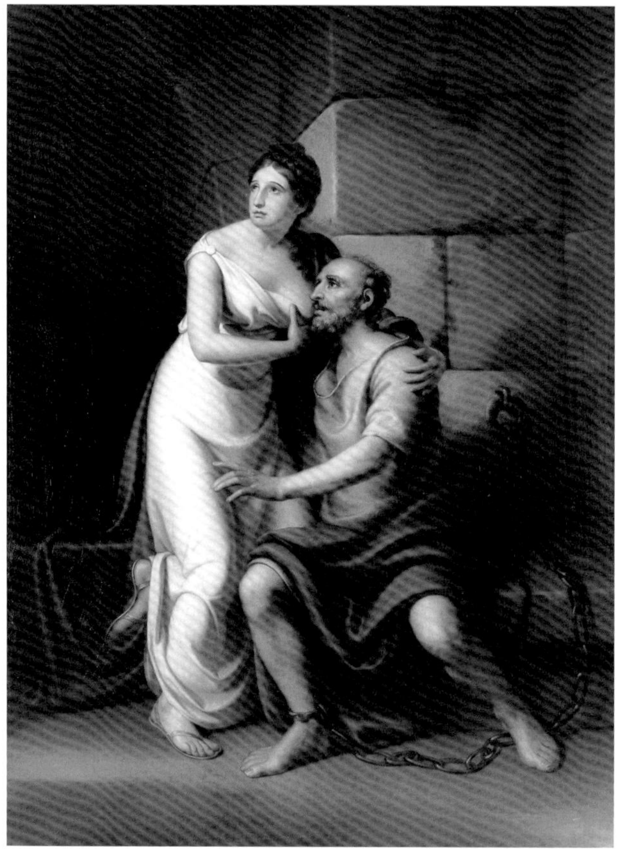

Fig. 12. Rembrandt Peale, *The Roman Daughter*, 1811. Oil on canvas, 84⅝ × 62⅞ in. Smithsonian American Art Museum. Gift of the James Smithson Society.

Lover of the Arts" in Philadelphia to denounce "'the filth of mythology' that had worked its way into the 'quiet, decent, moral city.'"[47] The characterization seems a bit naive, considering that not far away, Charles Willson Peale was burdened by the daily chore of clearing "drunks and prostitutes" from the venerable statehouse yard.[48]

Much worse for Rembrandt Peale than the sensational newspaper columns (which had the principal effect of sending more business his way, as they had for Wertmüller) was criticism that *The Roman Daughter* was plagiarized from a version of the theme by François Gérard that Rembrandt had seen in Paris. The Philadelphia critics ultimately proved too much for the young artist to bear, and in 1814 he decamped for Baltimore, where he founded a museum of natural science and art modeled on his father's. Before long, he was showing an increasing number of "nudities" there as well, including *The Roman Daughter*. The challenge for Rembrandt Peale, as for the American artists who followed him, was to balance a fundamental tension between profits and morals that two centuries later still persists—the roots of this conflict run deep.

In 1811, Charles Willson Peale wrote to Thomas Jefferson to air his concerns regarding public display of the nude in America. At a time when national habits seemed malleable, he referred to an especially interesting exchange to make his point:

> My son Rembrandt took the portrait of a noted Indian Chief called the Bastard, of a tribe from the upper lakes—he is 70 years old, a fine head, but what led me to mention him is a striking trait of the Indian Character As is usial [*sic*] the visiting Indians are shewn [*sic*] every thing that is esteemed curious in the City—A Painting by Vertmullier, Dana & the Shower of Gold now exhibiting for pay—The Indians was led to see it, while the Conductor was arranging matters at the door, the Indian Chief & his Son was sent forward to the room of Exhibition, when the Conductor came to the Room he found the old man & his Son setting with their backs towards the picture conversing together, he then pointed to the piece which they were brought to see, The old man replied, "that was not fit to be seen" and they would not look at it. This exactly corresponded with another instance of Indian modesty that I noticed before the revolution War.[49]

Charles Willson Peale's interest in Native American attitudes toward the nude demonstrates his own philosophical grappling with the issue. Here, there seemed to be an odd justification for American prudery and censorship in the example of the continent's first inhabitants.

Undoubtedly, however, Peale's comments also were driven by his larger concern about how his children were dealing with nudity in the paintings they created and exhibited in the United States. Rubens followed his brother Rembrandt in Baltimore by also exhibiting paintings of nudes in a museum. In 1815, Charles Willson wrote in an agitated state to Rembrandt:

> I find by your letters to Rubens that you have made some important alterations in the Picture [*Niobe*] of Io., but do what you will with it, still I have my doubts that you cannot be safe in making an Exhibition of any kinds of *nudities*. You know very well that it is all important, to keep clear of every offence to religious societies; you must know that if they take it into their heads that such exhibitions are improper, their inviteracy [*sic*] knows no bounds, and your establishment of the Museum may suffer irreparable injuries—. Religious ilnature [*sic*] knows no bounds. You may be taxed until they oblige you to shut it up, I say they because the Corporation is chiefly composed of Prysbetereans [*sic*] & Methodists. If you do exhibit the Venes [*sic*] and the Io, I hope it will not be in your House. I have been much mortified by the Exhibition of them at Ruben's [*sic*] when I heard it said that it ought to be presented [prevented] as a public nuisance.
>
> Perhaps you may get them sold by a raffle, and let them be seen in some other place rather than your Museum.[50]

Interestingly, Charles Willson Peale seems not to have concerned himself with the morality of the displays themselves, even though both sons had been publicly attacked by critics in the press. Rather, the elder Peale was mortified only when he heard the practice described as a public nuisance that might result in the assessment of penuriously high taxes. Peale, ever the marketing strategist, suggested instead that the paintings be displayed at a more distanced location and using a different sales model.

As to the question of whether or not to paint such pictures in the first place, all three Peale men seem to have understood that there was no better way to demonstrate the skill and sophistication born of their European training than monumental neoclassical history painting. In America, connoisseurs for such paintings were hard to come by, so it also helped if the subjects stimulated the kind of interest that would bring paying viewers in the door, and in that regard, even in the first quarter of the nineteenth century, nothing sold so well as sex. The large number of viewers willing to look at "nudities" refuted what the "religious societies" would have liked to believe about the morality of the city's residents.[51]

In fact, the result of the moralizing diatribes of trustees and critics in the press—then as today—was opposite the effect they might have wished. In the first quarter of the nineteenth century, the absence of public institutions willing to display the nude resulted in private exhibition galleries that amounted to little more than highbrow peep shows. The Washington Museum in Philadelphia went so far in 1819 as to advertise an "Anatomical Room ... which will be found worthy of attention of medical gentlemen and connoisseurs" for an extra fee of twenty-five cents.[52] The term "medical" was used quite brazenly here to signify nudity, and conventions of viewing the body not otherwise allowable in polite society. It is doubtful that all the "medical gentlemen and connoisseurs" who showed up at the "Museum" were interested in high art.

The indictment presented against Henry Robinson of New York on charges of obscenity in 1842 stated that "he had a very large quantity of [obscene] prints on sale at his establishments ... in a room partitioned off for that purpose, and others of a less obscene character, though clearly so, publicly exposed in his principal store room."[53] Although records of pornography vendors before the wave of prosecutions brought in 1842 are difficult to locate, it is quite possible that this was a business mode employed for quite some time in America. Rembrandt Peale chose the same physical arrangement for the display of his erotic *Dream of Love* in Baltimore when complaints arose. The *Dream of Love* and a wax figure of Venus were set in a separate room for those inclined to pay the necessary admission fee to view naked flesh.[54] The boundaries between sensual art and its sexual cousin pornography were a matter for consternation throughout the century.

Although some methods of displaying paintings and sculptures of nudes and pornography may have been similar, it is of course important to point out the difference between works by Vanderlyn, Peale, and Wertmüller and the standard fare of nineteenth-century pornographers. Helen Lefkowitz Horowitz has done her best to reconstruct what pornographic images of the century looked like, although she also points out the difficulty of finding materials that purposefully never were registered with the Library of Congress. Based on a few surviving examples, we do know that these images included "explicit and emphatic representations of sexual excitement and varied sexual acts. Some books contain many prints, and these could be separated for distribution. Other prints were sold separately. Explicit images of coition, oral sex, anal sex, females urinating, and females embracing each other seem designed to arouse men and to supply them with a range of titillating visual material intended for varied tastes. In such prints, the genitals of men and women are often highlighted by tinting."[55]

Two points are important here. First, although painters and gallery owners like Rembrandt Peale may have toyed with the sales conventions of pornographers (and it is possible that they inspired them instead), the large-scale paintings they made did not look like the images Horowitz describes. Oil paintings never were difficult to distinguish from the kind of engraved and later photographic materials that were viewed and sold in a furtive manner in the backrooms of bookstores and newspaper stands. And, of course, neoclassical subjects were seldom as explicit as those described by Horowitz. Elements both of context and content were important differences.

A second point is salient as well, however. Whether or not artists like Peale and Vanderlyn consciously sought to titillate their audience in the manner of pornographers, their mere adoption of French subjects and styles could not help but signify carnal sexuality.[56] In Philadelphia and Baltimore, as elsewhere in the United States, condoms were alternately described as "French letters," "French protectors," or "French rubber goods," and, later in the century, readers seemed to understand what advertisers in popular magazines meant when they offered "Gay French photographs from Life."[57] In New York, the popular and tawdry *Police Gazette* advertised "books such as *Pauline's Caprice*—'daringly unique in its spiciness' and complete with colored illustrations, ... the story of 'a Young and Gay Girl's Life in the Whirlpool of Fast Parisian Gayety.'"[58]

When American artists boasted of their French training and sophistication, their countrymen understood that they had been exposed both to professional education and to a much more libertine society. This assumption was not new. Benjamin Franklin's success at mastering French manners as representative of the American colonies was largely credited with saving the revolutionary effort at a critical moment, while the habits he adopted abroad were seen as dissipated. The Americans who followed Franklin in bringing Parisian manners home found themselves holding the same double-edged sword in a scenario rife with both hypocrisy and opportunity.

As a student in Paris from 1866 to 1869, Eakins frequently commented on French manners in letters home, perhaps in an effort to assure his family that he was conducting himself well while abroad (and living on their financial contributions). In these letters, he took the opportunity to profess his virtue while admitting exposure to the seamier side of the city.

In his first year in Paris, Eakins wrote home to his father to describe an afternoon in the company of some of the French students he studied with in the Ecole des Beaux-Arts atelier of Jean-Léon Gérôme, presumably in a brothel: "The whole afternoon that I spent with them, I don't consider altogether wasted. I saw more of most characters and manners than I would ever have discovered by myself, nor am I ashamed to have accompanied them to the place. But I would be ashamed if I had been in the least attracted by the vice I saw there."[59] Eakins assured his father in this letter that his role in Paris was more akin to that of a cultural anthropologist than a young man drawn to "vice." In other letters though, Eakins also made clear his lack of aversion to nudity in art, and his acceptance of even the least moralizing displays of flesh offered in the Beaux-Arts tradition.

On the subject of one of Gérôme's most salacious paintings, *The Slave Market* (fig. 13), Eakins wrote: "I heard two fools say Gérôme painted that picture on the principle that Chaplin paints a girl with her clothes lifted up to interest only low people. It will interest very sensual people more sensual than those Turks who are yet hardly interested & they have nature while this is but a picture, but the sensual people are better than the fools. Above these only sensual, comes a higher class the thinking people & feeling ones who always want to see everything to know more."[60] Like Peale and Vanderlyn before him, Eakins carefully justified the erotic nature of French painting in order to make it more respectable, and acceptable, back home. Throughout his career, Eakins continued to insist that "thinking people" always wanted "to see everything to know more." In his mind, this simple quest was rationale enough for all the excesses others saw in his approach to the nude as an artist and teacher, including even disrobing and posing with his own students.

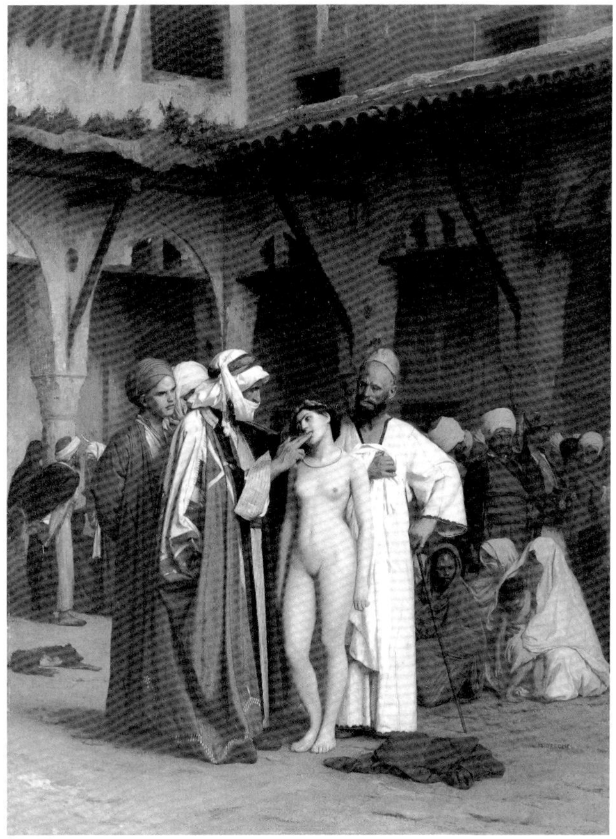

Fig. 13. Jean-Léon Gérôme, *The Slave Market*, 1866. Oil on canvas, 33 3/8 × 25 11/16 in. Sterling and Francine Clark Art Institute, Williamstown, Massachusetts.

As Eakins was to find out in especially stark fashion when he lost his job, however, nudity almost always was a fraught sell in nineteenth-century America. Despite even the most blatant, pandering efforts of profiteering artists and museum operators like Peale and Vanderlyn, the financial situation for ambitious Francophilic artists and for galleries like the Washington Museum ultimately faded. After the Panic of 1819, there wasn't much free money to be had even by a smart artist willing to brave censure.[61]

In 1820, Rembrandt made a last-ditch effort to save his enterprise, and his large and hungry family, with a bold and

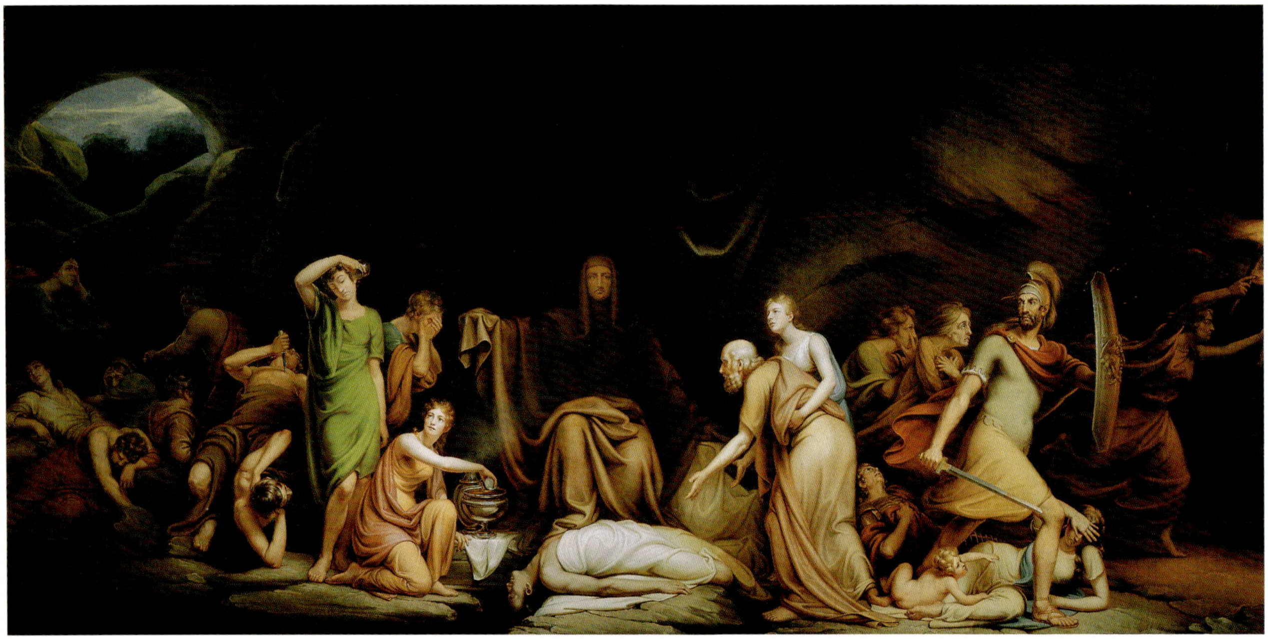

Fig. 14. Rembrandt Peale, *The Court of Death*, 1820. Oil on canvas, 138 × 281 in. The Detroit Institute of Arts. Gift of George H. Scripps.

ambitious new marketing strategy. If sexy paintings wouldn't sell anymore, then he would try their opposite, a thoroughly original painting predicting the dire fate of sinners—*The Court of Death* (fig. 14). If moralizing sentiment was what Americans really wanted, Rembrandt can have had little doubt as he went forward with his enormous and time-consuming project. This was, as Rembrandt advertised, "312 square feet" of preaching.[62]

Ever the businessman, Rembrandt smartly chose a type of religious message that both was newsworthy and benefited from fierce public debate in the press. The painting was based on a poem by the British abolitionist Bishop Beilby Porteus titled "Death, a Poetical Essay." Although Porteus was an Anglican, the underlying idea that man was responsible for his own sin was at the heart of Unitarianism, a denomination that was growing in popularity in cities like Baltimore and Philadelphia, and infuriating the more traditional faithful. Porteus wrote:

> 'Twas Man himself
> Brought Death into the world, and Man,
> Himself
> Gave keenness to his darts, quicken'd his pace
> And multiply's destruction on mankind.[63]

In his pitch to a large and paying American constituency, Rembrandt avoided portraying this moralizing theme with the kind of obscure classical references that had failed to impress audiences of *The Roman Daughter*.

Rembrandt's quite original conception instead was to tell the story of death with clarity—and clothes on. Death, cast as a hooded figure at center, is surrounded by twenty-one other life-size figures representing (from left to right) such themes as Despair, Fever, Consumption, Hypochondria, Apoplexy, Gout, Dropsy, Suicide, Delirium Tremens, Intemperance, Remorse, Pleasure, Pestilence, Famine, War, and Conflagration. A murderous warrior, an orphan, a corpse, and a widow complete the tableau of morbid horrors. In the foreground, hope is found in a figure of "venerable old age" supported by Faith.[64] Peale's use of his family as models made an even more direct appeal to viewers who came to understand the work as very much belonging to their own time and place. Charles Willson Peale, for example, appears in a filiopietistic display as the figure of virtuous old age.

Although Peale's enormous melodrama lost its public appeal long ago, it is hard to overstate the popularity of this work in the nineteenth century. In many ways, Rembrandt's bombastic painting was the opening salvo in the reform campaign that would come to dominate American religious and educational spheres in the antebellum period. The fact that the painting "was a huge success, viewed by more than thirty thousand people and earning more than nine thousand dollars in its first year of exhibition," was strong evidence that Rembrandt had struck cultural (and financial) gold.[65] The painting was still making money for its investors at midcentury, both in exhibition and through sales of engraved reproductions.[66]

In 1846, the painting's investors promoted Peale's money-making epic for a new generation of guilt-ridden viewers:

> Beneath the outstretched arm of Death, stoops the alluring semblance of PLEASURE. The smoke of her incense rises to soften and obscure the countenance of Death. Her hand prepares another intoxicating draught; and her animated features entice only to betray. A YOUTH, whose interesting form might promise a more honorable destiny, stands relaxed, the stupid and disappointed slave, rather than the participator, of pleasure.
>
> A companion of Intemperance lies at his feet, clasping his throbbing brain—another, at his left shoulder, hiding his guilty face, expresses the anguish of REMORSE—and another, behind him, is plunging the dagger into his heart. Like them, he must suffer the pangs of FRENZY, and the burnings of REMORSE; and were he to look back on his own shadow, he would perceive the form of SUICIDE. The hand of Intemperance is equally raised to take his own life.[67]

The torrid language the painting's investors used to describe the figures of pleasure and intemperance, and their results—remorse, frenzy, and suicide—matched the sermons of moral reformers who, by the 1840s, held sway among many Americans. This was the decade in which Thomas Eakins was born.

One of the most famous and influential of mid-nineteenth-century reformers was Sylvester Graham, who especially concerned himself with "self-pollution" (masturbation), a sin that he believed was responsible for physical and mental disease. The obsessive efforts of reformers like Graham to regulate American sexuality in the mid–nineteenth century explain a good deal about why Benjamin Franklin's indiscretions were so much better tolerated than those of Thomas Eakins. At the very least, the moral reform movement provides insight to the cultural influences that shaped Eakins' attitudes toward the body and its sexual nature—or at least to the influences he rebelled against.

Sylvester Graham did not invent the idea that masturbation was a danger to health, but he can be credited with bringing this idea to the attention of general audiences in the United States in 1833 with his publication of "A Lecture to Young Men." Graham had no medical training, but rather advertised himself as a "Public Lecturer on the Science of Human Life." In this capacity, he was able to earn a substantial living both through speaking engagements and sales of his printed essays.

On the title page of Graham's 1833 lecture, he began by quoting a variety of relevant religious tracts, including "For this is the will of God, even your sanctification, that ye should abstain from fornication: that every one of you should know how to possess his vessel in sanctification and honor; not in the lust of concupiscense."[68] Despite initial appearances, religion was not Graham's primary motivation for preaching abstinence. Building on a revised version of European medical texts that predicted doom for those who wantonly expended their health-producing reserves of semen, Graham instead believed that sexual stimulation itself was the cause of disease.

> The convulsive paroxysms attending venereal indulgence are connected with the most intense excitement, and cause the most powerful agitation to the whole system, that it is ever subjected

> to. The brain, stomach, heart, lungs, liver, skin—and other organs—feel it sweeping over them, with the tremendous violence of a tornado. The powerfully excited and convulsed heart drives the blood, in fearful congestion, to the principal viscera,—producing oppression, irritation, debility, rupture, inflammation, and sometimes disorganization;—and this violent paroxysm is generally succeeded by great exhaustion, relaxation, lassitude, and even prostration. These excesses, too frequently repeated, cannot fail to produce the most terrible effects.[69]

By locating the problem of poor health in the "convulsive paroxysms" of sexual desire and orgasm, rather than the loss of semen, Graham had authored a perfect justification for the censorship of images and texts deemed to cause "agitation." Although Graham did not refer to visual stimulation much in his lectures, he did include "obscene conversation or talk, lewd books, and lascivious images" along with "improper diet," "want of exercise," and "disproportionate exercise of the brain" as the "principal agents" that could lead to "self-pollution."[70]

Graham's prescriptions for health were different for married and unmarried men. For married men, there was a beneficial relief to be found in the "diminished" effects of sexual excitement. When the married couple became "accustomed to each other's body," then "their parts" would "no longer excite an impure imagination" and intercourse thankfully would occur "very seldom."[71] Some unhappy couples might have been surprised to hear this effect of marriage spoken of as a good thing. Graham's program for boys and young men was much more extreme, and set the stage for a climate of sexual repression that informed the education received by boys of Thomas Eakins' generation.

Sylvester Graham was optimistic that boys could be saved, despite his hysterical reporting of the frequency of masturbation among schoolboys, many of whom "went to the still more loathsome extent of an unnatural commerce with each other!"[72] Both for boys and for any men suffering from "nocturnal emissions," Graham believed that the remedy lay in strict adherence to a program of diet, exercise, and a lifestyle that avoided any possible sensual pleasure. Feather beds were to be avoided, baths were to be cold, and vegetarian food was to be the centerpiece of each meal, principally including "Farinaceous food" such as "good bread made of coarsely-ground, unbolted wheat, or rye, or Indian corn … taken with a little molasses or sugar … and freely masticated."[73] The perfect food, of course, was the "Graham cracker" the lecturer himself invented in 1829. In contrast, the most popular sex manual of Benjamin Franklin's era, *Aristotle's Masterpiece*, taught that pleasurable sex was necessary for the health of both men and women, and in fact that conception was ensured only if both parties experienced orgasm.[74]

Although it is impossible to know if Thomas Eakins was raised on a diet of the supposedly health-promoting crackers, we do know that he and his father spent a great deal of time engaged in "active exercise" while enjoying "free and copious draughts of the pure air of heaven!" both of which were heartily recommended by Graham.[75] Eakins' most well loved paintings depict the outdoor sports he and his father and friends engaged in and enjoyed watching—rowing, sailing, hunting, baseball, and wrestling.

Thomas Eakins may never have read Graham's lectures, or heard him speak, but we do know that the ideas of moral reformers were ubiquitous in public schools at midcentury. At Central High School, Eakins' required courses included "moral hygiene," a phrase redolent with overtones of the reform movement. A book of class notes written during this course in 1859 records passages from a "Lecture on Delirium Tremens" given by E. W. Vogdes, M.D., at the school: "Delerium Tremens. There is no form of evil so universal as the partaking of alcoholic drinks. Alcohol leads to insanity." Professor Vogdes' lectures on the dangers of alcohol, which included mental and physical decline, extended for several weeks.[76]

The following year, Eakins and his classmates had the opportunity to see the perfect illustration of the lecture subject. Another Eakins classmate, Joseph Boggs Beale, kept a diary in which he recorded his visit to see Rembrandt Peale's grand, moralizing sermon in paint on display in Philadelphia on June 30, 1860. He wrote: "I went next door to the Concert Hall to see R. Peale's great & beautiful painting of 'The Court of Death.' … This picture is 13 by 24 ft. long & contains 23 life size figures representing Death, Corpse, Old Age, Faith, Pestilence, Famine, Victim of War, Orphan, Widow, War, Conflagration, Pleasure, Remorse, Intemperance, Suicide, Delerium Tremens, Gout, Dropsy, Apoplexy, Hypochondria, Consumption, Fever, Despair."[77] Beale's attentiveness to all the figures in the painting indicates that he took its message seriously enough to record each detail for posterity.[78]

Although there certainly were important American subcultures that scorned such moralizing sentiments, Eakins largely was educated by those who were in agreement with reformers. Even in the medical arena in which Eakins soon circulated, the ideas of "lecturers" like Graham had yet to be refuted by any better science. The years Eakins spent in Philadelphia following graduation from high school are largely undocumented, but we do know that he purchased a ticket of admission to the clinical lectures at Jefferson Medical College, where he might have heard echoes of Sylvester Graham's ideas in the addresses of the famed surgeon Dr. Jacob Mendez DaCosta, a later portrait subject. Harry Jacob's student notebook recorded DaCosta's discussion of the dangerous symptoms caused by passion:

> A person Being in a *great passion* may have apoplexy. *Anger* may produce slippage of the action of the Heart. A Person who gives way habitually to his *Veneral Passion*, a person of *loose habits* in this respect may from the *constant exhaustion* of this produce Paraplegia ... *Love* may cause disease and death. Constant *agitation, sorrow,* Excitement of even *pleasurable excitement* which those people in *Love* are supposed to undergo, will produce at first a certain amount of functional disturbance and by this continuing will produce some organic disease.

DaCosta generally advocated celibacy as a vaccine against every manner of illness.[79]

Popular treatises on sexuality written after the Civil War continued to agree with Graham and DaCosta. In 1866, William A. Alcott, M.D., declared in *The Physiology of Marriage* that "the young man who has fallen into the habit of self-pollution will, almost of a certainty, be found greatly attached to hot and exciting food and drink." Alcott's remedy, like Graham's, required plain food, uncomfortable bedding, and reduced "excitement."[80] Central High School's faculty may have been aware of such recommendations as they enforced a rigorous curriculum that made sure the boys in its charge—including Eakins—had little time for "excitements."

Central High School was founded in 1836 as the first "high" school in the state, intended specifically to educate the most gifted (male) children of the working and middling classes.[81] During most of the nineteenth century, "only about 1 percent of male lower-school students in Philadelphia" were admitted.[82] Entrance requirements were based on performance in elementary school, the recommendation of its principal, and an examination that 50 percent of Philadelphia's best elementary students routinely failed.[83]

The anxiety produced by such stiff competition could be overwhelming. George Alfred Townsend, a student two years ahead of Eakins, recounted the following entries in his diary:

> January 2, 1856: "All my thoughts are bent on one thing,—to reach the High school."
> Monday, 21st: "if I fail to get in, nothing is left but to go to work."
> Friday February 1: "Vowed this morning that if I were allowed to enter the High School, I would forsake everything but my studies, and be a better boy."

And following the exam:

> February 6: "The algebra exam utterly unfit for boys so little prepared as we are."
> February 9: "Admitted to the Central High School to-day at about one o'clock; average 75.5. Number sixteen in one hundred and forty-two admitted. The greatest day in my life."[84]

Although Thomas Eakins left no records of his thoughts at the time of his admission to the high school, one can imagine similar feelings of pride and excitement.

Once these students were admitted, Central's founders made an especially concerted effort to avoid educating them in the manner of upper-class boys who studied classical languages and literature at private academies in preparation for college. Here the continuities between the lives of Franklin, the Peales, and Eakins are most direct. Benjamin Franklin's grandson, Alexander Dallas Bache, designed the school's curriculum and served as its first principal. Bache in turn chose Rembrandt Peale to design the drawing curriculum and teach art at the school.[85]

Bache's experience as a student at West Point largely influenced his decision to create a curriculum and disciplinary code designed to produce useful citizens—not only as soldiers, but also as engineers, surveyors, and scientists. Bache also had seen and admired this type of curriculum during a two-year tour of Europe's schools as president of Girard College. This trip resulted in his publication of a massive tome titled *Report on Education in Europe.*[86] Following various examples, Bache's program at Central High School aimed "to furnish an education preparatory to the pursuits of commerce, manufactures, and the useful arts," and featured a curriculum heavily weighted toward advanced study of the sciences and technical skills, including optics, calculus, and surveying. Bache's emphasis on science was perhaps particularly appropriate in Philadelphia, whose civic heroes included Benjamin Rush, Benjamin Franklin, and Charles Willson Peale.[87]

Professors at Central, chosen from among the city's best teachers and scholars, were divided between the "Literary, Mathematical, Scientific, and Technical Departments."[88] In his first year of attendance, 1857–58, Eakins studied general history, Latin, algebra, and physics five times per week, phonography three times a week, and composition and writing once a week. In the second semester, the writing course included instruction in drawing. In his second year, Eakins' program was more complicated; it included composition and elocution, trigonometry, geometry, Latin, surveying, writing, drawing, bookkeeping, moral science, French, chemistry, and German.

Eakins' third-year course schedule included differential calculus and engineering, mechanical and perspective drawing, and political economy. In the fourth year, Eakins learned integral calculus, astronomy, organic chemistry, and mental philosophy. Throughout his four years, Eakins followed the program mandated for the entire class; there were no electives available to students.[89]

The inclusion of drawing in the four-year program Bache designed at Central High School might seem surprising given the school's emphasis on useful education, but in fact some type of drawing course was included in every semester: first- and second-year students practiced writing and drawing; third- and fourth-year students learned perspective, mechanical drawing, and ornamental writing. This long-lived curriculum influenced generations of prominent future artists including Joseph Boggs Beale, Thomas Eakins, and William Trost Richards. All three men began their high school education in drawing by studying Rembrandt Peale's *Graphics.*

Peale's popular drawing book provided only slight introduction to art, but his influence in the educational arena went beyond conveyance of basic techniques. Peale was among the most vociferous of the nation's "art crusaders," arguing publicly that drawing instruction would raise the aesthetic standards of the country and provide skilled draftsmen for a host of industries. In agriculture, better sketching and planning could establish more efficient crop layouts. In manufacturing, American industries would more effectively compete in design and production with European goods. And in a true egalitarian and meritocratic spirit, following in his father's footsteps, Peale guaranteed success to any student who would only "TRY," promising that "nothing is denied to well-directed Industry."[90]

Decades later, Eakins followed Peale both in writing a drawing manual for art students and in asserting that its lessons were of "great simplicity and easy comprehension" if students would only "strain their brain rather than their eye."[91] Eakins also followed Peale in incorporating drawing techniques applicable to fine art as well as industry in his text. Eakins' inclusion of chapters on mechanical drawing, optics, and camera lenses demonstrates the ongoing influence of Central High School and Rembrandt Peale in Eakins' own definition of a useful life teaching and creating art, and inventing new devices.[92]

John Hart, principal of Central High School during Eakins' years there, was so enamored of Peale's *Graphics* and its potential for the nation's students that he bemoaned that it had not been adopted by all the elementary public schools, despite the artist's concerted efforts: "Could the plan have succeeded, and could the entire youthful population of that great city, which is pre-eminently a mechanical and manufacturing center, have grown up with a familiar practiced skill in the use of the pencil in ordinary off-hand drawing, there can be no question that it would have added untold millions to the general wealth."[93] Hart's quote is good indication of the importance assigned to art, industry, and education by Philadelphians at midcentury. The foundation Charles Willson Peale had laid for future appreciation of the arts in Philadelphia paid off in the lives of his children and grandchildren.

Thomas Eakins clearly lived in a time when many more educational opportunities were available in America than had been a century earlier, but it also is clear that not all of the changes between 1780 and 1880 were improvements. An excellent example of the era's increasingly frigid climate can be found in the treatment of its mythic hero Benjamin Franklin: his bawdy "Advice to a Young Man on the Choice of a Mistress," written in 1745, is now quite famous, but it was suppressed by Franklin's grandson and other compilers of his papers throughout the nineteenth century as being "too indecent" to print.[94]

Benjamin Franklin surely would have scoffed at such censorship, and at the prudish and pompous lectures of Rembrandt Peale, Sylvester Graham, and E. W. Vogdes, but both he and his era had passed, and the men of Eakins' generation were subjected to sexual information that consisted of little more than terrifying prognostications of death and disease. It was in this environment that Eakins would try to make his own contribution to the history of the nude in American art using French models as examples. The effort wasn't new, of course, but the language and conventions that formed the context for that project had shifted and hardened.

Anti-obscenity reformers won legislative and prosecutorial victories in the 1870s and 1880s that ushered in new reasons to fear censorship. In Eakins' day, Congress and the courts—rather than the "Prysbetereans and Methodists" who condemned *The Roman Daughter*—were the ones who attempted to enforce strictures against public exhibition of the nude. The mechanics and intensity of censorship had changed between 1810 and 1880, but the similarities among Franklin, the Peales, and Eakins demonstrate that the role played by intellectuals and artists as social provocateurs had not lessened. Definitions of culture and progress changed a great deal between the time Franklin and Eakins were depicted so imprudently in sketch and photograph, but the act of negotiating boundaries between the uplifting and the prurient in America stayed the same.

Despite the compelling corollaries between the Peales and Eakins, it is useful to close this chapter with one profound difference: the relative quality of their paintings. Eakins grew up in a city whose institutions were already built, their walls already stocked with portraits by his predecessors. The paintings of the Peales surrounded and undoubtedly motivated Eakins, but not necessarily only for their celebration of American heroes and moral tales. As someone who had studied anatomy from an early age, what must Eakins have thought of all the slouching, boneless shoulders, awkward imprecise renderings of contracted and extended limbs, and taxidermist-stuffed busts and britches in paintings by the Peales? Thomas Eakins took as his agenda not only the continuance of Philadelphia's tradition of artist-scientists. He also took as his mission the goal of doing it all much better than it ever had been done before. It was his unswerving and unflinching pursuit of that goal, in dissection halls, surgical clinics, and art studios, that brought him crashing up against the mores of late-nineteenth-century Philadelphia.

CHAPTER TWO

The Agnew Clinic, *The Gross Clinic*, *The Crucifixion*, and *Swimming*
Dissecting Eakins' Paintings

When Charles Willson Peale painted *Exhumation of the Mastodon*, he intended it as a backdrop for the bones of the beast, installed in his encyclopedic museum. Both the painting and the bones were impressive and tangible evidence of the artist's accomplishments and legacy. Eakins created several works with that same impulse, but the three that stand out most prominently in his career are *The Gross Clinic*, painted expressly for the Centennial Exhibition of 1876 in Philadelphia; *Swimming* (1885), intended to hang in the Pennsylvania Academy as a demonstration of the school's pedagogy; and *The Agnew Clinic*, painted in 1889 as a form of reentry into the Philadelphia scene following three years of punishing scandals and recovery.

It is significant that medical students commissioned Eakins to paint their famous and well-loved professor of surgery in 1889. Despite his diminished reputation in Philadelphia's art community, Eakins always was held in high esteem by doctors as a dynamic and skilled portrait painter who understood the milieu. The occasion for the portrait was the impending retirement of D. Hayes Agnew from the University of Pennsylvania Medical College. Perhaps sensing the possibility for his own "exhumation," Eakins launched into this project with great ambition, and insisted on composing a surgical clinic complete with portraits of each student in the background—a much more grandiose painting than the students had envisioned, but offered at the same price.[1]

The resulting *Agnew Clinic* is a true tour de force, exhibiting the artist's mature pictorial skills and his profound respect for his subject, and the science his painting celebrated (fig. 15). At 84 by 118 inches, this was a painting designed to impress—it was the largest canvas of Eakins' career. The composition is suitably grave: Agnew, his patient, and attending staff reside within a horizontal, arching niche—set vertically, the composition would resemble a lamentation scene with Agnew as God the Father. The gravity of the faces in the arena as they gaze intently and directly at the open breast of the patient is matched by the seriousness of the learners set above them—these are men (and one woman) with great purpose.

Like other nineteenth-century painters, in particular Jean-Léon Gérôme, Eakins' Parisian master, the artist used touches of red in *The Agnew Clinic* to move the eye across the broad horizontal canvas from left to right: we see brilliant strokes of crimson in the ears of the subjects who nearly bisect the canvas at its midpoint—the man leaning on his hand at left, Agnew himself, the seated listener at his flank, the anesthesiologist, surgical assistant, nurse, and then in the two men above and below her at the right edge of the canvas. One of those two men is Eakins himself—his wife, Susan, painted the portrait of her husband standing in the gallery, listening to the commentary of the physician beside him. The artist is first an observer, his eyes clearly focused on the patient, but we also are compelled to consider the importance of hearing in this situation as equal to (if not greater than) the importance of seeing. For most of the onlookers, sight of the work inside

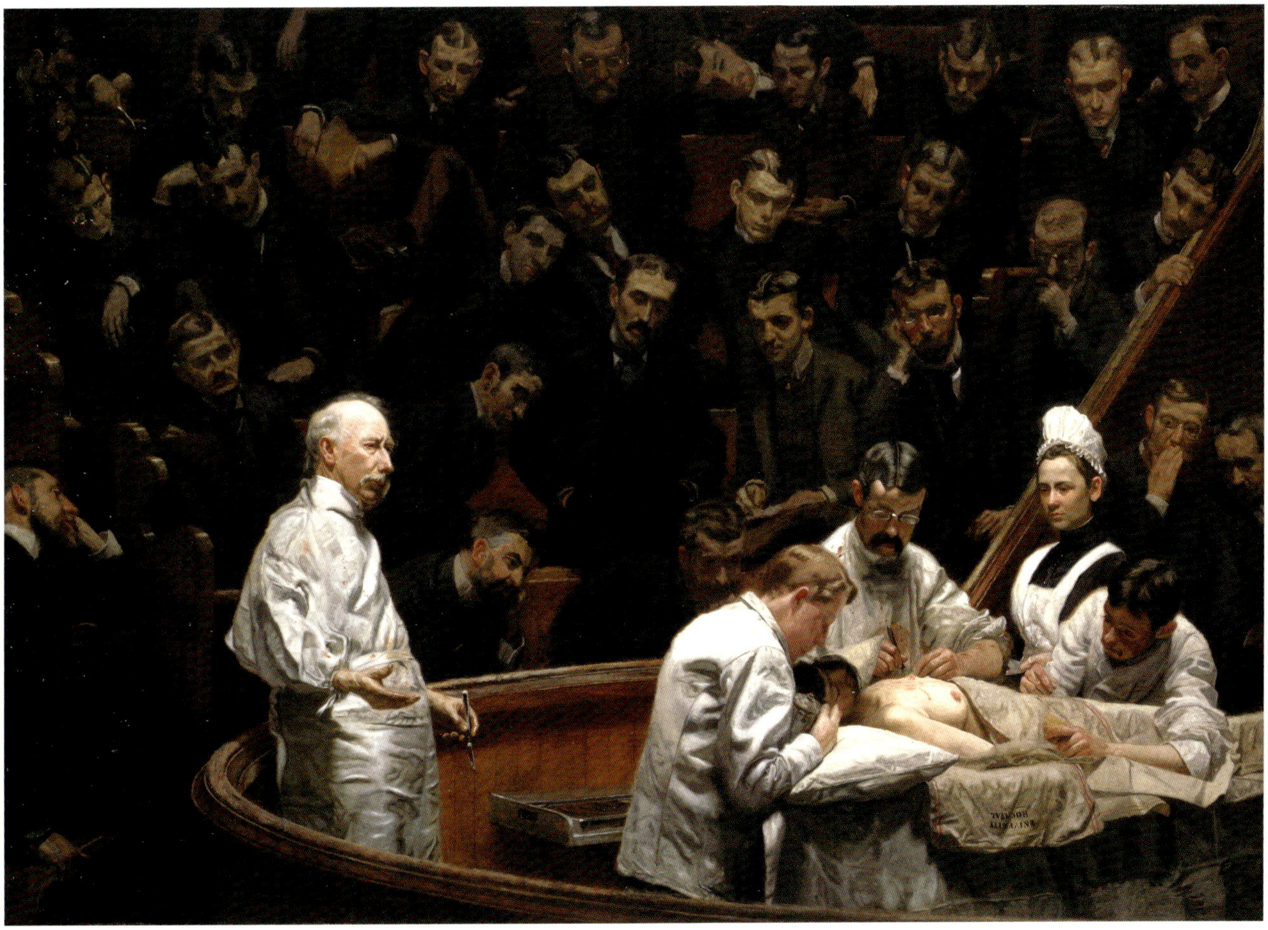

Fig. 15. Thomas Eakins, *The Agnew Clinic*, 1889. Oil on canvas, 84⅛ × 118⅛ in. Courtesy of the University of Pennsylvania Art Collection, Philadelphia, Pennsylvania.

the wound indeed would have been quite limited, and Agnew made no effort to enable or direct their vision as he operated. Agnew's surgical assistant in Eakins' painting, Dr. J. William White, wrote of the aging professor:

> His habit at his clinic was to precede his operation by a brief statement of the history of the case, and by some remarks upon diagnosis and prognosis, and upon his reasons for choosing the particular operative method he was about to employ. During the operation itself he said but little. Afterward he would usually leave some of the final details, the arrest of hemorrhage, insertion of sutures, application of dressings, etc., to his assistant, while he explained more fully what he had just done, and described what he had observed.
>
> He possessed to a remarkable degree the power of interweaving with his admirable descriptions of surgical diseases and injuries the underlying anatomical facts upon which accurate diagnosis and successful treatment so commonly depend. Indeed, as a practical surgical anatomist he was in this country without a peer.[2]

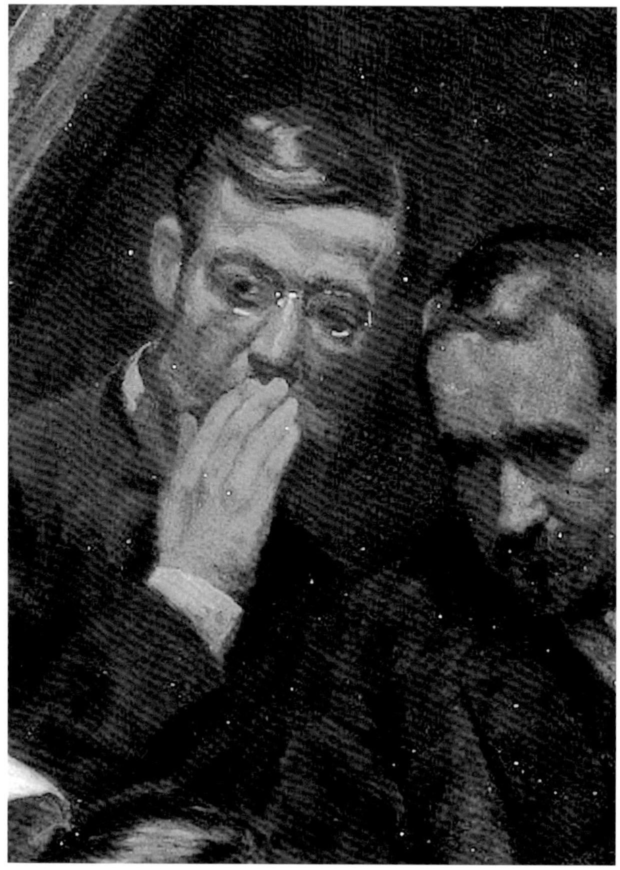

Fig. 16. *The Agnew Clinic* (detail).

Eakins' choice of this moment in Agnew's clinic—the surgery completed, the master now lecturing—is later in the course of the procedure than the moment he had chosen to memorialize Samuel D. Gross fourteen years earlier. Now, there is no bloody knife, no gaping wound. Agnew is in a less vigorous pose than Gross, having already completed the intense work of removing the cancerous tumor. The drama here lies in the educating taking place—lighting now plays evenly across the canvas, highlighting the reception of knowledge as much as its production. Agnew has already transitioned from his role as a surgeon, responsibility firmly with the patient, to his role as a professor, imparting his knowledge to a new generation of physicians who soon will stand in his place.

At this point in the clinic, Eakins is free to engage in hushed conversation about the case—Susan Eakins pictured him taking instruction from Dr. Fred H. Milliken (fig. 16).[3] This chapter focuses on this particular image within *The Agnew Clinic*—attempting metaphorically to eavesdrop on Eakins' conversations in the medical arena—the ways he talked about and looked at human bodies with his colleagues in this insular environment. My intention also is to compare these conversations with the historical and modern dialogues provoked by *The Agnew Clinic* and Eakins' other controversial images depicting anatomically correct bodies: *The Gross Clinic, The Crucifixion*, and *Swimming*. The contrast between Eakins' intentions and the public's reception of his work reveals a wide gap of understanding akin to conversants speaking different languages. Until we look at these canvases with a medical gaze, they continue to offer only a partial explanation of the artist's meanings.

In the effort to recapture Eakins' medical conversations, it makes sense to begin with that corner of *The Agnew Clinic* in which Dr. Milliken is whispering into Eakins' ear. Most likely, as White describes, Milliken was discussing the "underlying anatomical facts" Agnew considered so important to teaching surgery. Eakins was well prepared to take instruction from a "peerless" surgical anatomist in 1889, and to fully understand the biological intricacies related. By 1889, the artist already had been a dedicated student of anatomy for at least twenty-five years. Writing home from Paris in 1867, Eakins recalled that he had missed the recent graduation of his high school dissecting companion—presumably from medical school. He wrote to his father: "I am afraid diploma time is over and I just remember Cliff. Beecher who was my companion in the dissecting room. If his diploma is not yet filled give him a good skin & an extra flourish around his name."[4]

It may well have been Eakins' Central High School chemistry teacher, Benjamin Howard Rand, who first introduced these young students to anatomical study—Rand was a physician specializing in toxicology who left Central to join the faculty at Jefferson Medical College in 1864, three years after the artist's graduation. Eakins' classmates T. Guilford Smith and Joseph Boggs Beale recorded their attendance during those years not only at the Philadelphia School of Anatomy but also at surgical clinics at Jefferson.[5] Surgery was an exciting and public spectacle in mid-nineteenth-century Philadelphia, and it is hard to imagine Eakins not joining in. We do know that in 1864 he purchased an admission ticket to the anatomy course offered by Dr. Joseph Pancoast at Jefferson Medical College—a ticket that entitled him also to attend the surgical clinics taught by Samuel Gross and to take part in dissections.[6]

Surgical clinics were just as much an exciting public spectacle in Paris from 1866 to 1869, when Eakins studied there, but surprisingly the artist never mentioned attending them in his lengthy and numerous letters home. Nonetheless, it is possible that Eakins was inspired by the world-famous surgeons of Paris.[7] Upon his return to Philadelphia, records show that the artist once again purchased a ticket of admission to anatomical and clinical study at Jefferson in 1874.[8] In that year, Eakins also chose Dr. Benjamin Rand as his first large-scale portrait subject. By 1875, when Eakins began painting the surgical clinic of Samuel D. Gross, it is clear that Jefferson Medical College was a milieu the artist understood.

Twenty years later, Eakins still was dissecting, teaching anatomy, and researching on his own; in 1894, for instance, he presented a paper to the Academy of Natural Sciences in Philadelphia entitled "The Differential Action of Certain Muscles Passing More than One Joint." The author introduced his paper with humility: "It is not without diffidence that I, a painter, venture to communicate with a scientific body upon a scientific subject."[9] Eakins was unnecessarily humble; he had been communicating with scientists about scientific subjects for decades, as presumably he did with Dr. Milliken in Agnew's clinic. In sum, it is hard to imagine that Milliken would have needed to translate any terms for Eakins' benefit—the artist spoke the anatomist's dialect.

Both as a student and as a mature painter, Thomas Eakins undoubtedly spent hundreds of hours in conversations similar to the one he depicted in *The Agnew Clinic.* Discussions with the many world-renowned medical professors Eakins painted at Jefferson and the University of Pennsylvania Medical Colleges infused him with medical attitudes toward the body, and with clinical culture generally. Other prominent Philadelphia medical professors, including William Williams Keen, Harrison Allen, and S. Weir Mitchell, were important friends and professional colleagues.

The preeminent mission of these portrait subjects and friends, as Dr. White noted, was to study and research the underlying anatomy and physiology of the human body. Agnew began his series of anatomy lectures for students with an inspiring instruction: "At the very outset, therefore, of our subject we have medicine standing at the door of anatomy, like the ancient inquirer at the Temple of the Oracle, waiting for the voice within."[10] Lectures on anatomy and attendance at clinics were helpful to students, but no method of instruction was considered more valuable than dissection. It was here that students could take their places as conversants in a dialogue—it was here that they could speak as well as listen.

In a photograph of William H. Pancoast's anatomy dissection laboratory dating from the years of Eakins' attendance, we see Pancoast at center, surrounded by his students, scalpels in hand, dressed in aprons with sleeve guards over their suits, prepared diligently and unflappably to delve into the cadaver laid out in front of them (fig. 17).[11] The body on the table—half-flayed and eviscerated, and posed to look out at the photographer—seems a gruesome subject of study, but this was the daily pedagogical fodder of medical students. In

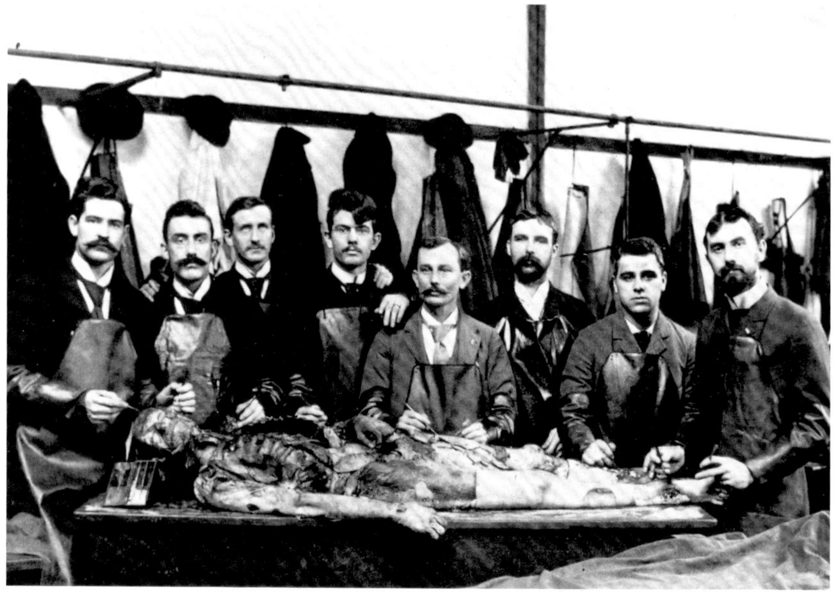

Fig. 17. Unknown photographer, *Dr. William H. Pancoast's anatomy dissection laboratory*, 1862–74. Photograph mounted on card, 6 × 8 in. © Courtesy Thomas Jefferson University, Philadelphia. All rights reserved.

this environment, learning could not take place without touching, so it is not surprising that all the students pictured rest their hands on the body. Eakins, like the medical students surrounding Pancoast, became inured to the look, the smell, and even the feel of dissected cadavers.

Outside the dissection hall, however, touch was not a sense used by students in their medical education. Eakins' emphasis on *ears* in *The Agnew Clinic* is no accident—the artist was drawing our attention to, or at least simply depicting, the didactic teaching methods of the nineteenth-century medical college. For the physicians-in-training stacked in rows above Agnew's surgical amphitheater, listening and observing were the central activities of their education outside the dissection laboratory—most would graduate without ever having touched a living patient. Students attended between four and six hour-long lectures each day, Monday through Saturday, nine months per year, a schedule purposely "leaving the afternoons free for dissection."[12] A sharp distinction was clear: live bodies were for looking at and hearing about, dead bodies were for talking about, touching, and probing.

In 1877, following the European model, the University of Pennsylvania moved to an expanded, "scientific" curriculum, but, even in this updated course of study, patients were seen but never touched or spoken to—the modern program, with its new emphasis on scientific research in fields such as biology and chemistry, included fourteen hours per week of "practical instruction" in the laboratory, and twenty hours in the lecture hall.[13] The process of medical education, then as now, was grueling. Agnew's students, as Eakins portrayed them, are watching and listening, principally occupied with the serious work of memorizing the words of their mentor. For the students in the audience, it would be years before they would attempt to heal patients on their own in the context of later apprenticeships. And they could qualify for this next phase of their education only by passing lengthy examinations testing their memorization of lectures and texts.[14] The dissection laboratory proved in this scenario an important outlet for free exchange, in which aspiring doctors could not only share information but also form professional and social bonds.

Humor was an important vehicle in the formation of both these types of bonds. Several of the doctors Eakins painted and worked with wrote memoirs late in their careers that reveal the macabre sense of humor and glib attitude toward the body shared in the medical community. Just as Eakins knew how to take instruction in clinic, he also knew how to understand and enjoy the jokes anatomists told, which often relied on specialized knowledge of the body and always demanded an inured audience. Agnew's biographer, for instance, related a story the surgeon undoubtedly, proudly, told himself many times: "His zeal to learn anatomy and surgery led him to a rather desperate scheme. He purchased bodies in Philadelphia, had them delivered to a dissecting room at his home, then engaged a farmer to sink the remains in a local pond, where the eels finished the dissection and prepared perfect bone specimens. The eels were said to be noted locally for their flavor, size and snappiness—until the secret got out."[15] Agnew's anecdote hardly would have made acceptable dinner conversation in a mixed crowd, but it was refined compared with other stories told by the physicians with whom Eakins associated.

William Williams Keen, Eakins' colleague in teaching artistic anatomy, in particular shared "humorous" anecdotes in his copious writings, and presumably in his conversation and teaching. In his "personal recollections," he recounts the story of his first fatality, and the post-mortem examination made to determine the cause of death:

> I should explain here how we remove the brain for examination. One sweep of the knife is made down to the bone over the top of the head from one ear to the other; the hair being previously parted in this line so that when brushed again into its ordinary place the incision is completely hidden. The whole front half and the back half of the scalp are then detached from the skull, the first being drawn as a flap over the face and the other low down on the back of the head. On the temples—this is a very important point in this narrative—are two strong muscles which pull the lower jaw tight against the upper jaw. By placing one's finger on the temple and "chewing" repeatedly—one can feel them contracting. As soon as they are uncovered by displacing the scalp as above described, these two muscles are divided by knife at the level at which it is intended to saw all around the skull. This detaches the entire top of the scull [*sic*] from the lower part and makes easy the removal of the brain.
>
> My assistant—he who had given the chloroform and himself therefore quite nervous—was stooping and steadying the head while I used the saw.... With the first full sweeps of the saw to and fro suddenly the patient loudly champed his jaws at us several times! My assistant instantly dropped the head and leaped backwards holding up both hands in horror and exclaimed "Good God! Isn't he dead"! I stood trembling and aghast.... Consider all the circumstances ... —the scalp on the top of the head wholly torn loose and the top of the skull half sawed off—in those pre-antiseptic days a surely mortal wound if the man wasn't really dead.... In a few moments we had sufficiently regained our self command to realize that the man was surely dead and to continue this post mortem.... Finally when I rolled the brain out of the skull into my left hand my assistant with a sort of ghostly smile and a sigh of relief turned and said "Well, Doctor, he's dead now anyhow!"[16]

Keen's willingness to share amusement at the gory vision of a sawed-off head, jaws chomping, and the comic relief of the brain finally "in hand," indicates his expectation of an appreciative audience. Eakins would have been amused, but his acculturation among Philadelphia's medical elite did not necessarily serve him well in more general social circles.

The contrast between the way men like Keen talked about the body and the way artists and art critics talked about the body could not have been starker. Part of this rift was due to a general concern expressed by popular art theorists like John Ruskin, who wrote under the heading "Science desiccates nature": "Every archaeologist, every natural philosopher, knows that there is a peculiar rigidity of mind brought on by long devotion to logical and analytical inquiries. Weak men, giving themselves to such studies, are utterly hardened by them, and become incapable of understanding anything nobler, or even of feeling the value of the results to which they lead.... The man who has gone, hammer in hand, over the surface of a romantic country, feels no longer, in the mountain ranges he has so laboriously explored, the sublimity or mystery with which they were veiled when he first beheld them.... In his more informed conception, they arrange themselves like a dissected model."[17] Ruskin's phrasing here is pregnant with references to the practice of anatomical study, and his verdict is clear. Exploration of the "dissected model" could only ruin appreciation for the "romantic" terrain of the body.

Ruskin was even more strident in his condemnation of Darwinism, about which he wrote: "In all probability the race of man is appointed to live in wonder, and in acknowledgement of ignorance; but if ever he is to know any of the secrets of his own or of brutal existence, it will assuredly be through discipline of virtue, not through inquisitiveness of science."[18] Eakins was not a fan. He wrote from Paris that he would take Gérôme's advice "quicker than the work of a writer who knows nothing about painting such as Ruskin."[19]

Although Eakins certainly would have preferred otherwise, echoes of Ruskin's sentiments are rife in criticisms of his paintings. These comments are a good reminder that the two principal subcultures the artist worked in offered vastly different conversational styles and shared assumptions. One can hardly imagine Ruskin being amused by Keen's story of chomping jaws.

Among others who are not likely to have been amused by such anecdotes are the cultivated fine arts critics who scorned *The Agnew Clinic*, a painting that not only placed a "dissected model" at its focal point, but clearly devoted itself to a celebration of the "inquisitiveness of science." At the University of Pennsylvania Medical College, Eakins' canvas generated celebratory praise from its patrons, who hung the painting prominently and recorded the names of its many subjects for posterity. In later years, the painting was used to illustrate the covers of several medical school textbooks.[20] Unlike the medical school colleagues and clients of Eakins, however, art exhibition juries and reviewers were not impressed. Comments expressed at the time indicate that, like Ruskin, they felt that art should elevate through "virtue," rather than scientific accuracy.

To say that reception of *The Agnew Clinic* in the art world was disappointing would be a vast understatement. Margaret Supplee Smith writes that when the Pennsylvania Academy declined to exhibit *The Agnew Clinic* in 1891, "publicly, the painting was rejected on the technicality that it had been previously exhibited in Philadelphia and was therefore ineligible.... Privately the directors revealed the real reason for their rejection of the painting: 'Some thought the picture not cheerful for ladies to look at.'"[21] The jury at the Society of American Artists simply refused to hang the painting, prompting an infuriated Eakins to resign his membership in an organization that would dare to reject "a composition more important than any I have ever seen upon your walls."[22] In Chicago, an art critic reprimanded the selection committee for choosing to hang the work at the World's Columbian Exhibition of 1893, warning that "delicate or sensitive women or children suddenly confronted by the portrayal of these clinical horrors might receive a shock from which they would never recover."[23] As another critic put it, although the portraits and composition were "really excellent," the "surroundings and accessories" were found to be "scarcely in good taste." And for another reviewer, the painting was little more than an excuse for "depicting the horrors of the dissecting table."[24]

The difference between this artistic rhetoric and the conventions of medical dialogue are both striking and telling. Whatever Dr. Milliken and Thomas Eakins may have discussed as they observed the surgical clinic of D. Hayes Agnew, the concepts of "horror" and "good taste" were certainly not among the terms bandied between them—criticisms like these would have seemed patently absurd in Agnew's amphitheater. Eakins had reason to expect a better response—here was his *Exhumation*, the culmination of so much study of anatomy, paint handling, and pictorial space. This was Eakins' magnum opus.

Eakins also could reflect on the fact that he already had made concessions to public taste. Certainly, this was a much different painting from *The Gross Clinic*, which had shocked audiences fifteen years earlier through its inclusion of the red, glistening wound and bloody knife. Agnew is reported to have asked Eakins to leave the blood out of his portrait, but it is possible too that the artist hoped to avoid the same virulently negative critical response that his first surgical painting generated.[25] Then, almost every reviewer had expressed shock at the subject matter of the painting, with one critic going so far as to claim "although vigorously treated, it ought never to have left the dissecting room."[26] There is no question that Eakins' skill in *The Gross Clinic* was noticeable, and several critics were impressed. William Clark, writing for Philadelphia's *Daily Evening Telegraph* in 1876, stated that "nothing finer" than the explosive Gross portrait had ever been attempted in the country.[27] At the same time, more conservative artists and critics refused the painting a place in the art galleries of Philadelphia's Centennial Exhibition for which it was intended.[28]

Perhaps hoping for a more favorable response in New York, Eakins tenaciously entered *The Gross Clinic* three years later at the Society of American Artists' second annual exhibition. Most city newspapers reviewed the work extensively. The *Herald*, for instance, termed the painting "decidedly unpleasant and sickeningly real in all its gory details, though a startlingly life-like and strong work"; others found it "powerful," "horrible," "compelling," "nauseating," "revolting," and "fascinating."[29]

Fourteen years later, Eakins was a more subtle painter. Even if Agnew did not specifically ask him to leave blood out of the scene, it makes sense that the artist chose not to include a gaping surgical incision at the fulcrum of his later painting—it would have been a jarring disruption within the classically masterful composition of this more mature work. In *The Gross Clinic*, Eakins had chosen a palette of deep contrasts—strong blacks, whites, and, at the crux of the work, the red blood on the opened thigh and on the scalpel and fingers of the surgeon. In *The Agnew Clinic*, light plays more evenly across the canvas in muted tonal contrasts: the frieze-like composition, with its parabolic niche inscribed within, directs the gaze with much gentler subtlety than the dramatic diagonals and jarring color composition of the earlier treatment of the surgical clinic theme. Now, the focus of the painting is the pale white breast that faces us, attracting attention by virtue of its connotative rather than its compositional shock value.

In spite of the significant differences between the two pictures and the startling elements in each, their reception was similar—they were largely condemned in the art world, but accepted and praised in the medical settings they depicted and for which they were painted.[30] The medical and artistic communities of late-nineteenth-century Philadelphia could not have presented two more different audiences or two more different visual languages. Eakins' anatomical view of the body as expressed in *The Gross Clinic* and *The Agnew Clinic*, informed as it was by the community the paintings were created for, translated poorly outside that realm—just as Agnew's and Keen's anecdotes could not have failed to cause an irrecoverable "shock" to "delicate or sensitive women," or even to "delicate" male art critics. The patient's guardian cringing at the left edge of *The Gross Clinic* was perhaps meant to embody the irrational response Eakins knew many viewers would have, inviting his audience instead to mirror the calm and rational students above her. Like them, we are meant to take instruction from Eakins' grand lecture with composure.

But Eakins' view of the human body was far more acute than his gaze at the body politic. Given the startling nature of their subjects for uninitiated viewers, it is hard to imagine a set of circumstances in which *The Gross Clinic* and *The Agnew Clinic* would have met with general praise in the art world of the late nineteenth century. It is also important to understand that it was not just the artist's paintings expressly about medical anatomy that caused discomfort. Eakins not only spoke the anatomist's language, he developed a painting style that gave artistic form to this unwelcome voice and then applied it to a variety of subjects. As one critic wrote in an otherwise scathing review of *The Gross Clinic*: "It is painted in a dry but highly technical manner, which, in one sense may be said to have agreed with the subject."[31]

The artist's desire to meld anatomical study and painting style is evident even as early as his student work in Paris. In 1868, Eakins wrote to his father, discussing the benefit of his studies in the medical arena: "My anatomy studies and sculpture, especially the anatomy comes to bear on my work & I construct my men more solid & springy and strong. It makes me catch forms quicker & the slightest movements of the model don't hinder or worry me, only show me plainer what I am doing."[32] The artist's first portrait subjects, soon after his family members and close friends, were the award-winning rowers Max Schmitt (fig. 18) and the Biglin brothers, chosen for their accomplishments on the Schuylkill River and also for the excellent condition of their bodies. Muscular definition, slim physique, and scant clothing allowed Eakins to use the knowledge he had gained of the proportions and actions of muscles, tendons, ligaments, and joints. After finishing his series of rowing portraits, the artist turned to baseball players, whom he praised as "very fine in their build. They are the same stuff as bull fighters."[33] Later in his career, Eakins photographed a variety of track and field athletes and painted wrestlers and boxers.

In contrast to the reception of the clinic pictures, anatomical clarity was forgiven, overlooked, or even admired in reviews of Eakins' paintings of athletes. Critics praised the rowing scenes in particular, with one writing: "The representation of splendid muscular development and the suggestions of great physical power in excited exercise [are] perfect. The force of drawing can no farther go." Another wrote: "Biglin Brothers Practising [*sic*] is an oil painting with a strong effect of late golden light playing around the knotted muscles of the oarsmen."[34] These paintings clearly presented fewer challenges to their audiences: the subjects are healthy, uncut, and clothed, their reproductive anatomy kept private—these factors offer an obvious contrast with *The Gross Clinic* and *The Agnew Clinic.*

One might assume from this contrast that the difference lay chiefly in Eakins' startling exposure of titillating parts—the buttocks in *Gross* and the breast in *Agnew*. But no such easy rule can be extracted regarding allowable uncovering in high art. Reviewing the standard fare of exhibitions at the time, it immediately becomes obvious that it could not have been the mere presence of a naked breast that was at issue. Public galleries of the time had come a long way from Charles Willson Peale's era, and were filled with female nudes. Rather, it was the idea of the woman as surgical patient, her flesh diseased and now sliced open, that was the shocking transgression—the unallowable subject.[35] Certainly this was not the ideal woman portrayed as a waxy sexualized confection in such paintings as *An Eclogue* by Kenyon Cox (fig. 19), or in works by Abbott Thayer, Thomas Dewing, William Merritt Chase, and other American artists praised in the very same essays that condemned Eakins for his choice of subject matter.[36] The presence of the naked breast was never specifically commented upon in reviews of *The Agnew Clinic*—by the 1880s, it was a mark of intellectual and cultural attainment to accept the idea of nudity in art—but it is also true that few critics wanted to write the words "breast" or "cancer."

Reviews of Eakins' work make only one point clear: the rules regarding what anatomy could be depicted in art were hard to gauge, and both context and style were key. Nudity was allowable in nymphs but not surgical patients. This distinction may seem obvious and natural today, but we must remember that rules like these always are in flux, and often brighten into visibility only after they have been violated. In the 1880s, for example, Eakins' painting of a partially clothed single man presented as Christ in *The Crucifixion* received far more hostile rebuke than his image of a group of men naked outdoors together, *Swimming*. To modern eyes, however, the latter is far more provocative. The truth is that Eakins painted so much anatomy in his career, in so many different contexts, that he managed to transgress a sizable array of unspoken "rules" governing the presentation of the body in

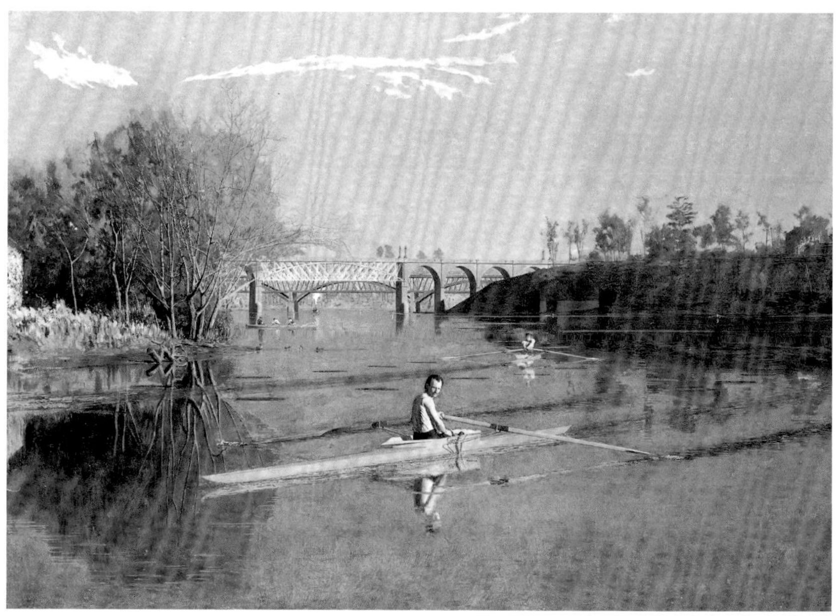

Fig. 18. Thomas Eakins, *The Champion Single Sculls (Max Schmitt in a Single Scull)*, 1871. Oil on canvas, 32¼ × 46¼ in. The Metropolitan Museum of Art, New York. Purchase, The Alfred N. Punnett Endowment Fund and George D. Pratt Gift, 1934.

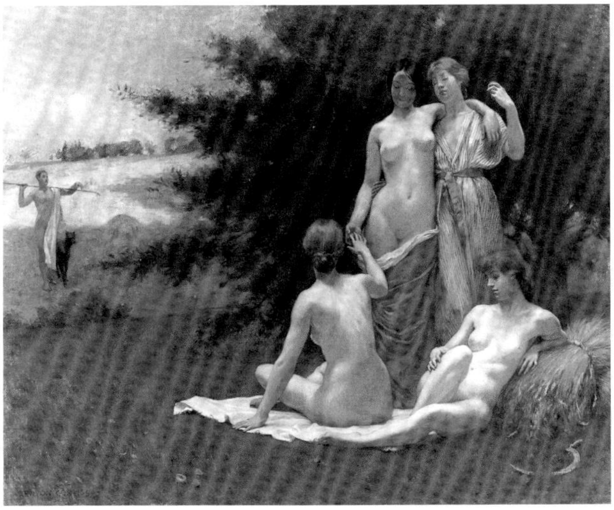

Fig. 19. Kenyon Cox, *An Eclogue*, 1890. Oil on canvas, 48¼ × 60½ in. Smithsonian American Art Museum. Gift of Allyn Cox.

art. Comparing historical and modern dialogues about Eakins' paintings makes clear the unstable ground on which such criticisms always rely.

In 1880, Eakins' *Crucifixion* hung in a New York salon de refusés where critics took turns savaging this canvas that already had been rejected by the Society of American Artists (fig. 20). One reviewer went so far as to title his essay "Christ Crucified by Eakins."[37] Another critic wrote: "To those who from deep sacred feelings invest the person of Christ with ideal characteristics and qualities, the manner in which Mr. Eakins has treated the subject can never seem anything else than offensively repulsive."[38] And yet another disgruntled writer in New York complained: "Mr. Eakins finds in this picture the worst possible excuse for making a study of the nude figure. His Christ is the subject of a dissecting-room table—sickening, repulsive to the last degree."[39]

As he did *The Gross Clinic*, Eakins saw this canvas as an important work and submitted it to a variety of exhibitions, but reviewers in other cities were no kinder. A critic for the *Boston Daily Advertiser* wrote: "Don't go to see Eakins' 'Ecce Homo.' You won't wish to buy it, and you will wish you had never seen the hard and impossible and extraordinary attempt at a picture of the cross and its Sufferer. If you do stumble upon this picture you may be relieved from the impression of its anatomical and artistic lifelessness by the amusing spectacle of some horses above and to the right of it."[40] Another reviewer of the Mechanics' Fair exhibition in Boston protested that "the figure is painted with painful minuteness from a living suspended model, and however able it may be, is a decidedly disagreeable affair."[41] Eakins' most supportive critic, Mariana Griswold Van Rensselaer, wrote that "after seeing a hundred crucifixions from modern hands this one seemed to me not only a quite original but a most impressive and haunted work," and she called the painting "more than a mere anatomical study." Even in Van Rensselaer's devoted praise, the prevalence of references to Eakins' work as an anatomist is striking.[42]

Given Eakins' outspoken agnosticism, his motivation to paint a crucifixion scene is frankly curious. Elizabeth Milroy explains the picture as Eakins' attempt to craft a grand history painting in the European manner with an "informed adaptation" of admirable sources.[43] Alternatively, in light of his familiarity with the body culture of anatomists, we may see Eakins' crucifixion project as fulfilling a prophetic hope he had overtly expressed early in his career, in a letter written from Paris in 1868: "I can conceive of few circumstances wherin [*sic*] I would have to make a woman naked but if I did I wouldn't mutilate her for double the money. She is the most beautiful thing there is except a naked man but I never yet saw a study of one exhibited. It would be a godsend to see a fine man model painted in a studio with the bare walls, alongside one of the smirking goddesses of waxt [*sic*] complexion."[44] Eakins' "godsend" is in fact this stark painting, which contains not even "bare walls," and hardly a single descriptive passage outside the painting of the body and the few props that support it (the artist probably could not have imagined painting an outdoor nude in 1868). Rather than an interest in spirituality, or history, which are harder to read in the finished work, Eakins' *Crucifixion* reveals, again, his fascination with human anatomy. The body itself is clearly the subject of this painting, presented in a manner that allowed the artist to consider the weight of the form in an extraordinary pose.

J. Laurie Wallace, the artist's model for *The Crucifixion*, had just the type of physique Eakins liked to dissect, draw, photograph, and paint. Wallace's lean adolescent body allowed him to see and then to represent interesting anatomical structures, including the crest of the ilium at the hip, the tendons of the wrist, the articulation of the complex bones of

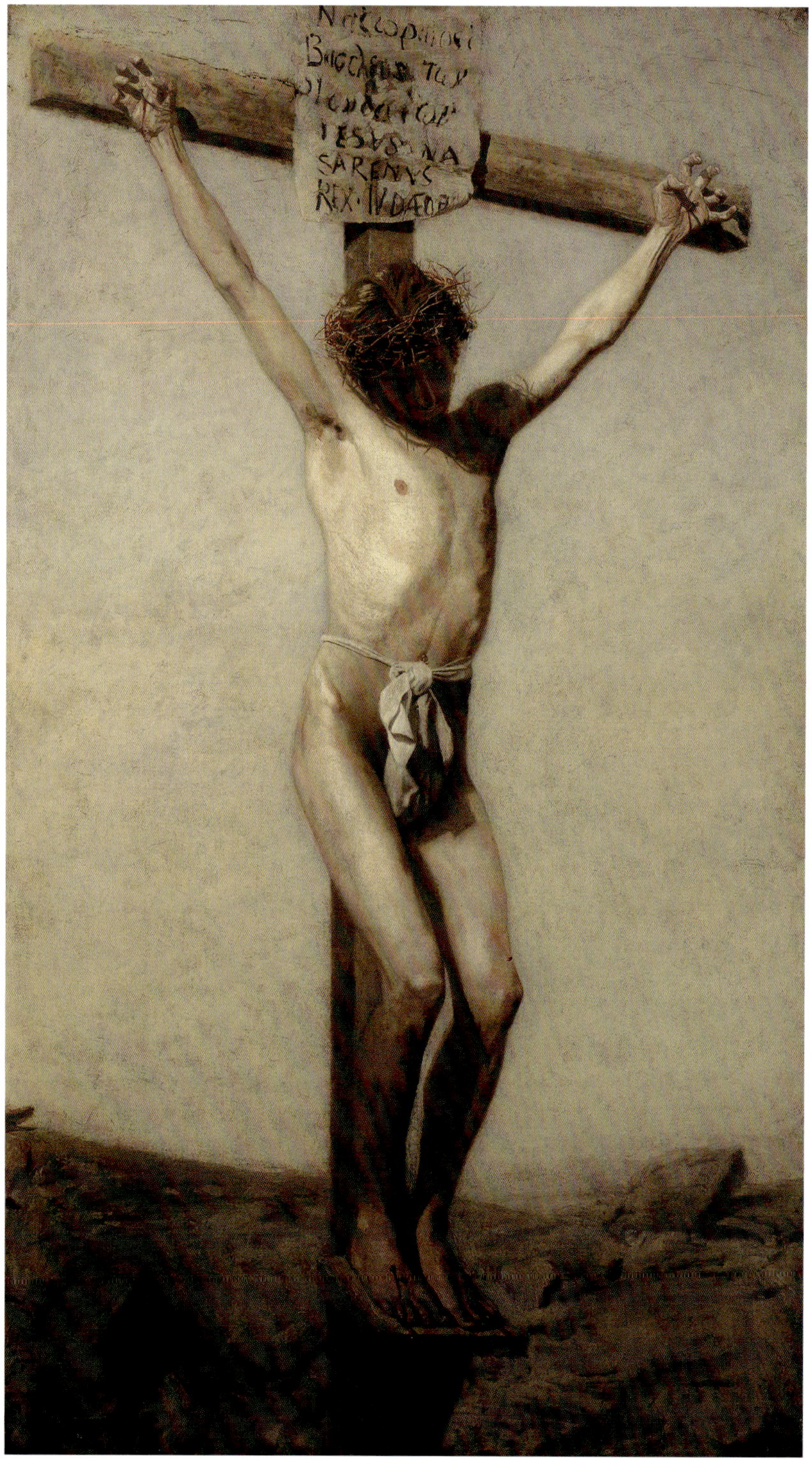

Fig. 20. Thomas Eakins, *The Crucifixion*, 1880. Oil on canvas, 96 × 54 in. Philadelphia Museum of Art. Gift of Mrs. Thomas Eakins and Miss Mary Adeline Williams, 1929.

the fingers and toes, the bony protrusion of the olecranon at the hinge of the elbow, and the corresponding patella at the knee joint. Eakins clearly tried to capture the look of a dead body hanging from its hands—the blood flows more freely from the feet than the hands, for example, illustrating the effects of gravity. The sternum and the ribs are subtly but demonstrably portrayed, along with a particularly fine passage of painting conveying the articulation of the armpit where the humerus is received into the cavity of the scapula. Surely, Eakins was influenced by the descriptive realism of the Spanish Baroque masters he had admired when studying in France and Spain years earlier; as Elizabeth Milroy points out, his *Crucifixion* is reminiscent of versions of the scene by Delacroix, Velázquez, and Rubens, along with many other popular scenes of martyrdom both old and new. Léon Bonnat, whom Eakins studied with for several months in France, painted an impressive version of the scene in 1874 with a similar emphasis on anatomical clarity and correctness.[45]

Nineteenth-century Philadelphia audiences did not see and admire the tradition of such venerable sources as Velázquez and Bonnat in Eakins' work. What they were looking for—and what was conspicuously missing from *The Crucifixion*—was a sign of divinity in the body of the martyred Jesus. Instead, they were confronted with proof of the knowledge that came from hands-on dissection, and they had little use for an anatomically correct expression of religious sentiment. As one succinct reviewer put it: "The artist who undertakes anything of the kind should endeavor to present it in a reverential light.... Mr. Eakins, on the other hand, paints as a student of the human body."[46] It is easy to imagine Doctors Gross, Agnew, and Milliken discussing the evident features on this body, but to the art world the painting was notably lacking elements that might make it a suitable subject for conversation about its obvious subject—Jesus.

Rather than reading scripture or looking to earlier prototypes in preparation for painting *The Crucifixion*, Eakins brought Wallace, his sixteen-year-old student, to a secluded spot in southern New Jersey where he dug a hole, raised a cross he had built himself, and then provided his model with a homemade crown of thorns. He later conducted more "sittings" for the painting on top of the roof of his home.[47] Eakins was especially interested in capturing the body as seen in brilliant, raking light. It is of course an amusing example of the artist's literal-mindedness that he felt southern New Jersey was a good approximation for the holy land—reviewers certainly did not. But Eakins' reason for going there at first may well have been more for privacy—Wallace recalled years later that he and Eakins had to move more deeply into the wilds of the marsh after hunters stumbled upon them as they set up the cross.[48] In the late nineteenth century, this context hardly mattered. Critics didn't seem impressed by the artist's attempts to be faithful to the context in which the scene occurred.

More than 120 years later, the merits or even the appropriateness of Eakins' blend of anatomy and art are no longer much questioned. The passions of the artist's own age long since have faded, and anatomical clarity is no longer derided as a ruinous element in his work. Today, passions are stirred by a set of concerns that, while not entirely new, are nonetheless much more differently articulated than they were in the 1880s. Today, Eakins' painting *Swimming* of 1885 is more provocative than *The Crucifixion.* In the slightly later work, Eakins chose a subject that allowed him to photograph and then paint a grouping of slender, fully naked men at a popular watering hole (fig. 21).

The inception of *Swimming* can be credited to Edward Hornor Coates, the new chairman of the committee on instruction at the Pennsylvania Academy of the Fine Arts—technically, he was Eakins' supervisor. Coates' idea, as best it can be recovered, was to commission a portrait from Eakins that would show the full flowering of the academy's pedagogy. Coates would then donate the painting to the academy where it could be admired by prospective and current students as well as city residents. Eakins spared no expense of time or resource in the venture—he created preparatory photographs and even wax models using the techniques he shared with students daily.[49]

Above all, this was a painting that flaunted the benefits of anatomical training. Bodies are seen in a variety of poses and perspectives: frontal, from the rear, left and right sides, vertically and horizontally, joints straight and bent, muscles bear-

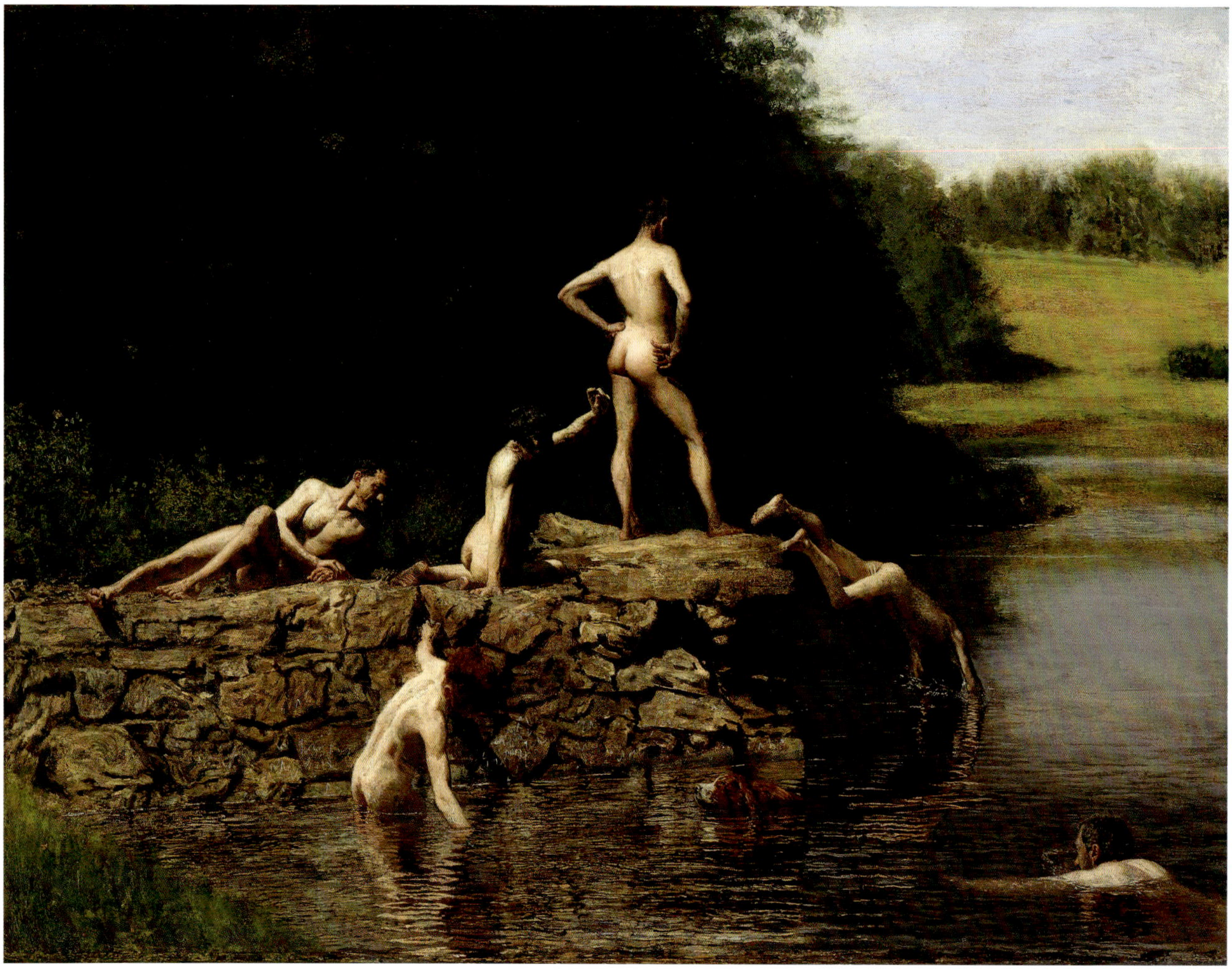

Fig. 21. Thomas Eakins, *Swimming*, 1885. Oil on canvas, 27⅜ × 36⅜ in. Purchased by the Friends of Art, Fort Worth Art Association, 1925; acquired by the Amon Carter Museum, 1990, from the Modern Art Museum of Fort Worth through grants and donations from the Amon G. Carter Foundation, the Sid W. Richardson Foundation, the Anne Burnett and Charles Tandy Foundation, Capital Cities/ABC Foundation, Fort Worth Star-Telegram, The R. D. and Joan Dale Hubbard Foundation, and the people of Fort Worth.

ing weight and relaxed, spines convex and concave. The raking sunlight crossing the scene helped Eakins prove his consummate understanding of the human body. From Eakins' point of view, *Swimming* must have seemed the perfect satisfaction of Coates' intent. He might have imagined himself standing before the painting in an academy gallery, leading a discussion with students, perhaps pointing out aspects of the curvature of the spine in various contortions. Instead, Coates allowed the painting to be exhibited at the academy but politely declined to accept it, taking instead *Singing a Pathetic Song*, which he termed "more representative, and it has been suggested ... perhaps more acceptable for the purpose which I have always had in view."[50] Eakins undoubtedly was disappointed—his preparations for *Swimming* were extraordinarily elaborate, and while *Singing a Pathetic Song* was a fine work, it was not nearly so useful for students as an illustration of anatomy and complex composition.

As usual, Eakins was undeterred by rejection, and he sent *Swimming* to the academy's fall exhibition of 1885, and then to Louisville, Kentucky, and Chicago in 1886. Not a single critic in three cities complained about the subject matter of the work. The effects of photography were mentioned in Philadelphia, and landscape elements were criticized, but the nudity of the subjects was not articulated as a problem.[51] Soon, the scandals of 1886 gave Eakins far more to worry about than bad reviews—he confined *Swimming* to his home and painted no more nudes until the turn of the century.

Scholars critiquing *Swimming* in recent years rarely have been as reserved as Edward Coates, and unlike earlier critics they certainly have found the subject matter a fruitful topic of discussion, in styles ranging from subtle to supple to hardcore. At one end of the scale, Kathleen A. Foster, the least speculative and most scrupulous of Eakins' modern biographers, concerns herself largely with issues of sequencing, dating, and historical fact in her extensive discussion of the artist's preparatory photographs of adolescent boys and young men wrestling, boxing, swimming, diving, and sunning themselves. Foster's willingness to speculate goes only so far as to say, "the fact that many of them feature [Eakins'] own naked body must also tell us something about the latent narcissism and exhibitionism indulged while the cause of art, science, or practicality was being pursued."[52]

That Eakins liked to be naked, or at least saw no shame in nudity, is confirmed by many accounts of his personal and professional life—and by numerous photographs. Eakins was surrounded by like-minded colleagues in this regard, including J. Laurie Wallace (who posed not only for *The Crucifixion* but also for *Arcadia* and *Swimming*) and George Reynolds (a frequent subject in photographs, and the diver in *Swimming*). Preparatory photographs for the painting offer evidence of many more students who were equally unabashed. Rather than speculating on the photographs and the painting as an indication of the artist's, or his students', sexual activities, Foster objectively discusses their impact on Eakins' career. She concludes that the painting was a professional miscalculation: "*Swimming* stood as visual confirmation ... of teacher-student nudity."[53]

Elizabeth Johns, writing with a more thematic purpose, views the painting as an example of Eakins' emulation of the Greeks. "At a period when there was much interest in bringing into modern life ideals from Greek antiquity, *Swimming* certainly alludes as well to such 'Greek' values fundamental to academic discipline as bodily beauty and mental control.... In this environment of mutual respect for the endeavors of the arts and sciences, Eakins might well have compared his leadership to that of Plato in the informal outdoor academy in ancient Athens."[54]

Although Johns might have wished to keep her discussion on a Grecophilic (and Platonic) plane, she goes on somewhat wistfully to admit that "a generation ago even to include sexuality in interpretations of the painting would have been unthinkable. The critical climate has changed, of course, and now the issue is not whether but how to discuss sexuality." Johns then posits Eakins as a sensualist whose life seems not so much "explicitly homosexual" as akin to the work of Walt Whitman in its "passionate devotion to the body and to the material manifestations of the spirit within it."[55] Johns quotes a suggestive passage from Whitman's poem "Twenty-Eight Young Men": "The young men float on their backs, their white bellies bulge to the sun, / they do not ask who

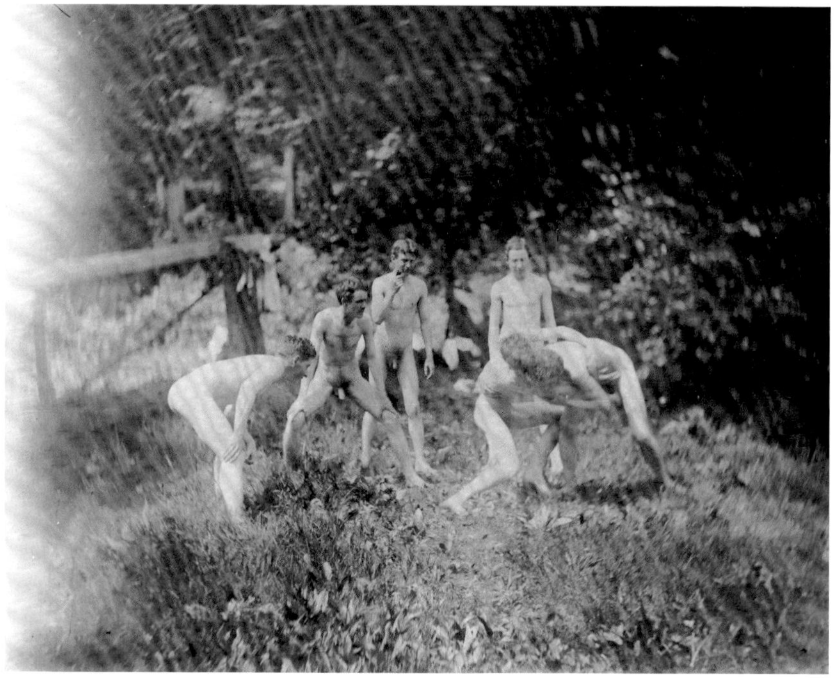

Fig. 22. Thomas Eakins, *Six males, nude, two wrestling at right*, c. 1883. Dry-plate glass negative, 4 × 5 in. Courtesy of the Pennsylvania Academy of the Fine Arts, Philadelphia, Charles Bregler's Thomas Eakins Collection. Purchased with the partial support of the Pew Memorial Trust.

seizes fast to them, / They do not know who puffs and declines with pendant and bending arch, / They do not think who they souse with spray." Comparing *Swimming* to this erotic poem, and calling Eakins Whitman's "twenty-ninth bather," politely hints that the artist may have thought about these bodies with more than a spiritual energy.[56]

Johns' somewhat allusive approach to questions of sexuality posed by *Swimming* was no doubt prompted by the publication in 1994 of an article on Eakins by Whitney Davis titled "Erotic Revisions," an essay that creates a sexualized narrative of what Johns later described as a "platonic" outdoor academy. Davis reconstructs the preparatory photographs made by Eakins as a serial fantasy of sodomistic couplings, followed by a dip in the water. As evidence for this approach, we are told that Eakins manipulated his point of view to maximize visibility of the genitals of the wrestling and boxing adolescents in the photographs. Davis also proposes that Eakins (at least subconsciously) experienced an erotic thrill by penetrating a maquette that the artist prepared to study the challenging, foreshortened view of the diver. Davis supports his interpretation by relying on Freud's theories of Nachträglichkeit: the painting evinces a "continuity of eroticized revision in relation to earlier wishes."[57]

For Davis, *Swimming* is proof not that Eakins necessarily did anything sexual with (or to) his students, but rather that he created the painting as a means of articulating innate, long-standing, and "surging desires" so that he could repeat, reject, reroute, and replace them.[58] This argument was almost certainly intended to expand upon Michael Fried's essay on *The Gross Clinic* eight years earlier, wherein Fried viewed the surgical scene as containing "elements of what Freud in the Schreber case history calls a 'paranoiac' scenario based on the homosexual fantasy of being sexually possessed by a man," in which "there too the threat of castration is said to play a constitutive role." For Fried, the suggestive positioning of the patient's body, the father figure (Gross), the knife, and the cringing, clawing female all lend themselves quite nicely to Freudian interpretation as evidence of repressed desires and anxieties.[59]

As these modern texts make clear, conversation about Eakins' work has radically shifted since the artist ceased exhibiting *Swimming*. If the painting had circulated more widely in its own time, it undoubtedly would have faced complaints about anatomically correct bulging muscles and knobby knees. Today, those issues are relatively uninteresting. The fact that a male artist photographed and depicted naked men now in and of itself raises a question never asked (at least publicly) more than a century ago. In addition, these men touch and gaze at one another in a manner that today seems quite provocative. In the photographs, the men's bodies are intertwined in wrestling poses (fig. 22); in the painting, they gaze at each other's buttocks in a manner that could be construed as sexually suggestive. In lieu of any written documentation of homosexual love affairs or longings, repressed or realized on Eakins' part, these elements of the series instead have been pressed into service as evidence.[60]

Looking at *Swimming* and its preparatory photographs for evidence of Eakins' yearnings in a cultural rather than psychosexual framework yields quite another conversation. Rather than speculate about what Eakins and his students may have sexually thought or did (or repressed—an even harder claim to research), it is more feasible to ask what those choices would have meant in that time, place, and culture. Carroll Smith-Rosenberg, in her writing on lesbian relationships in the nineteenth century, presents a model for analysis that is applicable to the study of men as well.

Placing the history of intimate same-sex friendships "in a larger world of social relations and social values," Smith-Rosenberg shifts "the focus of the study from a concern with deviance to that of defining configurations of legitimate behavioral norms and options."[61] More than in modern times, "deeply felt same-sex friendships were casually accepted in American society" in the nineteenth century. This certainly was the case for Eakins and his close friends J. Laurie Wallace and Samuel Murray, among others throughout his life.

Plumbing the evidence of the nineteenth century, it is clear that spheres of male and female life were profoundly segregated, even within the nuclear family, resulting in conceptions of friendship and marriage far different than ours today. When we cast the discussion of Eakins and homosexuality back into nineteenth-century terms, we find both a more intense repression, and perhaps a more liberating freedom. Eakins didn't experience a different public dialogue about the meaning of homosexuality when compared with modern scholars; rather, he experienced the absence of a public dialogue altogether.

In the 1880s, part of the security that men could feel in bathing, wrestling, and more generally consorting with one another naked, even on camera and canvas, is that homosexuality was almost completely nonexistent in public discourse. If a practice or desire could not be named, it could not be impugned. At the time Eakins created and took part in his bathing scene, men (or women) could enjoy close physical relationships with their same-sex friends without danger of provoking suspicion or derision.[62] Men swimming, boxing, and even wrestling together naked simply were not an unusual occurrence in the nineteenth century, and casual references to these practices are easy to find.

Eakins' own biography bears good witness to this claim. In November 1866, for example, Eakins wrote in a matter-of-fact tone to his father, describing life in the atelier of Jean-Léon Gérôme: "There was a dispute in the studio between two of the fellows as to which was the strongest. It was decided they should wrestle as soon as the model rested. So they stripped themselves and fought nearly an hour, and when they were done, they were as dirty as sweeps and bloody. Since then there has been wrestling most every day and we have had three pairs all stripped at once, and we see some anatomy."[63]

Another example of the unremarkable nature of group male nudity in Eakins' circle is Fairman Rogers' explanation in 1881 of the gender balance of models at the Pennsylvania Academy: "Because the male figure is more familiar to the male students, at least, than that of the female, through opportunities afforded in swimming and the like, for the past two years the sexes have been alternated so that the class sees the same number of each during the season."[64] The habit of men to swim or wrestle naked together, which today seems unusually evocative of sexualized relationships, was so common then that it was taken for granted.

In these regards, *Swimming* and the easy circumstances of its production marked the end of an era, for not long after Eakins completed the work the language of sexual discourse shifted, with the publication in 1887 of Richard von Krafft-Ebing's *Psychopathia Sexualis*, an extensive and extraordinarily explicit examination of hundreds of case studies of a variety of sexual practices considered to be "pathological"—including, for the first time, homosexuality.

At the time of this landmark publication, Krafft-Ebing was director of a sanitarium in Austria, and the most famous neuropsychiatrist in Europe. In following years, Krafft-Ebing debated the proper emphasis and approach to the study of sexuality with his younger colleague Sigmund Freud. Academic conversations like these firmly established the topic of homosexuality as a legitimate subject of discourse among respectable doctors, and with fifteen thousand Americans studying medicine in nearby Munich following the Civil War, it did not take long for such discussions to reverberate in Philadelphia clinics as well.[65]

Krafft-Ebing's experiences in publishing his groundbreaking study demonstrate just how limited public conversation was about homosexuality in the years leading up to 1887. Hoping to avoid prurient interest and any readership outside of doctors, lawyers, and jurists, Krafft-Ebing translated all the explicit case material from the original German text into Latin, prompting rumors of "a marked increase in the sale of Latin dictionaries in Germany and Austria" in following years as circulation grew.[66] Krafft-Ebing remarked that discussion of "sexual relationships" prior to his time were "so thoroughly incorrect and illogical that, so far as science is concerned, empirical psychology and the metaphysics of man's sexual existence are simply virgin soil."[67] As a final note to his introduction, Krafft-Ebing adopted "the saying of *Tardieu* ('Attack upon morals'): 'No physical or moral misery, no wound, no matter how infected, should frighten someone who has dedicated himself to the science of man; and the sacred ministry of the physician, while obliging him to see everything, also permits him to say everything.'"[68] This plaintive statement reveals Krafft-Ebing's awareness that he was breaching a taboo—in fact an enormous number of them. Unfortunately, his plea was mostly ignored.

Although psychiatrists and psychologists today consider *Psychopathia Sexualis* a groundbreaking tome, at the time the eminent physician was shunned from nonscientific circles.[69] Among modern sympathizers, Krafft-Ebing is credited with beginning a relatively compassionate and "scientific discussion of homosexuality" that argued that the practice should be legalized and that "therapies" for the "condition" could induce at most celibacy, not heterosexual inclinations.[70]

One certainty in the discussion of the nineteenth-century context for Eakins' *Swimming* is that Krafft-Ebing's work proves that men at the time did engage in a wide variety of homosexual practices.[71] Eakins might have been introduced to Krafft-Ebing's tome after its publication, when *Swimming* already was gathering dust—he certainly knew how to translate Latin from his years at Central High School. Even if he had access to the text, however, it is doubtful that the artist ever would have seen his painting as "pathological."

As fruitful as *Swimming* has been for modern scholars, it is only one of many of Eakins' pictures that have served as veritable "field days" for au courant academic dialogue. *The Agnew Clinic*, for instance, also has provided ample fodder for art historians to consider the meaning of yet another Eakins painting in which men mill about together, albeit in this case clothed.

Modern discourse on *The Agnew Clinic*, in contrast to *Swimming*, has centered on the relationship of men not to each other but rather to the half-naked woman at the center of the painting. Gender and sex relations in this painting are both more complex than in *Swimming*, and a more inviting subject for feminist interpretation. Agnew—and by association Eakins—are obvious and easy targets for linguistic salvos in this interpretive vein.

The University of Pennsylvania Medical College was without doubt a profoundly sexist educational environment in the nineteenth century, and for much of his life, Agnew was without doubt an atrocious sexist. His biographer J. William White writes:

> He never approved of the co-education of the sexes, nor of the medical education of women under any circumstances, believing that any possible advantages to them were far more than counterbalanced by what he thought would be the inevitable loss of dignity and delicacy resulting from the association of the sexes under such conditions and from the character of their studies.... He was never an advocate of what is now called the higher education of women in any direction. He admired the domestic virtues, and at one of the last dinners he ever gave, he remarked that a woman should be taught housekeeping, hygiene and belles-lettres. After that, he said, the more she knew the worse off she was.[72]

Agnew's rabid sexism extended beyond offensive remarks to his colleagues. In 1871, Agnew resigned his teaching position at the Pennsylvania Hospital rather than lecture before an audience including students from the Woman's Medical College of Pennsylvania, one of the first institutions of its kind in the nation.[73] The board of the hospital, somewhat more graciously, accepted Agnew's resignation and allowed separate clinics to be held for the women students, but even then "dissatisfaction arose," this time from the women who were offered only limited, inferior opportunities compared with those given to the men.[74]

Although this evidence has been used to support interpretation of *The Agnew Clinic* as a misogynistic work, replicating the prejudices of its day, in fact the historical record is much more complex than previous authors have acknowledged. Bridget Goodbody, for example, discusses Agnew's speeches and actions of the 1870s, but then fails to account for the marked evolution of his ideas and practices in the years immediately preceding Eakins' painting of the clinic scene.

Returning to the theme of the artist's conversations in the medical arena, co-education hardly could have been avoided as a topic. While the students of the Woman's Medical College faced enormous opposition and inadequate educational opportunities in the 1860s and 1870s, over the next decade they were rapidly accepted into clinics in Philadelphia's hospitals. As Clara Marshall, dean of the college, recalled in 1897: "The desire of the faculty was gratified, when during the session of 1882–1883, the students of the College were admitted to the regular weekly clinics. It is interesting, in this connection, to note that Dr. Agnew, six years after his resignation, was invited by the Managers of the Pennsylvania Hospital to resume his place on the staff, that his letter contains no reference to the vexed question of women students and that he lectured to a mixed class during this second connection with the Hospital whenever women chose to attend his clinics. In the latter part of his life Dr. Agnew accepted invitations to consult with women physicians."[75] Times had changed, and by the time of his memorial portrait even D. Hayes Agnew had changed with them.

There is no doubt that rabid sexism was rife in the world of nineteenth-century medicine, and following chapters explore those themes in some depth, but interpretation of *The Agnew Clinic* requires a more nuanced understanding of the events and realities of the day. As in the case of *Swimming*, the language of modern scholarly response offers a striking contrast to the dialogues surrounding production of the work.

The worst review received by *The Agnew Clinic* to date was penned not by the admonishers of "horrors of the dissection table" in Eakins' own day, but rather by Bridget Goodbody, who in 1994 claimed that the work portrays "a surgical initiation ceremony, through which a hierarchy among the initiated was established to promote the continuity of the dominant homosocial order."[76] In her essay "The Present Opprobrium of Surgery: *The Agnew Clinic* and Nineteenth-Century Representations of Cancerous Female Breasts," Goodbody describes the painting as celebration of a surgery that Agnew performed knowing there was no possibility of cure, but only of unnecessary pain and disfiguration.[77] Ultimately, she concludes that "the Hippocratic Oath seems to have been brushed aside and replaced by what appears to be hysterical attempts to maintain power and control over the bodies of female patients."[78] For Goodbody the painting exists as both documentation and active agent of oppression.

Although there is no doubt that works of art often convey and promote prejudices of their day, nevertheless scholars should be careful in their assignation of blame—even to the dead. The title of Goodbody's essay, for example, relies on a text by J. William White, Agnew's biographer, assistant, and successor, in which he discussed the "opprobrium" of surgery. Goodbody builds her argument on the idea that treatment of breast cancer, in particular, was undertaken in that spirit of "disgrace resulting from shameful conduct" represented by the term. White in fact wrote: "[Agnew] believed, for example, that just as surgical tuberculosis is slowly but surely coming under the control of the surgeon, so carcinoma, the present opprobrium of surgery, would in time yield to methods of treatment yet to be discovered."[79] The "opprobrium of surgery"—the shame that Agnew humbly and sorrowfully acknowledged—arose not from his treatment of breast cancer specifically, but rather from all surgical treatments of carcinoma.

As Diana Long points out, surgeons of the late nineteenth century had no effective means of dealing with advanced breast cancer patients like those who were admitted to the Pennsylvania Hospital. Surgery was palliative, in removing the "foul and disabling" tumors, but Agnew himself admitted that "the permanent recoveries fell far short of 9.05 per cent," the figure given by Samuel W. Gross (son of Eakins' portrait subject). Unfortunately, it was also true that the cancer, if left alone, "inevitably" killed, and by removing the tumors Agnew felt he could provide at least a "moral effect" on the patient.[80]

Certainly no historian of medicine would disagree that many nineteenth-century surgeries were ineffectual and conducted primarily for the purposes of research and teaching, and sometimes for the palliative of providing empty hope to desperate patients and their families. But to suggest, as Goodbody does, that Agnew operated with misogynistic desire to preserve dominance over women is to deny more profound truths and, in the process, to obscure the complex and interesting conversation of the time.

White also wrote of Agnew that "no surgeon ever lived and attained eminence who was more careful to throw around his patients every safeguard, or who strove more earnestly after successful results." Agnew was revered for his authorship of the massive *Treatise on the Principles and Practices of Surgery*, the standard text used by medical school students for decades, and also for his surgical abilities "made most manifest during the removal of a deep-seated growth of the neck or of a mammary tumor."[81] White's florid prose is typical of the inflated literary style of his day, but even hyperbolists deserve to be quoted fairly.

As to why Agnew chose to be depicted performing this surgery, and why Eakins chose to paint it, we may in partial answer refer to the artist's past precedent: as with *The Gross Clinic*, Eakins chose to paint a surgery for which his portrait subject was justly famous, and he inserted into the scene his trademark element of provocation. Patricia Hills explains the choice of breast surgery by referencing Edmund Burke's concept of "the sublime," with the breast representing the fearful "irrationalism" of nature and its awesome power to make victims of any human.[82]

There is no doubt that the presence of the exposed breast in *The Agnew Clinic* inserts a challenging element into the scene that Eakins certainly could have avoided had he chosen to depict Agnew's other famous surgery—a "growth of the neck." David Lubin probably goes farthest of the painting's critics in emphasizing the power of the breast: "Not only does this bosom suggest a human eye, but also a bull's-eye—the term used to denote the center of a target. The nipple occupies the exact center of the semicircle or open curve described earlier; it is the nodule in the midst of the gap that our gaze has sought to penetrate. If we were to drop a line from the nipple to the bottom edge of the canvas and use this as a radius with which to trace a circle on the picture plane, its arcs would travel close to or through the crown of each attending physician."[83]

Lubin rightly points out that the diseased breast of the patient is exactly at the crux of the painting, its unmarred twin splayed toward us as the patient lies on the table, vulnerable and etherized. The connotative shock of the "sublime" breast follows the vulnerable exposed buttocks of the young patient facing the audience in *The Gross Clinic*, and of course the "declarative ass" at the center of *Swimming*.[84] Eakins was an equal-opportunity provocateur. No one sex, or body part, escaped exposure or "declaration" in the artist's oeuvre.

In the context of the time, there was another shock in *The Agnew Clinic*. Perhaps the most radical inclusion in the painting was in fact not the naked breast at its epicenter but the nurse, Mary V. Clymer. Eakins not only included Clymer in the somber scene, but he placed her in a position equivalent to Agnew's at the opposite side of the canvas; Nurse Clymer's size, scale, and even the contrast of light and dark in her figure are equal to the emphasis given to the famous surgeon opposite her. In dramatic fashion, Eakins asserted her presence in the arena, at the heart of the scene.

The fundamental lesson of *The Agnew Clinic* in its own context is that times had changed, and both Agnew and Eakins had changed along with them. In *The Gross Clinic*, the sole woman represented in the scene was the recoiling guardian, disparaged by virtue of her depiction as the only individual not involved in teaching, healing, or learning. In fact, she is shown to be the worst kind of viewer—a hysteric.[85] Yet between 1875 and 1889, the cultural and professional shifts involved far more than just the recognition of germs—the "little living bodies" Clymer so scrupulously would fend off in Agnew's clinic. In 1875, the hospital that eventually employed her wouldn't allow nurses in the door—even under the most providential economic circumstances. Around the time Eakins painted Gross, "Pauline Henry, a wealthy invalid, offered $1,000 to the new University of Pennsylvania Hospital for nurses' training. The men refused her money, so Henry gave $3,000 in 1875 to the Woman's Hospital to send their trained nurses to other hospitals.... Undaunted, Henry also tried to place trained nurses in the Jefferson Hospital for the insane, but men balked at providing even a minimal monthly salary of $10 and a separate dining table for the nurses."[86]

Although we may rightly praise Agnew as an important and dedicated medical pioneer and at the same time condemn him for his earlier virulent sexism, it is important to distinguish the artist from his portrait subject in the latter regard. Mary V. Clymer's presence, in fact, marks a momentous and quite recent historical advance—she was among the first, if not the very first, nurse to perform specialized duties in the surgical amphitheater. A graduate of only the second class of the Training School for Nurses of the Hospital of the University of Pennsylvania, Clymer also was at the top of her class and a recipient of the Nightingale Medal for general excellence. At the moment of her graduation, Clymer was "nursing in the flooded district of Williamsport."[87]

Mary Clymer kept a detailed record of her "ward notes" and "lecture notes" the year Eakins painted Agnew, in which she describes the constant washing, administration of medicines, and dressing of wounds required of her position. She may have felt the weight of history as she sat down to write in an era in which women were making nearly daily strides in opening up professional opportunities. On a Wednesday, undated, she wrote: "Allowed to prepare table for operation. Saw and assisted with two operations. Saw ... diseased bone removed without much loss of blood and prepared antiseptic dressing for the wound."[88] Later in her "ward notes," Nurse Clymer recorded that she was taught to catheterize patients. All this may not seem far removed from older duties of nursing, which historians describe as glorified domestic chores, but in fact this was all revolutionary—Nurse Clymer, as documented in *The Agnew Clinic,* was now a working woman in the very public (and very masculine) realm of surgery.

Scholars have observed in the past that the existence of germs was discovered in the intervening years between *The Gross Clinic* and *The Agnew Clinic.* Whereas Gross wore dark street clothes to operate in 1875, by 1889 the surgical team knew better—white clothes helped display dirt. Nurse Clymer describes boiling and "carbolizing" as major elements of her job. In discussing the breast specifically, she wrote: "The skin of a breast case contains hundreds of these germs and should be cleansed the same as surgeon's hands, some hours before the operation and a towel wet in the solution ... placed over it and kept there."[89]

On January 8, 1889, Mary Clymer recorded specific notes about her duties in preparing a patient for breast surgery. She was responsible for preparation of "room and patient." Light was to be strong but not direct, heat was to be adjusted to "70 or a little above," and "superfluous objects" were to be removed (although the "brandy and whiskey" that were to be provided as "stimulants" for the doctors were not considered superfluous). Sterilization was of chief importance, but so was attention to the patient, who was to be purged, cleansed, calmed, and dressed. "Have clothing loose and if necessary cut out the sleeve. For a breast case only put one in the night dress and be sure and have the one exposed that is to be operated upon."

Scholars including Bridget Goodbody have commented on Eakins' depiction of both diseased and healthy breasts in *The Agnew Clinic.* Here, in Nurse Clymer's diary, we have an important piece of evidence—it seems likely that Eakins' climactic "bull's eye" was a choice all his own. Recollections of participants, and a photo of Agnew's clinic dating from 1886 (fig. 23), offer no further insight on the question of whose decision it was to point that healthy breast out at us.

If Eakins did make the decision to more fully disrobe the patient in *The Agnew Clinic,* it is possible to imagine various reasons why he chose to do so. A cloth nightshirt cutting across the chest would have blocked our view of the fine work of sewing up the wound and obscured the anatomy undergoing surgical treatment—or the artist might simply have wanted to provoke our response. There is no bloody wound at this focal point of the painting, but a bare female nipple serves just as well to direct our attention.

Another conversation also is relevant to this decision. Eakins' conceptualization of paintings clearly was often guided by paradigms operable outside the world of art. Eakins almost certainly spent a great deal more time with Henry Gray than Edmund Burke. Gray's description of the mammary glands Eakins painted at the focal point of his work is remarkably free of references to the sublime, the misogynistic, or the homosocial: "In the female, they are two large hemispherical eminences situated towards the lateral aspect of the pectoral region corresponding to the interval between the third and sixth or seventh ribs, and extending from the side of the sternum to the axilla. Their weight and dimensions differ at different periods of life, and in different individuals.... The *nipple* is a cylindrical or conical eminence, capable of undergoing a sort of erection from mechanical excitement. It is of a pink or brownish hue, its surface wrinkled and provided papillae, and it is perforated by numerous orifices, the apertures of the lactiferous ducts."[90] Gray's version of the "excitement" associated with the mammary glands reminds us that the language with which medical practitioners discussed the body was both more neutral—and more shocking—than contemporary discussions by art critics, and even farther removed from the discourse of modern scholars.

Returning to the image of Milliken whispering in Eakins' ear, and the photo of Pancoast's dissection laboratory, we must ask how physicians and students of anatomy talked and thought about the sight of carving into the breast, or shoulder, or pelvis. A photograph of the dissection room at the University of Pennsylvania in these years makes this point even more dramatically. Tables in this cavernous hall are filled with flayed breasts, elbows, genitals, and skulls, all rendered equivalent through the paradigm of medical training (fig. 24). This kind of visual experience could not have failed to change the way it feels to look at bodies.

Julie Berkowitz, writing about the reception of *The Gross Clinic* at Jefferson Medical College, offhandedly remarks that "even today the monumental painting still has the power to shock, and many lay viewers react viscerally."[91] The term "lay" is invaluable for understanding what Eakins' surgical pictures really represent. The truly "bonding" experience demon-

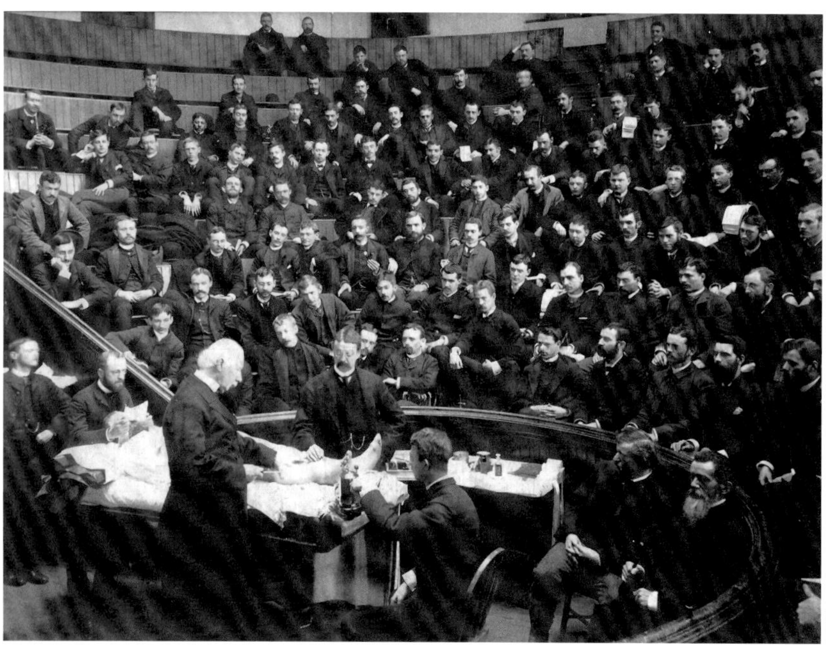

Fig. 23. George Chambers, *Agnew clinic*, 1886. Black and white photograph. From the Collections of the University of Pennsylvania Archives.

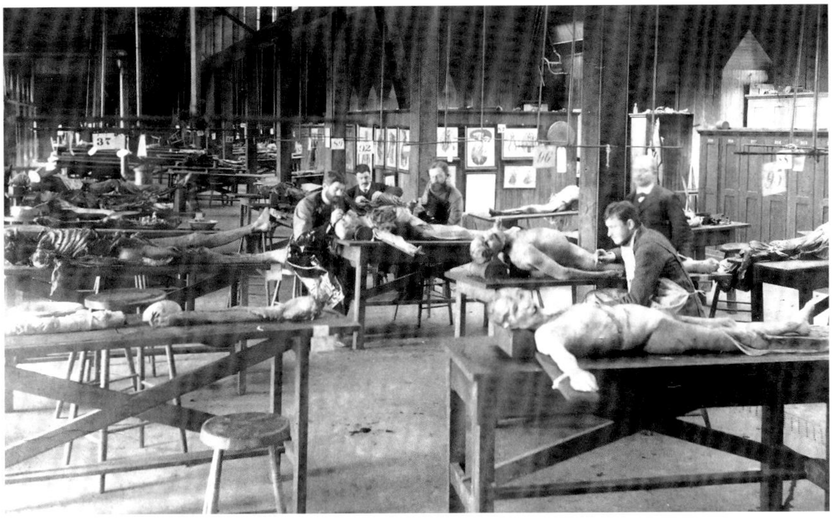

Fig. 24. Unknown photographer, *Dissecting room, University of Pennsylvania School of Medicine*, mid-1880s. Black and white photograph. From the Collections of the University of Pennsylvania Archives.

strated in *The Agnew Clinic* was only homosocial when medical training was segregated. The bonds much more obviously involved a new approach to the body—and in the 1880s, with even Agnew's help, women were beginning to share the experience of viewing the body through dissector's eyes.

Not only did Eakins disrupt a long tradition of "homosocial" medical portraits through his prominent inclusion of Nurse Clymer, but he also incorporated into the painting the educated labor of another woman—his wife, Susan. Metaphorically, by asking his wife to paint him into the scene, Thomas Eakins asserted her right to be in the amphitheater of listeners in this stimulating educational environment. Then, by exhibiting the painting in places where women would see it, he invited them in as well, despite the assertions of male reviewers that they might faint from "horror."

Given all the artist's conversations in the medical arena, and his presence in previous clinics, he certainly would have been aware of the significance of Mary Clymer's presence in the room and her place in the heroic progress of the age. Clymer's private notes testify to the slow but momentous desegregation of the surgical clinic; Eakins' enormous canvas makes that testimony public and powerful.

The exercise of viewing Eakins' images as psychosexual, homoerotic, or misogynistic—or some mélange of the three—still leaves us without an assessment of these works that acknowledges Eakins' project in their own ontological framework. In the terms of Eve Kosofsky Sedgwick, we rob Eakins of the right to "self-definition" if we fail to take his perspective seriously as well.[92] While Johns is right that it has become impossible to talk about paintings like *Swimming* without plunging into an exegesis on sexuality—which this chapter itself demonstrates—an examination of the influence of anatomical training on the way Eakins conceptualized the human flesh before him provides us with an additional paradigm for understanding his contributions.

Modern aficionados may scorn those nineteenth-century critics who failed to see the glory of Eakins' works, terming them instead repulsive "horrors" from the dissecting lab, but we should not deny that these men and women understood exactly what Eakins was doing. He *had* spent an enormous amount of time in dissecting rooms, and his vision of the body had been profoundly changed by that repeated visual experience. It could not have been otherwise. Both nineteenth-century and present-day accounts describe the powerful impact of dissection.

In the nineteenth century, students frequently complained of the "brutalization" that seemed an "inbuilt danger of medical education." Joseph Jones wrote in Philadelphia in 1853 that sessions in the dissecting room "have a manifest tendency to harden & corrupt the heart." Another student felt the practice rendered "the sensibilities Callous," and yet another worried that "anatomy, however indispensable it may be, tends certainly to freeze up the springs of human feeling."[93]

Three recent descriptions of the experience of attending first-year gross anatomy class add interesting insight to how Eakins' vision was formed by his conversations and visual experiences at Jefferson Medical College. These autobiographical accounts of the experience, in the explicit, modern language we speak today, demonstrate the profound distancing from conventional understandings of the body that emerge as an inevitable result of dissection, and also show how that transformed view of the body alters, at least temporarily, its usual ability to provoke arousal.

In *Getting Better: A Medical Student's Story*, Dr. Kenneth Klein recounts his first encounter with the new privilege of looking at sexual anatomy. A cardiology patient readily takes off her blouse in front of medical students in their first week to show the placement of her pacemaker, leading to a sense of shock. "I had been allowed to look at this woman's chest. Would she still have let me look if she'd known I hadn't learned anything yet? I felt like a fraud."[94] The sense here is of a privileged access to the body not yet earned.

Only after he pushes open "the door that bar[s] admission to the general public" and enters "the pathological world of the dead" in a morgue does Klein "feel like a bona fide medical student."[95] As Dr. Perri Klass writes of her experience entering the dissection lab: "For the first time in medical school, I have a sense that I am being initiated into a priesthood. This is something that 'normal' people never do." She goes on to reveal the elements of her initiation:

> And so we do the first dissection, opening up the chest of our cadaver. The skin, after long soaking in formaldehyde, is quite leathery; it doesn't look or feel like skin, which makes it easier to cut. Our cadaver is female, and when the time comes to cut away the breast, I feel a certain tremor in my own chest. In fact, none of the four of us, three women and one man, is eager to do that, and we find ourselves delaying until one of the teachers comes around and does it for us. The semester moves on. I do like anatomy. I find myself watching the muscles move under my own skin when I flex my arm, thinking about how they attach to bones, how they are nourished by blood vessels, how the nerves weave in and out. In fact, when the exam comes, we are all sitting there flexing and extending our limbs, trying to remember which muscle fits in where. One man with a very well developed upper body comes to the exam in a tight sleeveless teeshirt, and all the students sitting near him keep sneaking surreptitious looks at his biceps, his triceps, his pecs.[96]

The initiation is, by the end of the semester, complete. The bodies of others, even the students' own bodies, can be seen with that distanced vision—as evidence of anatomical attributes rather than in social terms as classmates, friends, competitors, or even potential lovers. And for Klein, that meant initiation also into the macabre sense of humor and willingness to shock others that resonates so strongly with stories about Keen, Agnew, and Eakins: "As we puzzled over the quadriceps muscles something flew across the room and hit Steve on the left shoulder. We both jumped—it was a morsel of fat. It stuck to his sweater. He picked off the foreign body, giggled, and threw it back to where it had come from. It hit an apparently innocent bystander on the chest and bounced to the floor. This new victim sliced some skin from his cadaver's arm and threw it back.... The cadaver room had become a free-fire zone."[97] To celebrate the end of the class, Klein cooked beef hearts using a recipe from *The Joy of Cooking*. To the horror of some of his guests, including one who went hungry that night, "the chef became an anatomy professor—I explained the coronary circulation, went over the cardiac chambers, and showed how the valves worked.... The anatomy lesson was delicious."[98]

For all involved, the anatomist's initiation into this other realm poses difficulties in integrating life with outsiders. Perri Klass worries that she smells like formaldehyde when she comes to bed with her partner, who frequently reminds her "that there are certain details he would rather not hear ('So we were cleaning the fat away from the stomach muscles when all of a sudden...')."[99]

The desexualizing effects of dissection described by these medical students are especially pervasive. Charles LeBaron talks about his experience dissecting his first cadaver alongside "a young woman whom I'd spent more than one lecture staring at":

> No lab coat, just a T-shirt and no bra. I stare in disbelief. I've never seen breasts that beautiful.... Around the room, other groups are at about the same stage we are, flaying back the skin of the chest.... Their corpse is male but seems to have an enormous amount of fat, lemon-colored fat globules are everywhere, they're scraping them off in huge, slimy cupfuls. Claudia's got the skin almost completely pulled back from ours now; flaps the color of old bacon hanging off; and the nipple that I cut around is left standing out on the underlying muscle, bizarrely

> orphaned of its surroundings, a lonely tuft of dimpled flesh in the midst of carnage.... We start turning the body to get to the armpit. Automatically, I cradle the head so it won't knock about. I realize it's absurd, but somehow it seems wrong to let a head bang and bounce, dead or not. Claudia pulls the arm out of the way. I take the saw and start cutting. The teeth bite quickly through the gaunt, waxy flesh, hit bone, start rocking the body back and forth. I pause for a moment. Claudia feels about the cut I made; I'm riveted again by those amazing breasts of hers, so close and naked under the T-shirt I have to restrain my hand from reaching up and cupping one. Yet even more I'm transfixed by the paradox of staring over the mutilated flesh of a corpse at live breasts and feeling a riot of contradictory impulses, nausea, and desire.... That body once had been round and plump and young, stubbed its toe and wept, fallen in love and been elated and made conversation, felt the slow creaky onset of age, now was inert upon a metal table.[100]

Breasts are not the only difficult terrain. Perri Klass writes: "There is the day we come in to do the dissection of the male reproductive system and notice that all the men in the class are looking pretty green. The women get to do a lot of dissecting that particular day; the men are not eager to do any cutting."[101] As these accounts demonstrate, the gender and sexual orientation of the viewer engaged in the process dramatically influence response, just as viewers of Eakins' provocative paintings will never see and experience all one thing either.

The initiation ritual of the anatomist does not necessarily desexualize its participants—although it is obviously possible that it could—but from these accounts it is clear that dissection makes attraction problematic, providing a new and not necessarily so arousing view of the body. In these descriptions breasts become "cheap cuts of meat" and pubic hair "sparse and stringy"; intestines lie "like a nest of enormous bloated earthworms."[102] Another medical student writes of the change in her feelings in gross anatomy class: "As well as those cadavers, something else will have to die, a coherent sense of what is human, an ancient shape in the mind."[103]

Now think about the bodies in *The Gross Clinic, The Crucifixion, Swimming,* and *The Agnew Clinic.* Just as Eakins' rowing paintings are perfect demonstrations of his perspective lessons, these paintings are perfect demonstrations of the artist's anatomy lessons, and his dissector's point of view. In *Swimming,* notice how many views are given of thighs and arms, for example, in a comprehensive summary of possibilities—flexed and extended, weight-bearing and relaxed, in motion and static—the painting teaches both anatomy and physiology. In *Agnew,* the display of the healthy breast allows us to view the operation under way and also provides a reminder of the exterior terrain that any medical student would need to know, both on exams and in actual practice, particularly before delving into interior realms. In *The Crucifixion,* there is little to distract our attention from the real show—the body itself.

From his high school days, Eakins had always stood like "the ancient inquirer at the Temple of the Oracle" of anatomy, as Agnew described medicine in his lecture. Whether he placed his subjects around a swimming hole or on the surgical table, dressed them in classical garb or suspended them from a cross, these bodies and this art were always about anatomy. To have an anatomist's view of the body was not a diminished vision, it was an expanded one—Eakins saw, because he had not only felt but actually delved into the inner core, the biological and pathological fact, of human existence. As Michel Foucault writes in *The Birth of the Clinic,* since the beginning of the modern medical era, "the gaze is no longer reductive, it is, rather, that which establishes the individual in his irreducible quality."[104] As profound as this gaze was, most Americans in the late nineteenth century were not willing to admire the body in that way—nor did they feel they had earned the right to do so.

As Michael Sappol writes: "Anatomical dissection served as the ritual that inducted young men into the cult of medical knowledge.... Dissection was dangerous and difficult. Its attributes were at once masculine and professional ... and not permitted to members of the public, who were required by long-established custom to respect and safeguard the dead."[105] The critics who wanted Eakins' clinic pictures, and even paintings like *The Crucifixion,* sent back to the "dissecting room" recognized how the exhibition of these works breached that important assumption of the time.

Eakins' deep involvement in displaying the "irreducible"

reality of the anatomical body was the guiding intellectual passion of his life. In standing before *The Agnew Clinic* in the University of Pennsylvania Medical College, or *The Gross Clinic* in Jefferson Medical College, we should realize that those paintings are meant to be seen not as art critics saw them in the Centennial Exhibition or the Society of American Artists, but rather from the perspective of the seasoned and initiated dissectors who filled the halls of those institutions and commissioned those works—and by their followers even today.

When Velázquez positioned his audience in the shoes of the king and queen in *Las Meninas*, looking out at the family, friends, and staff gathered for their entertainment, it was a vision any audience could delight in. But in Eakins' case, the dissector's eyes that he asked viewers to peer through were identified in the public mind with blood, gore, and death.

Eakins' construction of *The Agnew Clinic* certainly was shaped by his experiences as a student and painter in the medical colleges of Philadelphia, but it also reflected more deeply personal reflections on the nature of teaching. This is, after all, a painting of Agnew in his capacity as a pedagogue more than as a surgeon, and thus also an allegory of education. Susan Eakins' contribution to the painting makes this case even more poignantly: Agnew is depicted with his students; Eakins paints with the woman who was both an impressive student and then his wife. In 1889, this reflection would have been especially sanguine, for Eakins must still have been pondering the difficulties at the Pennsylvania Academy of the Fine Arts that had led to his removal from his position as director of the schools just three years earlier.

Whether historians believe that Thomas Eakins refuted or reified his subject's early, infamous sexism in *The Agnew Clinic* through his own pictorial choices, his actions as an educator in his own institution demonstrate the artist's profound distinction from his surgical counterpart. Eakins ultimately sacrificed his professional position, his personal reputation, and his teaching career for his insistence on creating an educational institution perfectly equal in its treatment of male and female students, and male and female bodies. He not only invited women in his classrooms to share in the professional conversations that for millennia had been reserved for men, he went so far as to *insist* that they participate. His paintings still force his audiences to participate as well. *The Gross Clinic*, *The Crucifixion*, *Swimming*, and *The Agnew Clinic* are still intellectually improving for their ability to make us challenge our assumptions—and engage in vibrant dialogue.

CHAPTER THREE

Body Casts and "Anatomical Eyes" Thomas Eakins, William Williams Keen, and the Curriculum at the Pennsylvania Academy of the Fine Arts

In 1893, Dr. William Williams Keen found himself in a distinguished, though presumably nerve-wracking, position. Floating on a private yacht in Long Island Sound, Keen assisted in the removal of a cancerous tumor from the mouth of Grover Cleveland. Because Cleveland was president at the time, and undoubtedly considered his condition nobody's business but his own, Keen waited until 1917 to discuss the secret operation. In that year, he proudly wrote about the procedure in the *Saturday Evening Post* and "presented the tumor and a laryngeal mirror and cheek retractor used in the operation" to the Thomas Dent Mütter Museum at the College of Physicians of Philadelphia. The tumor joined such treasures as the connected livers removed from the Siamese twins Chang and Eng at the time of their autopsy, and bladder stones removed from Chief Justice John Marshall.[1] President Cleveland's tumor still keeps very good company.

Although the museum was founded in 1849, it was small and relatively uninteresting until 1856, when Dr. Mütter donated 1,700 specimens of the anatomical and pathological materials he used in teaching at Jefferson Medical College, along with the funds necessary to expand the museum's facilities and hire staff. Today, Mütter's collections are shockingly bizarre; body parts, many of them deformed, float in glass jars of rutile formaldehyde that fill elegantly substantial cabinets lining the large exhibit hall. To those uninformed visitors to the College of Physicians who take a wrong turn and end up in the museum, the display is both completely unexpected and perversely fascinating.

A lesser version of this shock also may be felt by visitors to the Philadelphia Museum of Art who wander into the Eakins galleries and discover bronze casts made of dissected body parts. Formed with the same lustrous metal as the artist's relief sculptures *Spinning* (fig. 25) and *Knitting* nearby, the flayed fragments are at once at home and strangely ill at ease in this environment (fig. 26). The juxtaposition suggests interesting questions: How might we qualify the difference between a mold of a body and a sculpture of a body? Is a naked open body more or less shocking than a naked closed one?

The research notes composed by curators at the Philadelphia Museum of Art in the 1970s and organized in their object files do not record consideration of these large questions, but they do mark some ambivalence about the status of these unusual objects. Each cast in the collection was painstakingly reviewed for signs of handwork, as though in an effort to find some art—a right hand shows marks above the wrist "which must have been produced with a tool," while a shoulder seems to disappoint with "no signs of hand modeling."[2] A physician's assistance was deemed necessary to formulate titles for the "works."

A decade later, curators at the Pennsylvania Academy tackled the more overwhelming but similar challenge of labeling and cataloguing dozens of the artist's drawings of

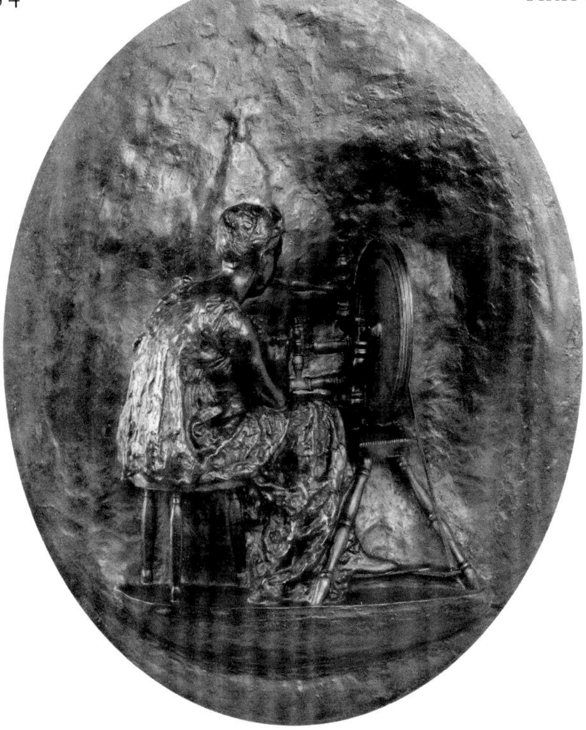

Fig. 25. Thomas Eakins, *Spinning*, 1882–83 (cast 1930). Sand-cast bronze, 18¼ × 14⅞ × 2¾ in. Philadelphia Museum of Art. Gift of Mrs. Thomas Eakins and Miss Mary Adeline Williams, 1930.

Fig. 26. Thomas Eakins, *Back of Male Torso*, 1880 (cast 1930). Bronze, length 30¼ in. Philadelphia Museum of Art. Gift of R. Sturgis Ingersoll.

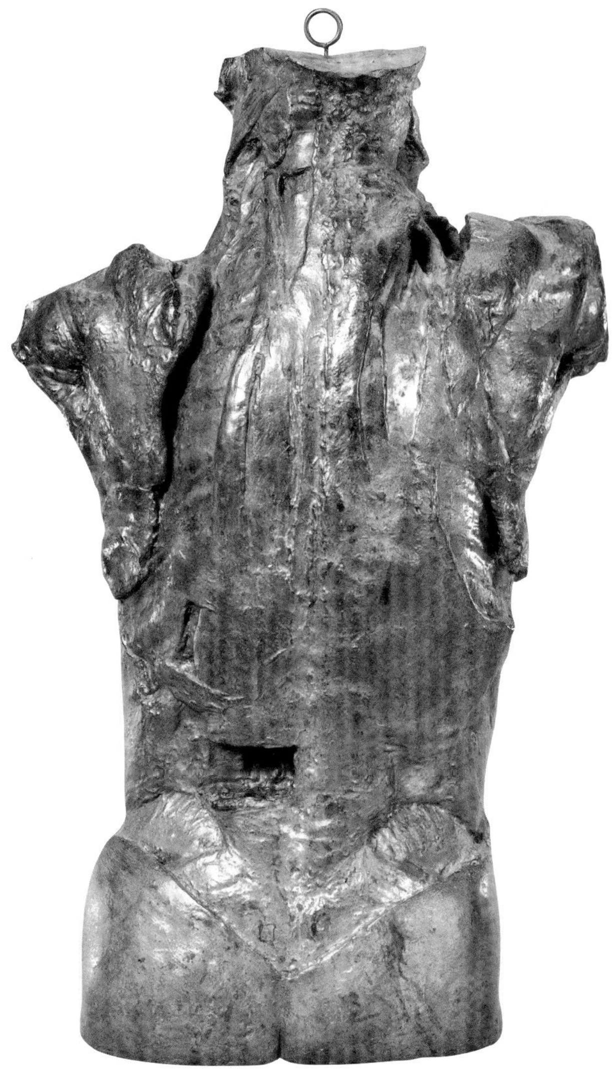

dissected humans and animals. According to Catherine Kimock, one of the researchers involved in the effort, "while many of the drawings are accompanied by detailed remarks and notes that identify the species as well as the anatomical features portrayed, just as many are not so conveniently annotated." After "careful comparison" with Gray's *Anatomy* and other sources relevant to animal anatomy, Kimock was able to group the forty-nine extant dissection studies into several categories by species: eighteen human studies, including cross sections and studies of muscles, and comparative anatomy studies including twelve of a cat, seven of a dog, two of a lion, and four of a horse.[3]

The difference between the drawings and the casts is not just one of numbers. Whereas Eakins clearly made the drawings, and annotated them in his elegant hand, the molds were made at the Pennsylvania Academy of the Fine Arts in the early 1880s with the assistance of students, and possibly Dr. Keen himself, who lectured on anatomy at the academy; the original plaster version was cast in bronze many years later.[4] The subject matter, and some might even say the style of the casts, should be credited to the "stevedore" who died suddenly near the academy and was immediately imported into the dissection rooms, along with the assorted other humans and animals whose anatomy all unwittingly became immortalized in museum displays and curatorial collections. Indeed, the artlessness of the casts at the time they were made was seen as their great virtue. Fairman Rogers, chairman of the committee on instruction at the academy until 1883, praised the casts in an 1881 description of the school: "They are much superior to the French casts usually sold for the same purpose, having been made from careful dissections by gelatine molds, possessing all the distinctness of the originals, free from all retouching, and therefore trustworthy."[5] One detects in Rogers' phrasing an air of irritation that the French prettified their corpses.

The distinction might have seemed subtle, but it reflects a core difficulty that Rogers and others had in defending Eakins' teaching methods. Much of the time, academy students didn't seem to be studying art. If the works art students create display scarce invention, are they artistic? If the human body is treated, and examined, as a biological organism, without regard to gender and with no more gravity than that offered horses, cats, and sheep, can that possibly promote aesthetic development?

Admirers of the artist's fidelity today should note that Eakins' late portraits across the hallway are in many ways similar in effect to the anatomical casts. The flaccid jaw and sagging cheeks of Mary Adeline Williams (fig. 27) are as carefully studied and observed as the tendons on view in the flayed shoulder. The powerful presence of anatomy in Eakins' casts, anatomical drawings, and paintings makes one thing clear. More than a century after his teaching of anatomy served as the (at least) nominal excuse for his dismissal from the Pennsylvania Academy, the artist is still forcing people primarily interested in painting and sculpture, including museumgoers and curators, to learn about the human body "in the manner set forth by [his] way of teaching."[6]

The story of Eakins' career in training artists to understand, depict, and sculpt the naked human body is multifaceted. Some facets have drawn much greater attention than others. The dramatic public scandals arising from Eakins' pedagogy and practices regarding nudity at the Pennsylvania Academy often overshadow the sheer magnitude of anatomical teaching in the artist's life—the academy, after all, was only one of seven institutions in which the artist lectured on the subject and directed dissections when he could. Eakins assisted Keen at the Pennsylvania Academy from 1877 to 1886, and later continued teaching anatomy independently at the Philadelphia Art Students' League (1886–93), the Art Students' League of New York (1885–91), the National Academy of Design (1888–95), the Drexel Institute of Art, Science, and Industry (1895), the Woman's Art School of the Cooper Union (1891–98), and the Art Students' League of Washington, D.C. (c. 1888–94).[7] Given Eakins' modest but independent means and the controversies often engendered by his efforts, all this travel hardly could have made sense as a paying job: teaching anatomy in his "manner" was a passion. At the Pennsylvania Academy of the Fine Arts, that passion bordered on obsession.

The extraordinary education in human and animal anatomy afforded to Pennsylvania Academy students in the early 1880s was partly a result of Eakins' philosophical bent and his own studies in Paris and at Jefferson Medical College. To a much larger degree, however, Eakins was influenced by his collaboration with Dr. William Williams Keen, who lectured on artistic anatomy at the academy and oversaw the school's dissection program in the years before removing President Cleveland's tumor on that steamer in Long Island Sound.

William Williams Keen is a truly extraordinary historical figure. In the narrative of nineteenth-century Philadelphia medicine, Keen is ubiquitous: progenitor of the Philadelphia School of Anatomy, beloved Jefferson Medical College professor of surgery, the author of fiction and nonfiction, and, in his spare time, outstanding innovator in the field of teaching medical and artistic anatomy. Keen, like Agnew, could not have helped but serve as an inspiration to Eakins; the two men were similarly hard-working and dedicated to rigorous study of the body, and to the goal of providing the finest education possible in a variety of institutions.

When the Pennsylvania Academy commenced art classes in 1875, following the construction of its new home at Broad and Cherry Streets, Eakins began his collaboration with Keen, who was then serving as the academy's professor of anatomy. Within a year, Eakins was teaching at the academy as well, as an unpaid substitute for Christian Schussele, who by that time was ill and often missed class. Early in 1877, the

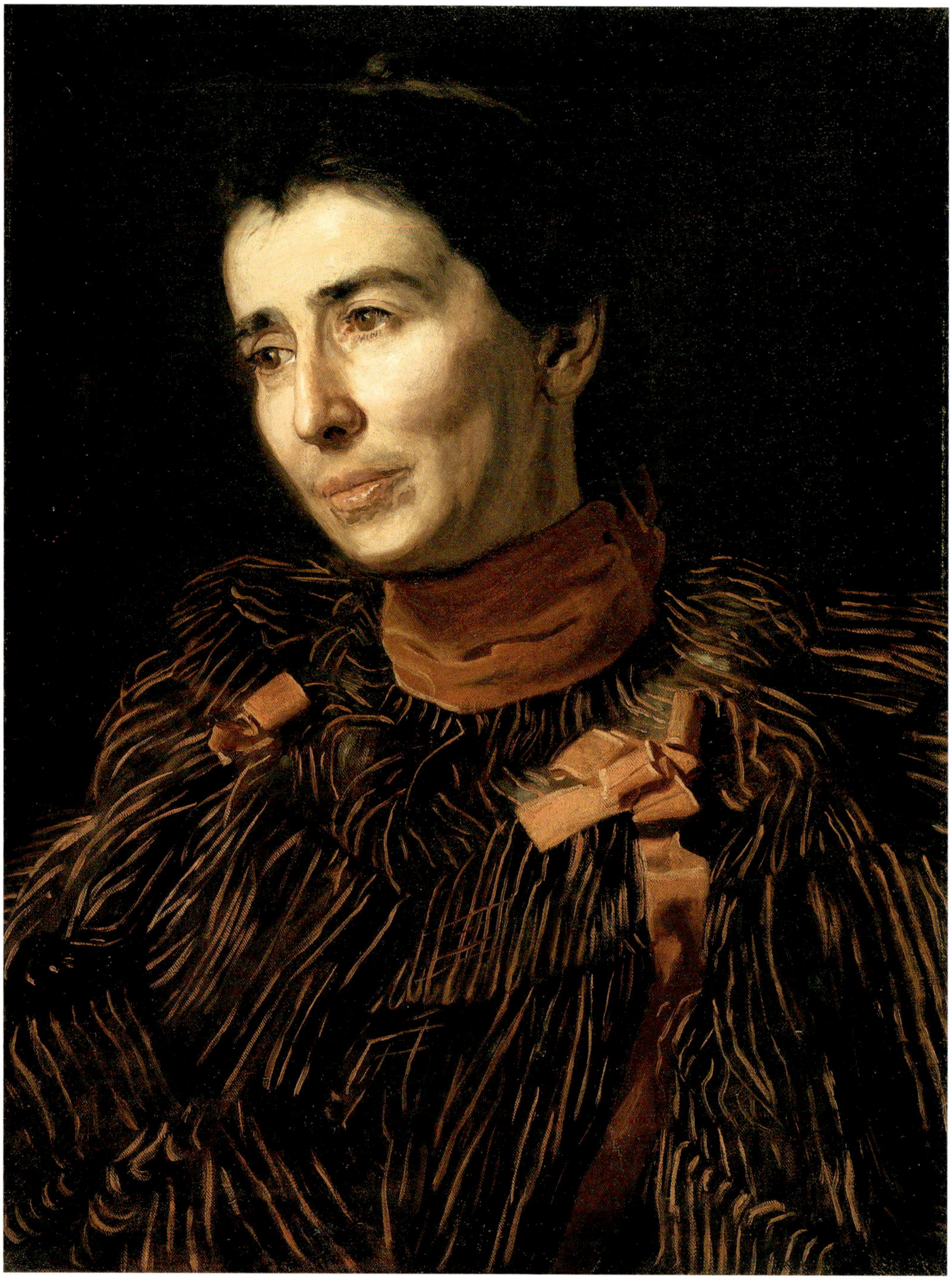

Fig. 27. Thomas Eakins, *Portrait of Mary Adeline Williams*, c. 1900. Oil on canvas, 24 1/8 × 18 1/8 in. Philadelphia Museum of Art. Gift of Mrs. Thomas Eakins and Miss Mary Adeline Williams, 1929.

artist expanded his teaching role at the academy to include serving as prosector for Keen's class, and giving guidance to advanced life students practicing dissection.[8]

Eakins' work in Schussele's class was suspended for the 1877–78 term, following the complaint of academy board directors that Schussele was wrong to delegate his responsibilities in the life class, but after this relatively brief hiatus, Eakins returned to the post of instructor to the life class. In the fall of 1878, Eakins was listed as assistant professor of painting, chief demonstrator of anatomy, and supervisor of the modeling classes. By any measure, Eakins was doing well, and shaping a coherent professional life; it made sense that the artist of the infamous *Gross Clinic* should teach painting and anatomy.

At the age of thirty-two, Eakins clearly had developed a strong sense of loyalty as well. When the board members threatened to fire Schussele and replace him with Eakins in 1879, due to the elderly artist's infirmity, Eakins stopped the plan by informing them that "it could not be accomplished without the loss of Mr. Eakins' services—he considering himself bound in honor to Professor Schussele."[9] When Schussele voluntarily retired not long afterward, his young supporter did take over, and from then on anatomy in various ways served as the principal element of the academy program.

The extraordinary emphasis on anatomy that led to the inclusion of dissection in the curriculum of the Pennsylvania Academy grew, in a sense, from deep roots. Eakins' anatomy program at the Pennsylvania Academy was uniquely advanced, but he did not invent the tradition in America. The earliest artistic study of anatomy in the colonies may be credited to John Singleton Copley, who was determined to learn about "mussels" and bones in Boston in the middle of the eighteenth century. In 1756, few educational resources were available in America for the study of art, but Copley did know that he would have to learn anatomy, and he determined to do so in a pragmatic manner. With no art academies or medical schools, Copley made his own anatomy book by copying plates from treatises owned by his artist stepfather, Peter Pelham.

Copley's *Anatomy Book, Plate IX* (fig. 28) demonstrates both his direct copying of previous examples—in this case an illustration by Jacob Van Der Gracht—and also the artist's earnest attempt to understand the parts of the body through explanatory notations. Jules Prown points out that Copley could not have made many of his notations without a physician's advice, indicating the artist's efforts to improve his understanding through every available means.[10] The anatomy books Copley relied on taught him two principles of artistic anatomy education developed in the Renaissance: first, that only external surfaces were of interest to the artist; second, that study of anatomy was never disconnected from the study of art. In this case, the emotion and pose of the

Fig. 28. John Singleton Copley, *Anatomy Book, Plate IX*, 1756. The British Museum.

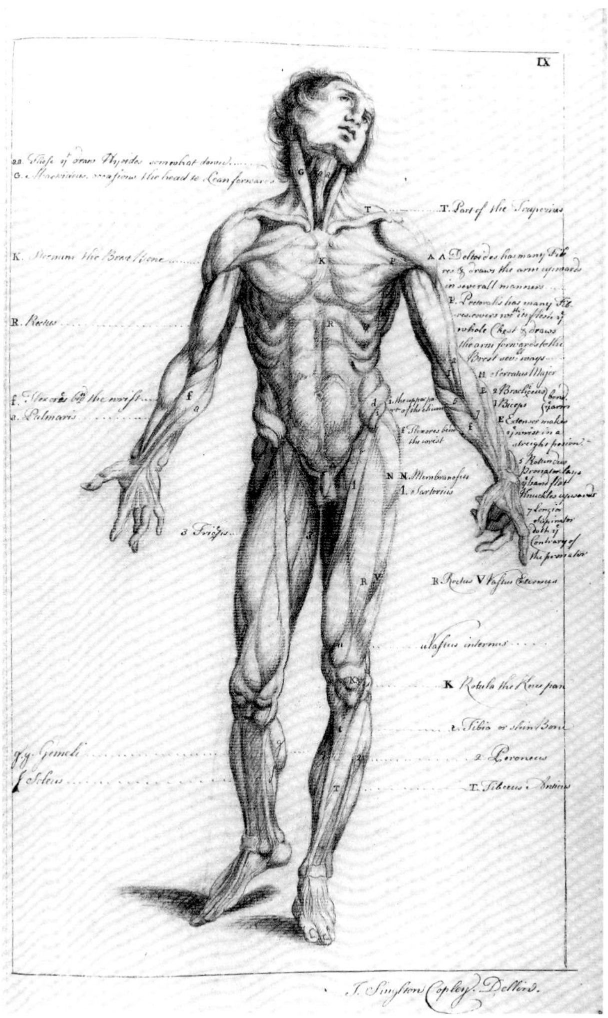

figure suggest a narrative context relevant to making art that tells a story. Notice too how Copley, following his predecessors, paid attention to the grounding of the foot using cast shadows—certainly an element of artistic study irrelevant to understanding muscles and bones. In his last anatomical plate, Copley included a measured drawing of a classical statue—the Medici Venus. This was standard practice in early anatomy books and a good reminder in neoclassical times that all venerable artistic roads still led back to Rome.[11]

A century later, William Rimmer, a former physician, may be credited with creating the first systematic program for the study of artistic anatomy in America at the Lowell Institute in Boston. Like Eakins, Rimmer used athletic models, advised clay modeling along with drawing from the nude, and shared experiences based on dissections in medical colleges (although the Lowell Institute did not offer the opportunity for art students themselves to dissect). Rimmer died in 1879, just as Eakins was beginning to formulate the Pennsylvania Academy curriculum, but Rimmer's work likely would have been known to the younger artist, both through his publication *Art Anatomy* and probably by reputation as well. In later years, Eakins followed Rimmer as anatomy lecturer at Cooper Union and the National Academy of Design.[12]

In Philadelphia, the roots of artistic anatomy training were somewhat less deep than in Boston, but still strong. The Academy of Fine Arts, after all, was founded not only by Charles Willson Peale but also by a group of Philadelphia luminaries largely composed of doctors. "The earliest actual evidences of an art school in connection with the Pennsylvania Academy … are found in the minutes of that institution for the year 1812. In the early part of the year, it was resolved that 'A Life Academy be at once started …' Subsequently, in the same year, it was recorded that 'Dr. Nathaniel Chapman was elected Professor of Anatomy.'"[13] The appointment of an anatomist to the faculty must have seemed entirely advisable in light of the prominent inclusion of anatomical training in venerable European art academies since the Renaissance.[14] By the nineteenth century in Europe, such study had become de rigueur. Even considering these many intellectual antecedents, however, Eakins' and Keen's anatomy program in Philadelphia was still unprecedented.

When William Brownell critiqued the program Eakins oversaw at the Pennsylvania Academy in 1879, he expressed admiration for the expansive facilities in the new building, and also remarked on the many innovative aspects of the curriculum. A student entering the Pennsylvania Academy after Eakins' arrival as a teacher in 1878 could look forward to a short "probationary" study of drawing from plaster casts of Greek and Roman sculptures in two courses, followed by relatively rapid admission to the life class.[15] In strong contrast to other art schools, Eakins reserved the right to drastically reduce this already shortened period of copying casts. Several student accounts record rapid promotion—including Francis Petrus Paulus, who recalled spending "only one week in the drawing from the Antique" before being plucked out for admission to the life class.[16] Louise Lippincott wrote that Eakins "visited [antique] classes only to urge students to begin painting."[17]

In some ways, Eakins' academy was not much changed from the system he had inherited from his predecessor, Christian Schussele. Students under Eakins' direction clearly spent less time drawing from antique casts than was customary in other art academies and under Schussele, but the course was still required. Eakins' attitude toward the value of Greek and Roman study for modern art students was an interesting modification of more usual practices.[18] Rather than spending their time drawing classical statuary, Eakins wanted his students to copy the manner in which those artists had worked themselves. He told Brownell in 1879: "I don't like a long study of casts…. The Greeks did not study the antique … the draped figures in the Parthenon pediment were modeled from life, undoubtedly. And nature is just as varied and just as beautiful in our day as she was in the time of Phidias…. Did you ever notice, by the way, those circus tumblers and jumpers? … They are absolutely beautiful, many of them."[19] Eakins exhibited his devotion to study of the human body and athletes in particular throughout his teaching and professional career.

After being elevated from drawing casts, academy students under Eakins' direction embarked on an extraordinarily comprehensive study of the nude—in painting, modeling, and anatomy classes. No course was strictly required once admission to life drawing was permitted, but ambitious students were left with no doubt that shortcuts were frowned upon. Advanced students could not expect to be treated seriously unless they participated fully in Eakins' rigorous program, including hands-on work in the dissecting rooms. Here again, some aspects of Eakins' program were not especially revolutionary. As Kathleen Foster points out, academy life class drawings from the 1850s demonstrate that, even at midcentury, sketching from the nude was routinely practiced and free from "covered faces or coy postures."[20]

Nevertheless, it is impossible to deny that Eakins was a superb and revolutionary artistic anatomist. A reporter did not understate the case in 1886 when he or she wrote, "It is one of the distinguishing characteristics of his management of the schools of the Pennsylvania Academy of Fine Arts, that anatomy is more thoroughly demonstrated there than at any other art school in the country."[21] Eakins' knowledge of the subject made him an incomparable lecturer; his passion for it was obvious, and his teaching methods were inarguably the most coherent and rigorous ever developed by an artist. In many ways, academy students constantly studied anatomy. In 1884 the school's course catalogue described the "arrangement of classes" as follows:

> Men's Life Classes, painting and modeling, 43½ hours per week.
> Women's Life Classes, painting and modeling, 43½ hours per week.
> Antique Classes, every day and evening.
> Sketch Class, every day.
> Lectures on Art Anatomy, two each week for four months, commencing in October.
> Lectures on Perspective and Composition by the Director, one each week during the months of March and April.[22]

With the exception of the sketch classes, in which clothed students posed for one another on a rotating basis, and perspective lectures, art students enrolled at Eakins' academy looked at the nude constantly after promotion from the antique.

Printed "circulars" following Eakins' reorganization of the school are striking in the prominence of their advertisements for this aspect of the curriculum—promising "nude study," dissection, and an expanded course of thirty-five anatomy lectures. Fairman Rogers rationalized this aspect of the program by emphasizing that the academy focused its efforts on providing students opportunities they could not easily afford on their own.[23]

A few aspects of Eakins' new curriculum mirrored the arrangements at the Art Students' League of New York. In June 1877, the league announced a schedule that included life classes for gentlemen from nine to noon each day and seven-thirty to ten o'clock in the evening. The ladies' life class met from one to four each afternoon. Portrait and sketch classes were held, along with lectures on perspective and composition, and anatomy—nearly the same offerings that Eakins soon arranged in Philadelphia.[24] The comparison was less close in other respects. Although the Art Students' League offered lectures on artistic anatomy, they were less extensive in both quantity and quality, and on-site dissections were not available, although some teachers advised students to attend medical school clinics and occasionally accompanied them there.[25] In his lengthy review of the Pennsylvania Academy for *Scribner's Monthly*, Brownell summarized the case succinctly: "In dissections presided over and directed by the professor of painting, the school of the Philadelphia Academy is, so far as I know, unique."[26]

Even the academy lecture course itself—a standard component of many art schools—was extraordinary. Charles H. Stephens' *Anatomical Lecture by Dr. William Williams Keen* (fig. 29) demonstrates the character of these classes. Keen is shown in his standard practice of lecturing, accompanied by a skeleton, a wax model upon which forms could be built up, a partially dissected cadaver suspended from a grappling hook, and a living man. Moving back and forth between dead and living bodies, the doctor was able to make his points about hidden and visible structures with utmost clarity. "Galvanized batteries" and a variety of weights were often connected to the cadaver to show the effects of motion—an addition that might seem ghoulish to us today but at the time was not much commented upon. Mary Shelley's *Frankenstein* was already sixty years old in 1878.

Keen was so devoted to the cause of artistic anatomy education that he prepared a manuscript on the subject for publication sometime after Stephens' painting was made.

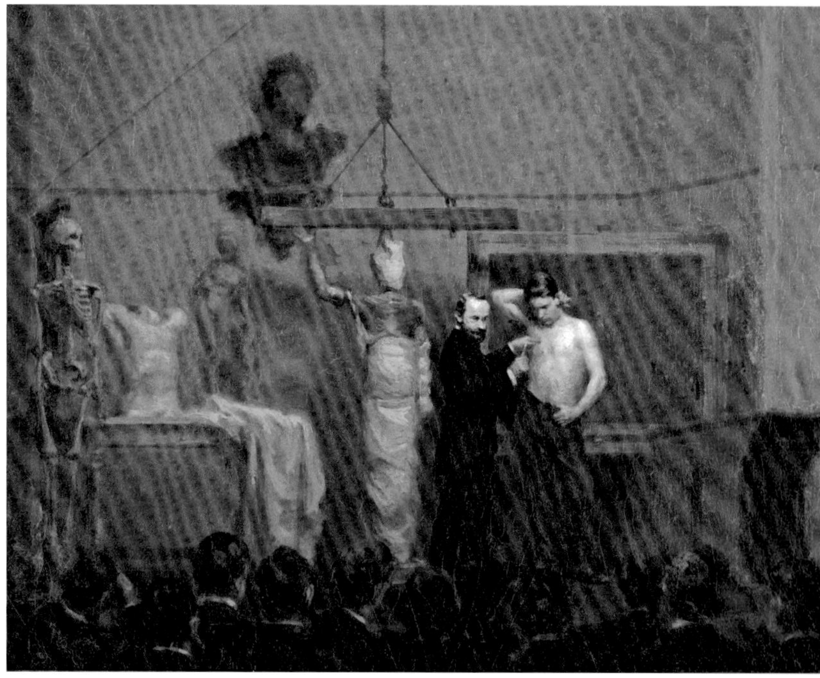

Fig. 29. Charles H. Stephens, *Anatomical Lecture by Dr. William Williams Keen*, c. 1879. Oil on cardboard, 8⅝ × 11 in. Courtesy of the Pennsylvania Academy of the Fine Arts, Philadelphia. Gift of the artist.

Professors commonly wrote the textbooks purchased by their students in nineteenth-century professional schools, and in this case the need was especially urgent, as there were no books available at the time that even remotely could have served Keen's purposes. General texts like Peale's *Graphics* and Chapman's *American Drawing Book* included scant instruction on the subject, although Chapman did concede the importance of anatomy. At the very least, he stated, "we would desire ... earnestly to impress upon the student the importance of a familiarity and knowledge of the structure, proportions, and action, of the skeleton, not only in its general characteristics, but as well in all its details." He went on to strongly advise that "no school where drawing is properly taught should be without [a skeleton], as well as approved plaster casts of complete anatomical figures and detailed parts in various actions." Chapman's minimal requirements clearly did not suffice for Keen—or Eakins.[27]

Other American textbooks were equally useless. The only two books specifically on art anatomy published before the 1880s in the United States were John Rubens Smith's *Compendium of Picturesque Anatomy, Adapted to the Arts of Design, Painting, Sculpture, and Engraving*, from 1827, and William Rimmer's *Art Anatomy*, each of which presented a rather different view of the subject than Keen and Eakins put forward.

Smith's enormous volume began with a flourish of "Recommendatory Certificates" by Washington Allston and Gilbert Stuart. Although the author's first plate provided drawings and summary descriptions of major skeletal and muscular features, he quickly moved on to his larger goal of helping artists to generalize forms, rather than to observe and understand individual manifestations. Confident that students had, by the completion of Plate IV (fig. 30), learned enough of anatomy, he wrote:

> Thus far is all that need be impressed on the mind of a student desirous of informing himself of the principles of motion as they govern forms; that imagination must be too feeble to hope for professional success that cannot go further into details without additional data or documents; in doing which, one must ever keep in the mind's eye the rules of proportion, which are here recapitulated in the form of a summary:
>
> The face of a man is no longer than the inside of his hand.
> The largest breadth of the body is the fifth of its height.
> The height of the forehead is the length of a nose.
> The nose is the third of a face and equal to the length of an ear.
> A man's length, when he stands upright, is equal to the distance between the tips of the longest finger of each hand, when the arms are fully extended horizontally.[28]

Keen certainly would have found Smith's rather dismissive attitude toward individual anatomical characteristics unacceptable, particularly since his predecessor provided scant description of the human body. And it is hard to imagine that

Eakins admired the grace with which skeleton "B" in Plate IV draped its gluteus muscles with a toga.

Dr. William Rimmer's *Art Anatomy* (1877) should have been much improved over its earlier competitor, but in fact Rimmer's text was even more eccentric than Smith's, and perhaps even less useful despite its greater heft. Like Smith, Rimmer included a few plates labeling major bones and muscle groups, but mostly filled his volume with a bizarre assortment of engravings, including plates such as "Hair—Female Form" in which Rimmer distinguishes between several illustrated hairstyles, labeling them "orderly" or "disorderly." At the bottom of this plate, he notes: "The vices and virtues of personal character stand in closest relation to the vices and virtues of personal ornamenture."[29]

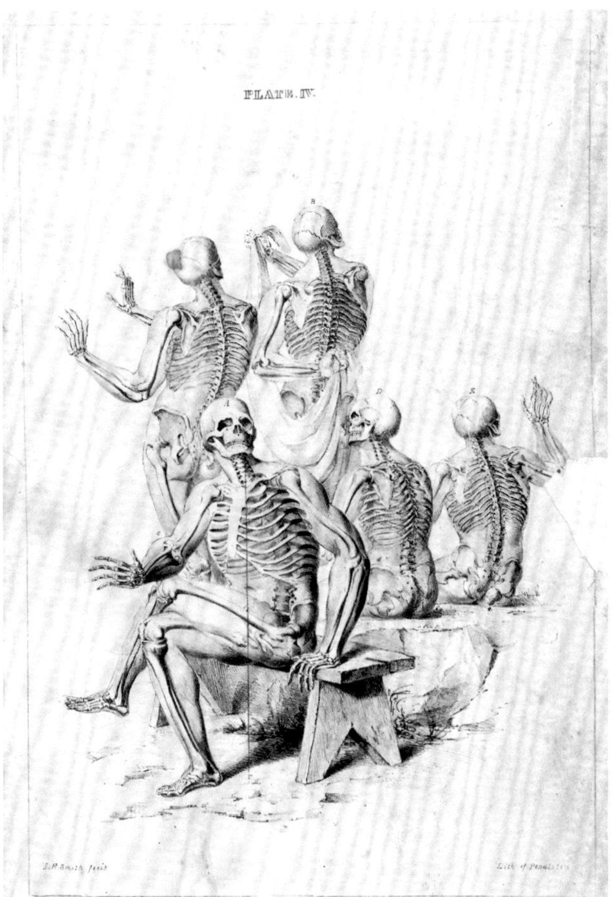

Fig. 30. John Rubens Smith, "Plate IV," published in *A Compendium of Picturesque Anatomy, Adapted to the Arts of Design, Painting, Sculpture, and Engraving*, 1827. Collection, Boston Medical Library in the Francis A. Countway Library of Medicine.

A newspaper obituary for Rimmer pasted to the frontispiece of his *Art Anatomy* text housed in the Countway Medical Library of Harvard Medical School defended the book's merits: "Casual observers of this work have charged him with copying the antique statues, but the writer, whose fortune it was to be with him during most of the time of its preparation, knows that not a single copy exists in the book. The drawing was done mostly during a vacation in the country, and most of the drawings were made by the doctor while seated upon the grass under a tree, without model, and without reference to anything whatever."[30] There can be little doubt as to why Keen felt it might be time to add a new text on artistic anatomy to the canon.

In strong contrast to Smith's and Rimmer's offerings, the text of Keen's unpublished and undated manuscript reveals the harmonious integration between artistic and medical study that the anatomist developed and imparted to Eakins and academy students in his lectures. Here, there was no discussion of "disorderly" hairdos. Instead, Keen's manual included chapters on the skeleton, bones, joints, spine, vertebral column, articulations of the spine, general remarks on the spine, head, cranium, face, general remarks on the head, and proportions of the human body.

Keen's text is remarkable for its clear, well-organized, and comprehensive description of the parts of the body of interest to artists, but even more so for its fluid interweaving of aesthetic and scientific commentary, in the tradition of art anatomy books generally but now much more rigorous: "The compact tissue ... is placed in the best position artistically as well as mechanically, for midway between the joints are the chief muscular masses and the beautiful contour of the limbs would be sadly marred were our bones of the same thickness throughout."[31] Keen's poetic descriptions of the body included more complex structures as well, often related to paintings his students would have been familiar with:

> Now having given you the important anatomical varieties and names and quite enough to weary you I fear let us add a word or

> two as to the artistic character of these various motions.... An excellent study of ... angular postures in varied handling may be had in the familiar pictures of Correggio's and Battoni's Magdalens.... The most beautiful of them all is the combined and multiplied slight movements of many small bones. The wrist is a good example but the spine is by far the best but this I shall again remind you of at length when we study that as a whole. Between those two extremes come the ball and socket joints and the rotary both of which produce effects very pleasing to the eye.[32]

As this text makes clear, art anatomy as taught by Keen was still a discipline removed from medical anatomy—there was no discussion of disease or injury, for example, and no review of organs and structures unrelated to surface appearances. In comparison, the Gray's *Anatomy* edition of 1878 included vast sections on arteries, veins, the lymphatics, nervous system, organs of sense, organs of digestion and their appendages, organs of voice and respiration, urinary organs, male generative organs, female organs of generation, surgical anatomy of inguinal hernia, surgical anatomy of femoral hernia, surgical anatomy of perineum and ischiorectal region, and so on.[33]

Although Keen's lectures at the academy clearly did not cover as much material as his medical school classes, this was also not as "artistic" an anatomical bent as that practiced by Smith and Rimmer. Keen was above all an anatomist and surgeon. Whereas Smith and Rimmer modeled their illustrations on Greek and Roman sculptures, Keen recommended that students use the academy casts as an extension of anatomy class, advising: "as excellent illustrations of rotation combined with the curves of the spine look at the Psyche, the Wrestlers, and the Dying Gladiator."[34]

Had Keen's lectures provided the sole anatomical study offered at the Pennsylvania Academy, they still would have been an extraordinary improvement over Rimmer's disjointed sermons, but they were merely the gateway to a field of study that in many cases occupied fully one-tenth of an academy student's time—dissection.[35] Following Keen's lectures, and with his assistance in obtaining cadavers, a variety of corpses were probed in academy rooms. Skeletons were lent by the Academy of Natural Sciences, and the University of Pennsylvania "assisted in obtaining material for dissection."[36] With characteristically varying temperaments, both Keen and Eakins put forth the case for such studies. The elegant anatomist wrote: "'While not wishing to give undue prominence to anatomy in the Course of Instruction I can but see that the only way really to *know* the anatomy of the *Human Figure* is to *dissect* it." Eakins phrased his opinion in a more direct way: "To study anatomy out of a book is like learning to paint out of a book. It is a waste of time."[37]

Eakins and Keen not only prepared a comprehensive series of dissections of human cadavers in academy rooms, they also frequently arranged for dissection of animal cadavers and even for field trips, including Eakins' annual excursion to "a suburban bone-boiling establishment." In summer, students visited Fairman Rogers' horse farm.[38] Although Eakins' chief purpose in studying animal anatomy was to assist students in depicting and sculpting popular artistic subjects, like Keen, he also valued the opportunity to compare and contrast a variety of structures. In his manuscript, Keen advised studying the bones of more than one human and comparing them with those of "lower animals" in order to be able to distinguish individual variations from constant forms. In his discussion of the cervical vertebrae, Keen demonstrated the value of such comparative studies: "The very name given to the seventh cervical vertebra is suggestive of this projection. The *vertebra prominensus*. Glance now for a moment at this skeleton of a horse which may serve as a type of horizontal quadruped with heavy head to be supported at the end, and with the leverage of the cervical spine instead of assuming the erect posture with the head nearly balanced on a vertical spine. See the immensely elongated spines not now only or chiefly the 7th cervical but several of the upper dorsal vertebrae. This is well seen even in the gorilla." Such lectures were a weekly reminder of the revelations of Darwin—man was not as distinct from animals as many would have liked to believe.[39]

To further such lessons and reminders, Eakins brought study of horses and other animals into both life and modeling classes, believing along with Keen in the profound educational value of comparative demonstrations. In the dissection laboratory, subjects included dogs, cats, sheep, a cow, and a lion, all examined both to contrast their forms and because they frequently were represented in art. Eakins' drawings of tendons crossing the joint of the little finger (fig. 31) and dissection study of a lion (fig. 32) demonstrate the "bare bones" approach to artistic anatomy Eakins and Keen developed in the dissecting room of the Pennsylvania Academy. One can hardly imagine the addition of graceful poses or shadowed ground lines in these summary studies, in distinct contrast to Copley, Smith, and Rimmer.

The curricular innovations developed by Keen and Eakins during the eight years of their collaboration owed little to the model of past art anatomy instruction, as these studies demonstrate. Rather, the chief influence on this program was Keen's work teaching medical students over a period of decades. Indeed, both the curriculum and the administration of the Pennsylvania Academy bear enormous similarity to Philadelphia's medical colleges.

In 1881, Keen published an essay in the *Transactions of the International Medical Congress* urging anatomy professors to adopt the system he was using at the Pennsylvania Academy:

> What I wish formally to urge upon teachers of anatomy, is not that the living model should be used occasionally, but regularly; not as a rarity, but as a constant means of illustration; as much so as the cadaver or the skeleton.... I have found it very useful to study the cadaver, not only horizontally, on a rotating table, as we generally do, but in the vertical position. I place two hooks in the skull, just above the ears, and suspend the body from the ceiling by a pulley, using also a cross-piece with cords and self-adjustment pulleys, by which arms can be raised at will, and the body easily rotated. The skeleton, cadaver, and model are thus all in the same posture, and no mental transposition of relations is necessary in passing from the one to the other.[40]

This system of demonstration, depicted in Stephens' painting, was considered so valuable in medical education that Keen was honored by publication of a longer essay, "On the Systematic Use of the Living Model as a Means of Illustration in Teaching Anatomy," in the 1887 American edition of Gray's *Anatomy*, already the most popular medical school anatomy text in the English language.

It is unclear whether Keen developed this system with Eakins at the academy or earlier in his own anatomy school.

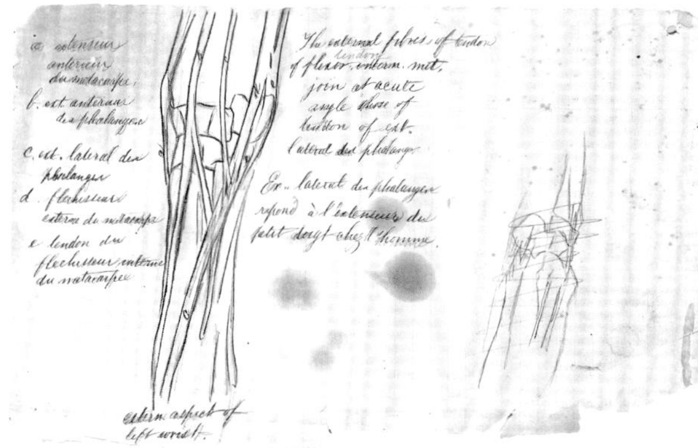

Fig. 31. Thomas Eakins, *Dissection Study: Human (Tendons Crossing the Joint of the little Finger, Left Arm)*, c. 1877–79. Black ink over graphite and blue pencil on foolscap, 7¾ × 12 7⁄16 in. (irregular). Courtesy of the Pennsylvania Academy of the Fine Arts, Philadelphia, Charles Bregler's Thomas Eakins Collection. Purchased with the partial support of the Pew Memorial Trust and the John S. Phillips Fund.

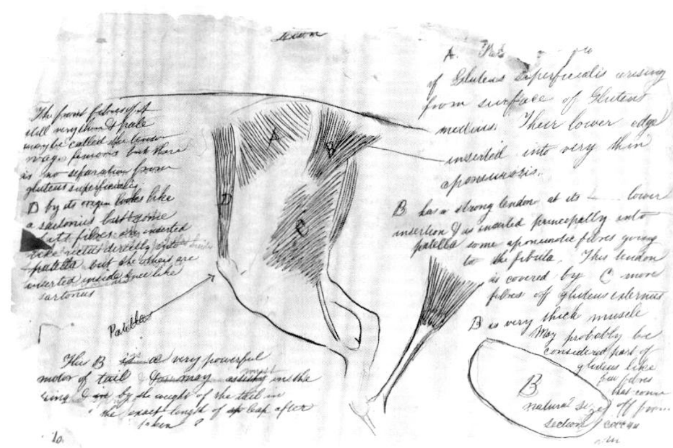

Fig. 32. Thomas Eakins, *Dissection Study: Lion (Muscles of Hind Quarters and Leg)*, 1885. Pen and ink over graphite on foolscap. 7¾ × 12 7⁄16 in. (irregular). Courtesy of the Pennsylvania Academy of the Fine Arts, Philadelphia, Charles Bregler's Thomas Eakins Collection. Purchased with the partial support of the Pew Memorial Trust and the John S. Phillips Fund.

Nonetheless, it is clear that he was largely complementing and expanding on an earlier inclusion to Gray's *Anatomy*—an essay by Luther Holden titled "Landmarks: Medical and Surgical," which taught students to use palpation as a diagnostic tool. Holden urged students to acquire the habit of examining the living body with "anatomical eyes":

> This habit is within easy reach of any one who has carefully dissected for himself, and acquired the knowledge of what to feel for....
>
> I would also invite teachers of anatomy to follow the example of Sir C. Bell, who was in the habit of introducing, from time to time, a powerful muscular fellow to his class, in order to show how much of the structure of the body, such as the articulations and the muscles, might be learned without actual dissection....
>
> Anatomy obvious to the eye and the finger depends in great measure upon the quantity of subcutaneous fat. In some it stands out beautifully clear; in others it is masked by obesity. [Select], therefore, for study a moderately lean person.[41]

It is almost impossible to imagine that this text did not influence Eakins as he designed the life classes at the Pennsylvania Academy.

Whether through Keen's suggestion or his own design, many aspects of Eakins' art curriculum bore the stamp of Holden's advice for medical students. The artist encouraged and indeed often badgered students to "carefully dissect" in the anatomy program, and, most notably, Eakins sought models in painting and modeling classes who offered a clear view of important anatomical structures. Unfortunately, another similarity between medical and art schools was the difficulty in following this advice.

In Europe, artists had their pick of models from a large group of uninhibited working men, women, and children, but in America conditions were different. William Sartain, Eakins' friend and fellow artist, recorded his experience trying to find models in the mid-1860s: "Before I went to Europe to study, models in Philadelphia were scarce. Once for the Penna. Acad. Life class—Daniel R. Knight and I went out to scare one up. We found a strong well built man and engaged him—When he arrived at the class room & found he was asked to undress he was furious & squared off at us—and the class speadily [*sic*] retreated out of harm's way. He hadn't understood he was wanted nude, and took it as a serious insult. Which reminds me that nearly 100 years ago Vanderlyn's studio in New York was mobbed because it became known he employed nude models. In those days evidently paintings of nude subjects were supposed to be products of imagination!" Later, in Europe, Sartain was able to report a vastly different situation: "Models at Rome are excellent and only cost 10 cents an hour against 20 in Paris and 50 in America."[42]

Eakins himself had traveled to Europe for education on the basis of similar earlier accounts, and as a teacher he felt it his duty to create improved opportunities for study of "good" nude bodies in the United States. When he tried to implement Holden's ideal, however, problems finding suitable models for the life classes began almost immediately.[43] On January 8, 1877, Eakins wrote to William's father, John Sartain, a family friend and chairman of the committee on instruction:

> The Life Schools are in great need of good female models. I desire that an advertisement similar to the following be inserted in the Public Ledger.
>
> Wanted Female Models for the Life Schools of the Pennsylvania Academy of the Fine Arts.
>
> Apply to the Curator at the Academy Broad & Cherry at the Cherry St. entrance. Applicants should be of respectability and may on all occasions be accompanied by their mothers or other female relatives. Terms $1 per hour.
>
> John Sartain
> Chairman of Com. on Instruction

The high fee was meant to assure a large applicant pool.

Eakins tried to appease the elder artists on the committee with some concessions to American manners and an explanation of the purposes for his desire to go public in seeking models:

> The privilege of wearing a mask might also be conceded and advertised. The publicity thus given in a reputable newspaper at the instance of an institution like the Academy will insure in these times a great number of applicants among whom will be

> found beautiful ones with forms fit to be studied.
>
> The old plan was for the students or officers to visit low houses of prostitution & bargain with the inmates.
>
> This course was degrading & would be unworthy of the present academy & its result was models coarse, flabby, ill formed & unfit in every way for the requirements of a school, nor was there sufficient change of models for the successful study of form.[44]

In Eakins' mind, "the present academy" was not a place that would any longer tolerate the unprofessional "inmates" who had posed in the past. Although the advertisement seems not to have been posted, nonetheless, as Holden recommended, Eakins' students were soon studying from more respectable "muscular fellows" and "moderately lean persons."

Medical schools in the United States experienced the same difficulties in procuring sufficient and appropriate human subjects for their students. This was not a new problem in the 1880s. Between 1808 and 1820, the sculptor William Rush created wooden anatomical models for Dr. Caspar Wistar at the University of Pennsylvania, "to make up for the lack of specimens available" to medical students.[45] Sixty years later, the situation markedly had improved. At the same time that Pennsylvania Academy circulars and administrators were actively promoting the school's abundant supply of models, the 1881–82 announcement of classes at Jefferson Medical College likewise boasted of its enhanced access to bodies—both clinically in the "twenty hospitals, nine dispensaries, and thirty-eight other charitable institutions with which infirmaries are connected" in the city, and in the "practical anatomy" course in which "a full supply of material is furnished at the small charge of $1 per part, and no extra or incidental charges are made."[46]

Both Eakins and his administrative colleagues at Jefferson shared the goal of procuring *good* bodies—thin in the case of living examples, and fresh in the case of the dead. Dr. John G. Lee, the Philadelphia coroner's physician, complained in 1882 that Jefferson College wanted "regular Apollos to operate on."[47] Eakins, still short of his hiring goals in the early 1880s, turned to his own students as models. Access to bodies, alive or dead, at medical and art academies was the draw. And success in this endeavor in both institutions was considered critical to financial well-being.

For both medical and art schools in the 1870s and 1880s, the impetus to change and improve came from ambitious and well-educated administrators like Keen and Eakins who sought to raise standards, advance progress, and elevate the credentials of their institutions. Another factor was constant worry over low enrollment as a result of overseas competition. In this sense, economic forces combined to set both these types of institutions on similar courses. Philadelphia competed for students not only with New York and Baltimore but also with Munich, Düsseldorf, and Paris. The flow of art students abroad from 1870 to 1900 is vast and well-documented.[48] Medical schools faced the same problem.

At the same time Thomas Eakins led a following horde of American art students into the Ecole des Beaux-Arts in Paris, American medical students were undergoing the same transatlantic search for superior teachers and facilities. One account of American medical students between 1870 and 1914 estimates that "some 15,000 studied in Germany, known for its progressive scientific education, as well as in Paris."[49] The reasons for the exodus in both instances had to do largely with the availability of bodies for study purposes. In the medical arena, European students reportedly enjoyed an "inexhaustible" supply of anatomical material.[50]

Famously cheap and available models both inside and outside the famous art academies of Europe offered similar enticements. When the Pennsylvania Academy highlighted the hours of study from the nude available in its circulars after 1879, it was following the marketing techniques of the Art Students' League in New York, which boasted "no less than 1377 hours … of study from the nude" in its 1878 annual report. A local newspaper publicized this statistic and added: "So far as is known, the greatest number of hours similarly devoted in any other American institution is only four hundred and thirty-two. These figures speak very clearly … and are in themselves the best testimony to the work and worth of the school."[51] Arts administrators—and prospective students—were clearly keeping score.

As is obvious from this example, competition within the United States was also increasing, as dozens of new regional medical colleges and art schools were founded in the post–Civil War period. In a volatile economic climate, medical schools in particular jockeyed for position to retain and enhance their prominence, lurching toward a modern standard four-year curriculum while struggling to balance their books.[52] When Harvard Medical School imposed more stringent standards and higher tuition in the 1870s, it saw a "temporary drop in enrollment" along with a "markedly higher caliber of student."[53] Entrance requirements, licensing examinations, and more rigorous curricula all led to better medical education in the 1870s and 1880s, along with higher status in the eyes of the general public. The Pennsylvania Academy was attempting to improve through similar changes in precisely these years. The curriculum was deepened and standardized, and the institution was expected to produce a "higher caliber" of student.

Administratively, another major shift also was taking place at both types of institutions. In medical colleges and at the Pennsylvania Academy, the concept of faculty was evolving. When Keen began his career as an autonomous anatomy instructor at his Philadelphia School of Anatomy, students paid him directly for education, and for body parts. Even at Jefferson and the University of Pennsylvania, medical students bought class "tickets" and textbooks that financially supported their professors until the early 1880s.[54] At that time though, as at an increasing number of medical colleges, both institutions acceded to the demands of faculty for more centralized governance, less financial risk to themselves, and standardized salaries. "Unlike before, when the faculty personally collected fees from the students and paid the operating expenses themselves, tuition was now paid directly to the university, which placed the professors on salary and assumed administrative responsibility for operating the school."[55]

Eakins, in effect, demanded and oversaw the same changes at the Pennsylvania Academy. On April 8, 1885, he wrote to the board of directors, demanding to be paid the $2,500 salary he had been promised by Fairman Rogers years before: "The number of classes has increased, the school is full, probably as full as it should be, its pupils are becoming known, its reputation is wide, and its standard of work is very high." According to Eakins, it was time for Rogers' promise to be fulfilled.[56] The board ultimately refused to do so, although it should have been capable of supporting the cost—the academy began charging flat tuition fees in 1881, at the same time as Philadelphia's medical colleges.

These enormous financial changes, all taking place during Eakins' years as director, meant both more autonomy for faculty everywhere, and less. While Eakins had a great deal of freedom to institute his reforms as a respected professional—for a while—he also was newly beholden to a board responsible for complex financial concerns that ultimately trumped loftier curricular ideals. Institutional reform, faculty professionalism, and curricular change were all controversial topics in many educational institutions in the 1880s. Eakins undoubtedly discussed these issues with his medical friends, colleagues, and portrait subjects, and in particular with Fairman Rogers, who was watching these changes evolve at both the Pennsylvania Academy as board member and chairman of the instruction committee and at the University of Pennsylvania, where he was an engineering professor before joining the board of trustees.

In spite of the relative turmoil of the period, the example of the medical colleges at Jefferson and the University of Pennsylvania as role models for the academy was sound. Not only were these programs acknowledged to be among the best in the world, but the excitement of medicine and science generally cannot be overstated. In an essay typical of the fervor of his colleagues, Keen wrote of the changes in surgery following the Civil War:

> We used only the ordinary marine or toilet sponges. After an operation they were washed in ordinary water to cleanse them of blood and pus, and were used in subsequent operations. In our ignorance of bacteriology we did not know that they harbored multitudes of germs which infected every wound in which they were used.... Before an operation nothing was rendered sterile by antiseptics, or by heat (boiling, baking). I have seen more than once, my old teacher, Professor S. D. Gross, give a last final touch to his knife on his boot—even on the sole—and then at once use it from the first cut to the last. When threading a needle, all of us

> pointed our silk by wetting it with germ laden saliva and rolling it between germ laden fingers ... it was seven times safer to fight all through three days of Gettysburg than to have an arm or a leg cut off.... What a contrast is the surgery of today![57]

Eakins too could have looked back at his own experiences as an art student in Philadelphia in the 1860s with a sense of great accomplishment. In place of the previous "program" of intermittent criticism by local artists, students now engaged in a coherent, full-time curriculum overseen by prominent experts in their fields. The progress of the age was thrilling, and striking. For many though, the value of all this change was somewhat arguable.

In 1879, William Brownell certainly wanted to embrace and celebrate change and progress when he set out to tour the nation's art schools and review them for *Scribner's Monthly.* He quickly comprehended just how radical and unique Eakins' and Keen's anatomy curriculum was, so much so that he devoted half his extensive article on the academy to describing this aspect of the program and to thoughtfully debating its merits. To consider its value, Brownell asked his readers to imagine themselves in the dissecting room, with its "dread-looking implements" and "the dead and dismembered semblance of what was once a human being. All one's feeling in regard to this is accentuated and emphasized by the thought that it is all to an end distinctly not utilitarian but aesthetic; and thus one's physical revulsion is re-enforced by an intellectual notion that it is, in its nature, paradoxical and absurd."

Brownell went on to report a lengthy conversation with Eakins about the rationale for the curriculum. He asked the artist:

> "And don't you find your interest becoming scientific in its nature, that you are interested in dissection as an end in itself, that curiosity leads you beyond the point at which the aesthetic usefulness of the work ceases? I don't see how you can help it?"
>
> "No," replies Mr. Eakins, smiling, "we turn out no physicians and surgeons. About the philosophy of aesthetics, to be sure, we do not greatly concern ourselves, but we are considerably concerned about learning how to paint. For anatomy, as such, we care nothing whatsoever. To draw the human figure, it is necessary to know as much as possible about it.... You don't suppose we pay much attention to the viscera, or study the functions of the spleen, I trust."
>
> "But the atmosphere of the place, the hideousness..! I can't fancy anything more utterly—utterly—inartistic...."
>
> "Even to refine upon natural beauty—to idealize—one must understand what it is that he is idealizing; otherwise his idealization—I don't like the word, by the way—becomes distortion, and distortion is ugliness. This whole matter of dissection is not art at all, any more than grammar is poetry. It is work, and hard work, disagreeable work.... As for [students'] artistic impulse, such work does not affect it in any way whatever...."
>
> Insensibly, the visitor begins to be impressed by the extreme sense of this ... and his surroundings to take on a different look. The "subject" comes to be but an organism of bones and muscles. The casts of arms depending from a swinging bar become interesting for what they show; the muscles being painted red, the tendons blue and the bones white, one is enabled to see at a glance their reciprocal relations. One "places" all the paraphernalia of the room; begins to appreciate first how much less liable the young men and women who study here are to draw impossible legs, arms, and trunks, than they were before; come to feel that, after all, it is the province of an art school to provide knowledge and training and not inspiration; and finally to perceive how wide of the mark it is to suppose that familiarity with scenes such as this of necessity dulls one's sensitiveness.... It quite takes one's breath away, does it not? Exhaustive is a faint word by which to characterize such a course of instruction. Must a painter know all this, one asks himself in a kind of awe-struck bewilderment.[58]

Brownell never answered his own question, but many in the art world in following years did—with a resounding no, a painter need not "know all this." This basic philosophical rift formed the basis for Eakins' subsequent ouster from his position at the academy, but another factor was at least equally to blame. Thomas Eakins clearly admired the doctors he painted and worked with and implemented many of the aspects of medical college pedagogy into artistic education as director at the Pennsylvania Academy, but unlike his esteemed medical colleagues he vehemently rejected the notion that women should be denied the same professional and educational benefits as men.

Eakins was not the first faculty member to admit women to the academy. They were allowed into antique cast drawing classes in the 1850s, and to anatomy lectures beginning in 1868. Courses for women at the academy in Schussele's day were quite limited, but during Eakins' years they rapidly expanded to include life and modeling classes with nude male and female models, anatomy lectures and dissections, and every other aspect of the curriculum available to men. European women would not enjoy such advanced opportunities in art study for decades to come.[59] The Pennsylvania Academy was not the only American art school to educate women, but opportunities elsewhere were always both separate and unequal.[60]

The situation was far worse for women hoping to become doctors. As in European art academies, the vast majority of medical colleges on both sides of the Atlantic refused women the opportunity to apply. "By 1893 only 37 out of the 105 regular institutions accepted them," and most of these were state-sponsored programs far from Philadelphia.[61] Most medical colleges that met the standards of the newly organized and increasingly powerful American Medical Association resisted integration until after 1910, including the University of Pennsylvania, Columbia, and Yale, which began accepting women in 1918. Harvard waited until 1946, and Jefferson Medical College refused entrance to women until 1961. Professional organizations like the AMA, even late in the nineteenth century, expressed their hope "that women would never embarrass us by a personal application for seats in this association."[62] As Eakins was to find out, pioneering improved anatomy training for art students generally was a far less dangerous course than making that education available equally to men and women more than thirty years before any accredited Philadelphia medical school would agree to do so.

The reasoning that most medical school administrators cited for their refusal to admit women presaged especially ill for Eakins and his curriculum. Repeatedly, it was dissection itself that was used as an excuse for barring women from medical practice. As Michael Sappol writes, "the cadaver, with its stench, gory disorder, and unveiled genitalia, was the antithesis of domesticity's aesthetic and ethos, of femininity itself."[63] Many male doctors of the era spilled copious ink demonstrating the numerous ways women's physiology could not endure a medical education. Authors in the 1870s and 1880s stressed that "while the male could withstand the rigors of healthy competition at all times, the female's education had to allow for periodical lapses to permit the construction of her reproductive organs. Overexertion in mental activity would cause females to suffer from 'ovarian neuralgia,' resulting in the inability of the body to supply both the brain and generative organs with sufficient blood." Smaller brain weights in women were seen as an additional impediment.[64]

In response to the disavowal of their cause by most medical colleges and the vast majority of the public in the second half of the nineteenth century, women went abroad or founded their own schools, but here, too, they faced enormous difficulties.[65] The first women's medical school, the Boston Female Medical School, founded in 1848, was followed by a scattered few others in the following decades.[66] In Philadelphia, women quickly followed suit with the establishment the Woman's Medical College in 1850, which proceeded to graduate many of the most famous women physicians of the nineteenth century. This was no easy accomplishment.

The chief difficulty faced by Philadelphia's early female medical students was the lack of access to hospital clinics. The organizers of the college had managed to build an adequate facility for classroom discussion, and to implement and staff a program of courses matching in nearly every detail the classroom requirements at Jefferson Medical College, but for a decade the school struggled to gain admittance for its students to clinics in any local hospital. Clara Marshall recorded the events when the barrier was finally breached: "November the 6th, 1869, was a memorable day in the history of the College. Permission having been given by the managers of the Pennsylvania Hospital for attendance upon the clinical lectures of that institution, about thirty women students were present on that day. The conduct of the male students was such as to raise a storm of public indignation in Philadelphia and other cities, and, as a consequence, the subject of clinical instruction to 'mixed' classes was discussed *in extensor* in the public press." The conduct that raised such a storm included insults and offensive language directed at the women as they left, "yells, hisses, 'caterwaulings,' mock applause, offensive remarks upon personal appearance, etc." Despite requests for the men to behave in a gentlemanly manner as the clinic proceeded, "missiles of paper, tinfoil, tobacco-quids, etc., were thrown upon the ladies, while some of these men (?) defiled the dresses of the ladies near them with tobacco juice."[67]

In a foreshadowing of later events at the academy, University of Pennsylvania medical professors in 1869 joined forces to adopt a "remonstrance" that declared "that their deliberate conviction is adverse to conducting clinical instruction in the presence of students of both sexes.... It cannot be assumed, by any right-minded person, that male persons should be subjected to inspection before a class of females, although this inspection may, without impropriety, be submitted to before those of their own sex." The "unanimous" faculty of the university medical college went on to assert that there were operations and classes of diseases suffered by men that would inevitably be "shocking to the sense of decency." If such "joint participation" by students were allowed, "that Barrier of respect" would be broken down and "that high estimation of womanly qualities, which should always be sustained and cherished," would be lost, "thereby entailing most serious detriment to the morals of society."[68]

The dean of the Woman's Medical College responded not as Eakins might have years later, by insisting that women would not be ruined by the sight of male anatomy, but rather that she was sure there were surgeries women could see that would "involve no necessary exposure" and, more strong-mindedly, that "wherever it is proper to introduce women as patients, there also it is but just and in accordance with the instincts of the truest womanhood for women to appear as physicians and students."[69]

The subtext of these literary salvos is not hard to read. Male physicians assumed the authority to view and display the bodies of whomsoever they chose. They had no cause to actively protest the female medical students attending patients in the Woman's Hospital (which provided far inferior educational opportunities), but the exposure of male genitalia to women was simply unthinkable. For Dean Ann Preston (one of the first graduates of Woman's Medical College), it was too soon to demand the right to see those parts-which-could-not-be-named, but not too soon to demand that the often "sensitive and shrinking—albeit poor" women "brought to illustrate the lectures" should have representatives of their own sex in the room, in professional capacities.[70]

The clinics that followed the drama of 1869 were segregated. Women viewed operations on other women without male students present, freeing them from harassment, but not from chronic annoyance. In 1878, women were still complaining that "it was trying to have brought before them a woman only to be told that at the following clinic for men a capital operation would be performed upon the patient, or to be shown a woman on whom an operation of magnitude had been performed before the male class." After thirty-two years of complaint, finally, in 1882 "the desire of the [Woman's Medical] faculty was gratified, when the students of the College were admitted to the regular weekly clinics."[71] Eakins followed suit immediately by instituting a women's dissection class in the same year at the academy. As mentioned previously, even D. Hayes Agnew was among the physicians who lectured to mixed classes, including Woman's Medical College students in following years.

It is impossible to imagine that Eakins was unaware of any of these developments—the controversies and progress of the age were prominent not only in newspapers but undoubtedly also in the artist's personal conversations with his many portrait subjects, colleagues, and friends in the city's medical community. Eakins was in Paris in 1869 when professors at Jefferson first refused to teach in coeducational clinics, but he may well have heard of these historic events as he went forward in establishing his own mixed classes in later years. After all, the surgeon lecturing that first "mixed" day at the Pennsylvania Hospital was the artist's professor and later portrait subject Dr. Jacob Mendez DaCosta. And the professor of surgery at Woman's Medical College from 1884 to 1889, just as Eakins was implementing the most radical practices of his own coeducational program, was Dr. William Williams Keen.

Female students remembered DaCosta as a brilliant lecturer, but they were annoyed by his purposeful use of the term "gentlemen" when addressing mixed classes. He continued the practice as late as 1893.[72] Keen, on the other hand, was revered for his gracious professionalism. "When Keen left for the (same) position he no doubt coveted at Jefferson Medical College, the WMC faculty thanked him for his 'unhesitating surrender of time in doing a generous share of faculty work' and added 'warmest wishes for his success and happiness.' He long remained sympathetic toward WMC."[73] Again, it is impossible to imagine that Eakins was not influenced by these events as he formulated policies at the Pennsylvania Academy regarding the same pointed issues.

At the academy under Eakins' direction, most class hours preserved the separate manner of education commonly found in the late nineteenth century. Women's life drawing and painting classes met from nine to twelve every day and four-thirty to seven-thirty on Tuesday, Thursday, and Saturday (fig. 33). Women's modeling classes met from three to six in the afternoon, Monday, Wednesday, and Friday. Men drew and painted from the nude from one to four each day, and from seven to nine-thirty Monday, Wednesday, and Friday. They modeled on Tuesday, Thursday, and Saturday mornings while the women were drawing and painting, and also from seven to nine-thirty in the evening on Tuesdays, Thursdays, and Saturdays. Dissecting room study for women was held "at arranged hours" separate from those of male students.[74]

With such careful coordination, women and men rarely had cause to be in the Pennsylvania Academy building at the same time looking at fully nude bodies, although their opportunities were far more equal than those in medical schools. The truly mixed classes included those that modeled from the horse on Mondays, Wednesdays, and Fridays, and those courses without nudity at all, including sketch and portrait classes, perspective, and composition. Students always dissected in separate sessions, apparently even when the subject was an animal. Eakins' progressive curriculum in this regard was separate and equal, rather than separate and unequal or truly integrated.

The real exception to the idea of separate and equal at the academy was Keen's series of anatomy lectures, in which men and women sat together as the anatomist pointed out the features of the various dead and living, vertical and horizontal, whole and flayed bodies on the stage. The only time Keen distinguished among students was when he "separated the male and female students for the last two lectures in which he pointed out differences between the sexes on male and female models standing side by side, "omitting only the generative organs."[75]

In all his lectures, Keen discussed the differences between men and women without any of the usual disparaging terminology of the day, and this approach undoubtedly influenced Eakins as he directed the relatively egalitarian programs of the academy. When Keen turned his probing and clinical eye to anatomy, there were no "delicate sensibilities" to point out. Instead, Keen's artistic anatomy manuscript discusses points of difference with neutral clarity: "Hayden in his delightful lectures on Painting and Design has so written that one would suppose that women not seldom had an extra lumbar vertebra and that this would account for their longer loins. Undoubtedly they have longer loins but not for this reason for a sixth lumbar vertebra is excessively rare. The bodies of these vertebrae in women are longer and their ribs are less oblique; hence their waist is higher, the chest shorter and the loin longer than in men."[76] Keen's gracious manner and neutral tone went a long way toward keeping controversy at bay in this element of the academy curriculum.

Just as Keen acceded to propriety by separating male and female students for some lectures, Eakins maintained other policies that were meant to preserve respectability as well. To ensure that only mature students were exposed to nude bodies, minors were "not permitted to enter the life class without the written permission of parents or guardians."[77] And "no one except the professor and the chairman of the posing committee was allowed to speak to the model.... There were also rules forbidding such things as smoking, whistling, singing, loud talking, spitting, and trimming crayons on the floor."[78]

In spite of the careful arrangements at the academy, they were not sufficient to allay concerns for long. The same sticking point emerged as had been paramount in the case of difficulties for female medical students—the right of women to see and study male genitals. A particularly telling incident

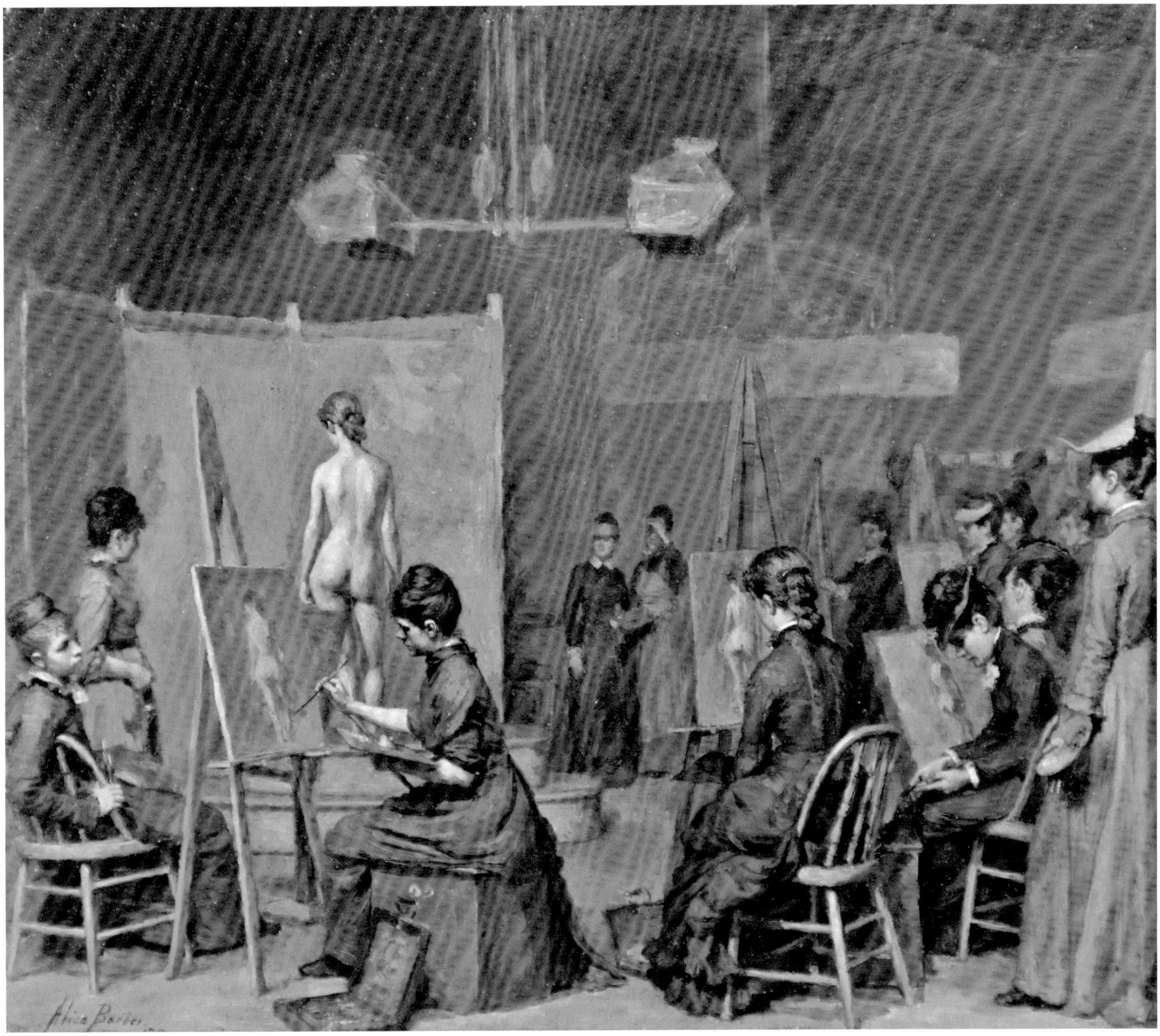

Fig. 33. Alice Barber Stephens, *The Women's Life Class*, c. 1879. Oil grisaille on cardboard, 12 × 14 in. Courtesy of the Pennsylvania Academy of the Fine Arts, Philadelphia. Gift of the artist.

occurred in the dissection laboratory just months before Eakins' dismissal. The artist wrote to the chairman of the committee on instruction in 1886 to relay his disgust that the genitals were removed from the male cadaver for the ladies' dissection class, stating with righteous indignation that "the mutilation of the male subject for the false modesty is to me revolting."[79] This extreme ploy to keep women from seeing and carving into a penis must indeed have seemed sacrilegious to an artist who had devoted himself to study of the body. And a significant percentage of the artist's female students were in agreement.

The situation for women students at the Pennsylvania Academy under Eakins' direction was complicated, and two factions emerged from their ranks. The female students whom Eakins had the most positive interactions with were vehement supporters of his brand of equal education—including his insistence that they study male bodies that were complete and naked just as the men did. These women respected Eakins' point of view and appreciated his efforts to equalize their educational experiences. In 1882, the year Pennsylvania Academy women first were permitted to dissect, Elizabeth Macdowell wrote to Eakins with a complaint and a request:

> I write to know if the mornings of our days in the dissecting room can be secured to us exclusively at once. Up to the present the boys have worked on the new subject, while we were at ours: but now beside the fact that ours is dried up completely, they have cut off the head, arms and scapulii so the back, about the freshest part, is about useless. This was done without consulting us and Miss Roberts and I had just prepared it for study ... the other girls are losing a great deal of valuable time having had no previous study to assist them with the old subject.[80]

Macdowell was one of two women Eakins appointed to supervise dissections for female students. She was clearly offended only by the unequal opportunities to which she and her classmates were subjected. Much the same annoyance was voiced by students at the Woman's Medical College who were forced to attend separate clinics and thereby miss out on seeing important operations.

Carroll Smith-Rosenberg would define the attitude of these female art and medical school students as in accord with the late-nineteenth-century ideal of the "New Woman": "In her own mind and the minds of her contemporaries, education constituted the New Woman's most salient characteristic—and her first self-conscious demand.... Many young women saw in higher education an opportunity for intellectual self-fulfillment and for an autonomous role outside the patriarchal family."[81] Many of the women attending the Pennsylvania Academy and the Woman's Medical College in the early 1880s could see clearly the opportunities available for study in their city—and they did not want a second-rate education. Other women were less certain of the benefits of "new womanhood." These women often wanted serious professional education as Eakins defined it, but they were not all, or always, comfortable with their new freedoms. And they had a former generation of parents and guardians at home to reconcile with.

Eakins was not the first academy administrator to deal with complaints from female students expecting accommodations that respected their refinement. Even before Eakins arrived at the academy, some female students were shocked when they found that they were supposed to draw from fully nude bodies. In 1877, Anna Sellers complained: "I have traveled considerable this summer and autumn, met and [conversed?] with many ladies, mostly married, several wives of physicians—All of whom *were shocked to find* we had introduced the European Custom of *the entire nudeness of our female model*, would it not be better to have some sleight drapery."[82]

Other American art educators faced similar difficulties. Peter Marzio notes that in 1831, John Rubens Smith was the only early drawing-manual author breaking taboos against nudity, insisting that one can't draw a clothed figure well without understanding its naked form, and that "tis in the mind of the observer all the evil lies."[83] Drawing-book authors declined to follow his example for decades.

Although Eakins and other academy administrators routinely received complaints similar to Sellers', some changes in the quantity and character of the bodies women were exposed to in the early and mid-1880s gave such complaints more weight and urgency. Fairman Rogers' 1881 article records that Eakins changed the balance of models in life classes to equalize the number of males and females, in addition to bringing in some athletes. This change meant that women were probably painting and sculpting from many more men than they had in the past.

Another policy shift was more difficult to negotiate. In reminiscences of his years as a student at the academy in the early 1880s, Joseph Pennell records: "If a student got hard up, and lots did, he disappeared or he posed to us; we thought nothing of that. Quaint things happened, but they concern nobody save those who lived and learned at the school."[84] Several female students were not so comfortable with analyzing the contours of their male classmates' physiques, and did not find the situation "quaint." In 1884, a group of women made clear to the board of directors that they did not want male academy students posing for them, and the practice was stopped.[85] All of this discussion took place at a time when the larger debate surrounding nudity in American culture was more rancorous and more dangerous than it ever had been, and administrators, faculty, students, and their parents undoubtedly were taking note.

Display of the naked human body, with all its unnamable parts, seems to have been the "red scare" of the late 1870s and 1880s, and art schools and institutions were by no means protected from the debate. In his chronicle of the Art Students' League of New York, Marchal E. Landgren writes: "The certain squeamishness in the United States on the subject of painting from nude models became a public issue in the 'eighties. The league naturally came in for its share of questioning. In February of 1881, Jennie June, the noted columnist, visited the league to report on the propriety of the classes. She seems to have been favorably impressed, noting that despite the skimpy attire of the man—simply 'a piece of striped cloth about his loins ... there was no suggestion of sex about the matter. The girls were students, not women; and their plain, short dresses of dark blue, or olive wool, or flannel—several of them covered with a long cotton blouse, or apron—possessed not the faintest tinge of coquetry.'" The columnist went on to note that she felt it was coarse to even raise the subject given the professionalism of the environment, but nonetheless, she asked a female student if she felt any "embarrassment of studying from the living model." The unhesitating reply included the remark: "We come here for a purpose, just as we might go to a hospital or dissecting room, and we see before us an anatomy which we have to study and reproduce with mathematical precision.... There is nothing indecent in act or thought."

Landgren goes on to report: "Later it was circulated that Anthony Comstock, whose raids have their ridiculous as well as their annoying side, was going to 'pull' the life classes of the League; and that the students lived in fear 'for they pictured themselves marched, handcuffed, perhaps, through the streets to Jefferson Market, where they would be kept in dungeons vile all night and brought to trial next day.'"[86]

Whether or not art students, and especially female art students, ever really faced any such danger, the perception was certainly real. Anthony Comstock threatened Americans, particularly on the East Coast, with jail time and seizure of property for violation of the nation's obscenity and decency laws throughout the last quarter of the nineteenth century. Serving simultaneously as a special agent of the federal postal service and secretary of the New York Society for the Suppression of Vice, Comstock "had the power to arrest those suspected of distributing obscene matter and to search for and seize those materials" from 1873, when he championed the passage of new legislation through Congress, until his death in 1915.[87]

Helen Lefkowitz Horowitz records that during the late 1870s and early 1880s in particular, arrests and property seizures by Comstock's forces went a long way toward making sexuality, and sexual parts, publicly unspeakable for fear of prosecution. Dr. Edward Bliss Foote, for example, who was fined $3,500 for distributing information and devices to aid birth control, kept up his publications on the subject by adopting more coded language. After Comstock, birth control was discussed only as a form of "'human weeding.' ... He imagined finding, as he put it, some 'harmless medicament' to prevent human ovulation." Ultimately, Horowitz writes, the impact of Comstock has been long-lasting. "I have long felt the inadequacy of understanding of America's sexual past. Now I know at least part of the reason why. Many of the sources potentially available to build a more accurate interpretation were rudely suppressed after 1873."[88]

Although few prosecutions under Comstock's law took

place outside New York State, the nation's hotbed for the dissemination of erotic materials, there is no doubt that for the female students at the Pennsylvania Academy in the 1880s, fear of prosecution was added to all the other anxieties associated with trying to acquire a professional education as a woman at that time. As Smith-Rosenberg notes, the situation was particularly difficult for women in mixed institutions. "Those women who dared to enter the formerly male strongholds of the newly coeducational universities faced a particularly alien environment. Their presence violated many more taboos than did women's attendance at an all-female college. And the co-eds' demands were far more radical. They sought not an equal but an identical education."[89]

In the larger American scene, the merits of such equality for women were fiercely debated, both by strident new feminists and by their nemeses. "To place a woman outside of a domestic setting, to train a woman to think and feel 'as a man,' to encourage her to succeed at a career, indeed to place a career before marriage, violated virtually every late-Victorian norm. It was literally to take her outside of conventional structures and social arrangements.... She thus made herself the intellectual peer of young men, and rendered herself socially questionable by that very act."[90] Becoming "socially questionable" was exactly what happened when women breached the taboo, preserved even at female medical schools, and painted, modeled, touched, and even carved into male bodies.

Fig. 436.—Vertical Section of Bladder, Penis, and Urethra.

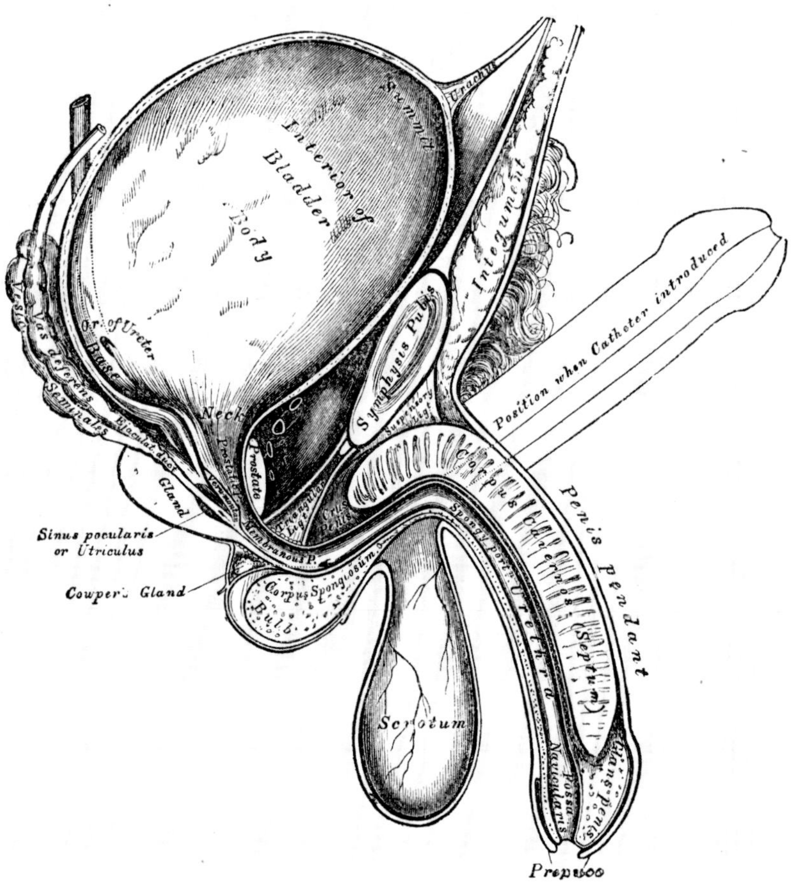

Fig. 34. "Vertical Section of Bladder, Penis, and Urethra," fig. 436 in Henry Gray, *Anatomy, Descriptive and Surgical* (Philadelphia: Henry C. Lea, 1870). Courtesy of the Dana Medical Library Medical History Collection, Burlington, Vermont.

In 1886, when Eakins wrote to the chairman of the committee on instruction to complain about the removal of the penis from the male cadaver for the sake of "false modesty," he enjoyed little likelihood of sympathetic response. For Eakins and Keen, this organ hardly could have meant the same thing as it did to non-anatomists. Gray's *Anatomy* provided the neutral language, and the neutral imagery (fig. 34), with which to describe it: "The Penis is the organ of copulation, and contains in its interior the larger portion of the urethra.... The mucous membrane covering the glans penis contains no sebaceous glands; but projecting from its free surface are a number of small highly sensitive papillae. The penis is composed of a mass of erectile tissue, inclosed in three cylindrical fibrous compartments."[91] As with the breast in *The Agnew Clinic*, "anatomist's eyes" gave dissection practitioners at least a temporarily desexualized view that equalized the value of every part of the body. All human components could be described in terms of their insertions and protrusions, attachments and membranes, compartments and eminences—even a catheterized penis.

The circumstances of Eakins' dismissal from the Pennsylvania Academy in 1886 are complex and recounted in more detail in following chapters, but it is of interest here that the particular offense believed by many at the time for the board's action was that Eakins had taken the loincloth off a male model before a group of women students during a lecture comparing male and female anatomy.[92] In so doing, Eakins took the practice of the "mixed class," already limited and professionally dangerous, to an entirely new level. Later, Eakins admitted that he had displayed his own pelvis to Amelia Van Buren "to demonstrate an anatomical point." She did not object, but the story became part of the proof of Eakins' disreputable character, and the artist wrote at length to Edward Coates in February 1886 in an attempt to salvage Van Buren's reputation—and his own.

> Having given you in fragments some account of Miss van Buren's studies with me I am moved to write it fully. She is a lady of perhaps thirty years or more.... She came to the Academy some years ago to study figure painting by which art she hoped to support herself, her parents I believe being dead. I early recognized her as a very capable person.... She soon surpassed her fellows, and I marked her as one I ought to help in every way. Once in the dissecting room she asked me the explanation of a movement of the pelvis in relation to the axis of movement of the whole body, so I told her to come around with me to my own studio where I was shortly going. There stripping myself, I gave her the explanation as I could not have done by words only. There was not the slightest embarrassment or cause for embarrassment on her part or on mine.... I do not believe she would have hesitated to undress herself before me any more than before her family physician.... The lady would hardly like to ask to see me, yet she was glad to do so. I think indeed she might have been embarrassed, if I had picked up a man on the street and endeavored to persuade him to undress before the lady for a quarter.[93]

Eakins' insistence on full display of the penis, dead and alive, his own and those of others, to women willing or not to see it can certainly be seen as a series of gestures whose intent was perverse or harassing. It also carried its own internal logic when seen through "anatomist's eyes."

Among the anatomical structures artists need to understand in order to represent the body knowledgeably, William Williams Keen believed that the pelvis and the spine were foremost. Fairman Rogers summarized this pedagogical principle in his 1881 article: "Great stress is laid upon the weight and solidity of the figure; it must stand upon its legs and show exactly what part of the general movement each portion of the body is bearing."[94] If students could not see the pelvis, how could they understand its role in the "bearing" of the body? Oliver Wendell Holmes shared this view in his newspaper column "The Autocrat of the Breakfast Table," writing that "the pelvis is the center of the body around which all the rest is built."[95] Despite the agreement among these intellectuals about the importance of the pelvis, however, few of these men would have agreed that it was a good idea to reveal their own to an interested female student.

Eakins again might have had a perverse intent in stripping down himself, or he may have been unable to see with any other than "anatomist's eyes." In his contribution to Gray's *Anatomy*, Keen advised medical students to look at and even touch each other's bodies. "Let a student examine his own body with a skeleton before him. Better still that two should work thus together, each serving as a model to the other."[96] Could there possibly be a more effective means of explaining the anatomical facts than demonstration on a (free and available) living model, as Keen had proven in his several articles on the subject?

Medical acculturation presented other problems for Eakins and his female art students as well. One of the most often cited complaints against the artist was his "coarse" humor, which many found offensive. Francis Petrus Paulus recalled: "One day in the women's modeling class … the cow started to answer a call of nature—Eakins was criticizing one of the young ladies, and when he saw this he jumped up and fairly yelled to Anshutz: 'Get the camera Tommy, I have discovered a new muscle.'"[97] Presumably, the "butt" of this joke would have been more obvious to listeners at the time.

Other jokes similarly reflected the dissection-room humor that dominated medical schools. Sappol writes: "In the eighteenth and nineteenth centuries, pranks involving body parts were common. Students courted disaster by throwing pieces of their dissections at visitors, displaying severed limbs in windows, of taking bodies and body parts home."[98] Margaret McHenry recorded similar pranks at the academy, including one episode in which students threw a dissected horse cadaver "down the stair well of the academy at a time when the Masonics were having an elaborate entertainment."[99]

Such pranks might well have been amusing to some of the students who took part in them, and they were in no sense especially outrageous given medical school behaviors of the day, but there is no doubt that they served even further to alienate some students and trustees at the academy. Eakins further appalled some students by asking models if they needed "to pea" [*sic*] and telling an unacceptable joke about "plums."[100]

In spite of his famous gentility, even Keen contributed to a culture of medical manners at the academy that may have been distasteful to many. He wrote: "Here as in many instances your own tables and kitchens will afford you frequent means of studying similar parts in the various meats we have. A chicken's leg will serve as an excellent means of studying both articular cartilage and synovia (the membrane is so thin as to require microscopic investigation)."[101] Some students may have followed their professor's advice, and no doubt appalled their family and friends with demonstrations performed at the dinner table. Keen, again unlike his predecessors, never pandered to the artists he taught, but rather treated them with the same seriousness with which he had taught medical students for decades. The consequences of such humor, however, were largely negative in the art arena, and especially so for the academy's female students.

Sappol's study of the "anatomical mayhem" in nineteenth-century medical culture is especially sobering when one imagines the experiences of women entering the previously male-defined realm of anatomical study. He writes that "cigar smoking, public consumption of spirits, [and] uproarious pranks, were all emblems of manliness" common in dissecting labs.[102] The culture established in dissecting rooms marked them as "homosocial" spaces, and there can be little doubt that this type of behavior, extended into the halls of the academy, was threatening and alienating to female students. As one woman wrote, "Our crowd didn't have much interest in studying with Eakins himself. He was so much concerned with anatomy that he thought a student was not serious if unwilling to carry home an arm or a leg to dissect in the evening."[103]

Eakins' obliviousness to or wanton disregard of the complaints of some of his female students was exacerbated by several factors. One was that he continued to be surrounded by a core group of faithful acolytes, including both male students who must have appreciated the "homosocial" aspects of the academy environment, but also Amelia Van Buren, Elizabeth Macdowell, his future wife Susan, and other "New Women" who largely agreed with his policies and methods and no doubt fueled his stubborn resolve with supportive comments and the comforting example of women at ease with his educational policies and methods. These women could look to the example of "New Women" like those in the city's medical colleges who formed their own sororal bonds of humor and hard work. Several of Eakins' female students, including Cecilia Beaux and Alice Barber Stephens, went on to successful careers as professional artists.[104]

After his teaching at the Pennsylvania Academy ended, Eakins was still in demand as a lecturer on art anatomy, but now he was more careful to explain his methods in advance, in detailed statements that reveal his most hard-fought philosophical beliefs. In 1888, he notified the Art Students' League in New York that he might be available to lecture, but he made it clear that his teaching methods were inviolate. His explanation was both difficult to argue with and defensive:

> The Nat. Acad. of Design has asked me to lecture. I am awaiting an answer to my terms and conditions. I should be glad to lecture at the League also if I can arrange convenient hours.
>
> In lecturing upon the pelvis which is in an artistic sense the very basis of the movement and balance of the figure, I should use the nude model. To describe and show an important muscle as arising from some exact origin to insert itself in some indefinite manner under the breech clout is so trifling and undignified that I shall never again attempt it....
>
> I am sure that the study of anatomy is not going to benefit any grown person who is not willing to see or be seen seeing the naked figure and my lectures are only for serious students wishing to become painters or sculptors.
>
> Adverse criticism could be avoided by announcement of when I intend to use the naked model.
>
> Those not wishing to come to such lecture could stay away or withdraw and lose nothing they could make use of, but would not hinder others wishing to learn.[105]

Despite his proposal of more careful notification, controversy over display of male genitals dogged Eakins throughout the remainder of his experiences as a lecturer on art anatomy. In 1894, the National Academy of Design called Eakins to task for some apparently unspeakable offense. Edwin H. Blashfield, a representative of the academy, wrote to him:

> The Council of the National Academy of Design have asked me to see or write to you before your next Anatomy lecture in reference to the same. Some member (or members) of the council has been informed that certain scholars have felt offended at something in the matter or the manner of one of the lectures.
>
> The Council appreciating the sincerity of your point of view, and the enthusiasm with which you treat your subject, is convinced that you will willingly avoid hurting anyone's feelings, and will be considerate of the point of view of any of your scholars if it differs from yours. This is simply a friendly request made to you, through me, by the council and school committee.[106]

By now, the unwillingness of so many Victorians to ever actually say what they meant must have infuriated Eakins. His response was somewhat less "friendly":

> I have no intention surely of hurting the feelings of any one & do not see just where can arise between me and my pupils, any serious or offensive difference of opinion in elemental descriptive anatomy.
>
> However, that we may know exactly what we are to discuss, would have you request [here Eakins crossed out "the lady"] the offended one [here he added "it must be a lady," but then crossed that out as well] to write down carefully for us the exact offense.[107]

In the following year, Eakins was forced to leave his lecturing position at the Drexel Institute for the same offense he had insisted on his right to commit in New York—display of the male pelvis with its attendant, undraped penis. The front page of the *Philadelphia Times* led with the headline: "A Revolt at Drexel Institute. Indignation Caused by a Nude Male Model Before a Mixed Class. Professor Eakins Removed." Eakins was paid his lecturing fee for the semester but was asked not to return.[108]

It may seem surprising that so many art academies continued to court such disaster by hiring Eakins following his first dismissal in 1886, but this is a good indication of how well known the artist was as a lecturer on anatomy. A sympathetic review of Eakins' class at the Art Students' League of New York in 1886 makes clear why he continued to be hired as an anatomy lecturer, and the loss students suffered when his methods were, repeatedly, found too controversial to institutionally abide.

> Professor Thomas Eakins, last month, began, at the Art Students' League, of which he is a member of the Faculty, a series of lectures unique in conception and character, and which, for practical utility, could not be improved upon. The professor is an enthusiast on the subject of artistic anatomy, and has mastered

> his subject by long and devoted study, and much experience …
>
> At the League, the lecturer's paraphernalia consisted of a skeleton suspended to a frame, a tub of modeling clay, an anatomical cast and a living model. The means by which he illustrated his remarks would have rendered the subject understandable to the least educated or intelligent person. By an audience as interested as that at the League the lecture was received with wrapt attention, and the hearers, instead of carrying away a few written notes, as is commonly the case at such a discourse, departed with a clear idea of the subject fixed upon their memories by a picturesque and lucid demonstration of it.
>
> Professor Eakins's plan is, first, to model a muscle in clay, and fasten it upon the skeleton in its proper place. Then, upon the plaster cast, he points out the location and appearance of the muscle as part of the whole form, and by the action of the living model he illustrates its general effect. Where the lower muscles do not appear in the entire mass, he demonstrates their influence upon it. Building up the figure in this way, elucidating his subject as he advances with it, showing from the first not only what muscular development is, but how it is created, what it is created out of, what its service is, and what it looks like when it is performing its service, his lecture has the double value of laying down the written law and explaining on what basis it has been written. For the purposes of the student the lecture possesses an undeniable advantage over the study of anatomy at the dissecting-table, since it presents him with the full fruits of that study and an additional instruction which only individual experiment upon the rudimentary lessons of the dissecting-room could provide for him. It is not so much the surgical knowledge of anatomy which is essential to the artist, as the ability to apply the discoveries of surgical dissection to the actual development and action of the human form. By combining these two departments in his ingeniously devised series of lessons, Professor Eakins condenses conveniently and forcibly two different sciences, which otherwise would have to be pursued independently of each other.[109]

But his enthusiasm, mastery, experience, and ingeniousness were not enough to rescue Eakins from those who simply could not accept that women should have the right publicly and professionally to look at a penis. Modern mores governing what can be seen in the media are in many ways no less slanted. Display of frontal female nudity is still far more accepted than the display of similar male nudity. This difference reflects vestiges of the power structures that operated to protect male professional prerogatives in Eakins' era.

In the larger scheme, there was much more than just prudery and power play at work in the many rejections Eakins faced in his teaching career, and in the art world more generally: the most benign cause of his demise was simply that gross anatomy was waning in popularity even among doctors. In the popular imagination, medicine was making strides in a host of new disciplines other than anatomical research, which unfortunately retained all of its negative associations with the dissecting room while losing its gloss.[110] At the very least, many in the art community were resolved that anatomical study, and indeed scientific inquiry of any type, was ruinous to the cause of art education. The era of the Peales in which art and science were inseparably intertwined truly had ended.

As early as 1879, when William Brownell reviewed the academy curriculum Eakins had reorganized, seeds of complaint already were in the air. After describing his "awe-struck bewilderment" at the "exhaustive" curriculum in anatomy, Brownell cautioned of the "dangers" it presented: "One is the danger of acquiring the habit of looking for anatomy and nothing else—which is practical enough; and the other, possibly none the less important, in that it is insensible and impalpable, the danger arising from constant association with what is ugly and unpoetic, however useful, instead of even occasional association with what is poetic and beautiful, however useless."[111] Eakins' opinion that anatomy was useful *and* beautiful simply had few takers, particularly among art critics. Three years after Brownell's article, such complaints were common, and resolute.

A critic of *The Crucifixion* in 1882 took the opportunity to denigrate Eakins' teaching methods, as well as his painting: "It is a fault of the Pennsylvania Academy of Fine Arts' system that the study of anatomy is so zealously pursued there that many of the pupils come away better anatomists

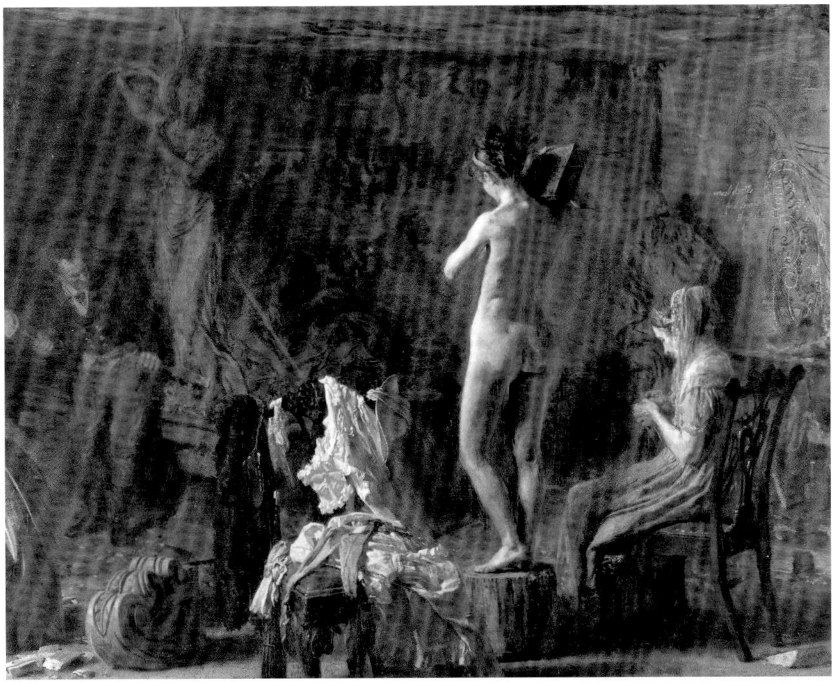

Fig. 35. Thomas Eakins, *William Rush Carving His Allegorical Figure of the Schuylkill River*, 1876–77. Oil on canvas, 20⅛ × 26⅛ in. Philadelphia Museum of Art. Gift of Mrs. Thomas Eakins and Miss Mary Adeline Williams.

than artists."[112] In his one dense article in the year Eakins began teaching, Brownell had presciently summarized the chief complaints that would follow the artist for the next twenty years. Both scientific and artistic winds had shifted in a dramatically different direction than Eakins was willing to sail.[113]

In the same year as Brownell's article, George Inness went even further in defense of aesthetics when he defined "good taste" as the "guardian of morality in Art-matters." How was an artist to determine the boundary between "objectionable" pictures that constituted unlawful obscenity in Comstock's world, and elevating, modern paintings? For Inness, speaking from New York to a writer for the *Art Journal*, the answer to the question was clear—it was the exact reverse of how Eakins had answered similar questions.

> All art in which the ideal predominates is pure. It is excess of realism in Art that makes Art-works disgusting. Here is a pencil-sketch of my own—a young girl about to slip into a brook from the overhanging trunk of a tree. She is disrobed, and proposes to take a bath. I did it with the purest kind of motive, feeling that it was a thing of beauty, and knowing that in no other way could I convey the sentiment which I wanted to convey. I shall put it on canvas, keeping the background cool and sweet, and trying to idealise [*sic*] the subject as much as possible. It seems to me that this subject, so treated, is as pure and beautiful as any other. If I should put coarse realism into it, it would be horrible.[114]

Inness' prescription for maintaining the elevating character of his nude study was fairly simple—he would view the subject from a distance, thirty or forty feet, for a "subdued effect." And in what may well have been a direct criticism of Eakins' *William Rush Carving His Allegorical Figure of the Schuylkill River* (fig. 35), which had recently been exhibited in New York, Inness continued: "Take ________'s *genre* pictures, for example. They are literal transcripts from the model who stands almost beside him. They are too sensuous. They are not art. The artist must never forget that in nude picture-making, when the ideal is ignored, the tendency is inevitably to the lustful. The nude human form should never be painted for its own individualities.... Otherwise the result is invariably something shocking to modesty. We don't need to contemplate individualities and peculiarities of the male or female figure, unless we are anatomists or surgeons."[115] Inness undoubtedly would have found ways to include "artistic sentiment" in an art academy curriculum, as opposed to Eakins who felt that such amorphous "art-matters" were extracurricular concerns. Instead, Eakins only promised Brownell that "as for [students'] artistic impulse, [dissection] does not affect it in any way whatever."

The idea of running an art academy that at best would not negatively "affect" students' "artistic impulse" was simply anathema to many in an era increasingly enamored of aesthetics. Cecilia Beaux, who went on to paint notably charming scenes, wrote: "Eakins found so much in bony structure, articulations, and balanced weight that could be expressed by Art, and Art only, that his finding and expressing these truths became a unique and precious revelation. He relished with high zest what he found, and in his hands it became Art, although he closed his eyes to all other pleasures of vision and equally veritable truths."[116] Beaux's commentary is telling. She appreciated her professor's achievements as an anatomist, but she ultimately found his approach limiting.

Eakins' portrait subjects often agreed with the assessment that what was a "precious revelation" to the artist did not necessarily provoke "pleasures of vision" in their eyes. Elizabeth Corliss didn't like the portrait of her father, George Morris, because it captured him "gritting his teeth," which he "did all the time" in those years. She wanted to see her father as the jovial and carefree person she had remembered him to be in earlier times. The daughter of Mrs. Helen MacKnight similarly complained about the portrait of her mother, who "was rather a sad person." She "couldn't bear to have the portrait around because it was too real and brought her mother back to her too much." Mrs. James Mapes Dodge was nursing a child at the time of her portrait. She complained that Eakins painted her with her "bosom simply bursting," "like a fishwife."[117]

None of these patrons wanted to see their loved ones through "anatomist's eyes" or to think about their bodies as examples of the lessons in Gray's *Anatomy*. Consider the artist's portrait of Amelia Van Buren (fig. 36), for example, in light of a lecture on the anatomy of the face by Dr. Keen:

> The *Superior Maxilla* or *upper jaw* is by far the largest bone of the face, except the lower jaw; but the latter is a single bone while of the former there are two, joined in the middle line. Its large size would make it too heavy were it not hollow in the centre. But the proceps are all stout and strong. This upper prolongation is called the *nasal process*, because it forms the nose along with the nasal bones. Accordingly, its flatness or prominence and its narrowness or its width are of the greatest importance to you. Especially to the portrait painters. Sometimes the soft parts are rather full and baggy over this process and the adjacent lachrymal bones which always gives an unpleasant expression to the face.... The body at or near the symphysis—that is the bony chin—varies considerably in its form and as the soft parts are quite adherent and fat does not accumulate here to soften or to alter it its form fixes largely the outline of the chin ... sometimes it is round and sometimes square, which causes not only a difference in the form of the chin, but where square it aids in bringing into prominence the two anterior folds in the skin of the neck especially in shriveled old women such as you will make your beggars hags or witches.[118]

Eakins undoubtedly found this explication by Keen more relevant to his pursuit than any writing by aesthetic critics or philosophers, but to Cecilia Beaux, and others, this clinical approach to the body was not only sadly uninspiring but also entirely at odds with the goals of art.

In the largest sense, rejection of Eakins' gaze was also rejection of the modern clinical view of the body as an appropriate vision for the artist. As Michel Foucault writes, with "the birth of the clinic,"

> an absolutely new use of scientific discourse was then defined: a use involving fidelity and unconditional subservience to the coloured content of experience—to say what one sees; but also a use involving the foundation and constitution of experience—showing by saying what one sees. It was necessary, then, to place medical language at this apparently superficial but in fact very deeply embedded level at which the descriptive formula is also a revealing gesture. And this revelation in turn involved as its field of origin and of manifestation of truth the discursive space of the corpse: the interior revealed. The constitution of pathological anatomy at the period when the clinicians were defining their method is no mere coincidence: the balance of experience required that the gaze directed upon the individual and the language of description should rest upon the stable, visible legible basis of death.[119]

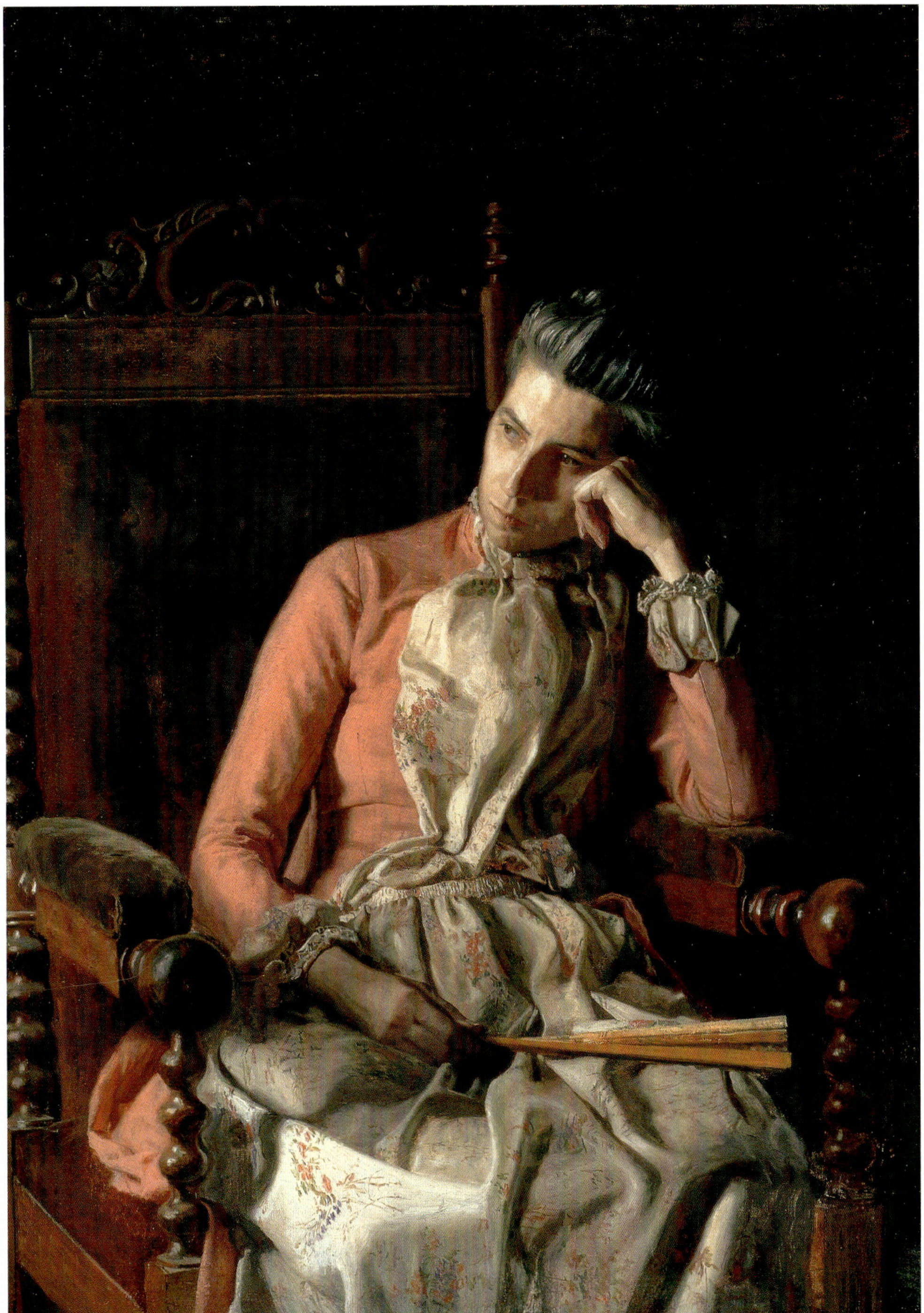

Fig. 36. Thomas Eakins, *Miss Amelia C. Van Buren*, c. 1891. Oil on canvas, 45 × 32 in. The Phillips Collection, Washington, D.C.

Eakins' anatomist's eyes—the eyes of the "clinician"—revealed the morbid truth of the body in a manner that seemed entirely inappropriate for art, which had long served to elevate through denial, to stand back far enough to capture the ideal.

Eakins' elevation of the body was no less profound than that of Ruskin, Inness, or Beaux, but it stemmed from a different source. From the perspective of a painter who worshiped the complexity and perfection of human anatomy and was bent on painting it right, there could be no better way to convey Amelia Van Buren's gracious and dignified demeanor in the face of a lifetime of disappointment and melancholy than by demonstrating the effects of those trials on her anatomical structures over time. For a portrait painter, it is always the actual work of painting the body through which deeper meanings can be communicated.

In his steadfast belief in the benefit of the clinical gaze even for art students, Eakins truly was a maverick. Even Dr. Gross in 1875 warned his medical students about ignoring the ameliorative effects of beauty: "There is nothing that a medical man should cultivate with greater earnestness than a taste for the sublime and beautiful in nature and in art, both on account of its humanizing tendency and the rational enjoyment with which it rewards the exercise. A reined and intellectual man never looks at a beautiful landscape, picture, child, woman, animal, bird or insect, without feeling the better and happier for the sight."[120] Gross was certainly among the most zealous advocates of modern clinical ontology, but like many in his profession, he placed strict limitations on the population he thought capable of joining in. The assumption implicit here is that women, like landscapes and insects, were objects for decorative and aesthetic pleasure, not subjects to discover the profound truths of their mortal existence.

Eakins' ideal of beauty lay rather in faithful, undistorted attention to the individual anatomy and attributes of each person he depicted. It was quite a different project than that of Inness, and one that required much closer proximity than thirty or forty feet. *Amelia Van Buren* is well painted *because* Eakins captured the "soft parts [that] are rather full and baggy over this [nasal] process and the adjacent lachrymal bones" and even the "anterior folds" in the sagging skin of her upper neck—he looked at her intently with full understanding of her "landmarks" and depicted, in Foucault's terms, "the interior revealed." In his teaching career, Eakins insisted that his female students strive equally to reach those depths of understanding as well.[121]

Standing in marked contrast to this strong argument for viewing Eakins as one of the great feminists of his era are the artist's own sexist remarks disparaging working women in letters sent home from Paris in the 1860s, particularly in his correspondence with Emily Sartain, who went on to become the principal of the Philadelphia School of Design for Women. While we may forgive the artist's early letters as immature bravado, there is another oft-quoted sentence fragment that requires examination. In 1886, Eakins wrote to Edward Coates: "I do not believe that great painting or sculpture … will ever be done by women." This letter to Coates—infused with the hindsight afforded by its being written seven months after his dismissal—merits quotation and analysis at some length, as it codifies his mature attitudes toward female artists with great clarity. He wrote,

> Although professional privileges are more tardily accorded to women than to men, and with reason, yet there is a decided advance making with respect to the education of women especially in America.
>
> And if women are to be taught at all I think they should have good teaching.
>
> I once knew a lady physician of some renown and large practice, whom I admired and greatly respected. She got a little troublesome sore on her master finger but did not recognize it as a venereal chancre, and delivering and examining many patients, she introduced the syphilis into a great many families who never deserved it, and died herself after great suffering from the effects of her ignorance.

The point of Eakins' story was clearly the danger that came from denying female medical students the same access to bodies as men. In this case, ignorance was not improving of the woman's refinement or delicacy—she and presumably many of her patients were dead. Eakins went on:

> But within the last few years the young women medical students attend the same clinics as the men. The most dreadful diseases are shown them, described, and operated on, much to the safety of those families who are afterwards to employ these students become physicians.
>
> And while students, these young women spy into each others' piddle with a microscope and do a hundred other unconventional things.

Eakins undoubtedly felt the time had come for the female students at the Pennsylvania Academy, like those at the Woman's Medical College, to do "unconventional things." The point of doing so was an acceptance of the realities of the "new" woman:

> I do not believe that great painting or sculpture or surgery will ever be done by women, yet good enough work is continually done by them to be well worth their doing, and as the population increases, and marriages are later and fewer, and the risks of losing fortunes greater; so increases the number of women who are or may be compelled at some time to support themselves, and figure painting is not now so dishonorable to them.

Earning a livelihood, as Eakins knew all too well from his own dealings with destitute female students, required great sacrifice and courage from women in the 1880s. Women who made that choice, willingly or by necessity, left behind the conventions expected of them. The self-sufficient woman would need to

> assume professional privileges. She must be the guardian of her own virtue. She must take on the right to examine naked men and women. Forsaking prudery, she locks her door whenever she wishes, and refuses admittance on the plea that she has a model. And without these privileges, she could not hope in any way to compete with men nor with the intelligent of her own sex, and a certificate of prudery would not in this age help sell a figure piece by a young lady.

Eakins may have revealed the limitations of his age in stating that he doubted women could accomplish truly great work as artists or surgeons, but his assumption that they should compete with the same privileges was progressive. And Eakins, always a keen intellectual and observer of his own times, saw through the chief limiting taboo of his own context:

> Should men make only the statues of men to be looked at by men, while the statues of women should be made by women to be looked at by women only? Should the he-painters draw the horses and bulls, and the she-painters like Rosa Bonheur the mares and the cows?
>
> Must the poor old male body in the dissecting room be mutilated before Miss Prudery can dabble in his guts? Such indignities anger me. Can not any one see into what contemptible inconsistencies such follies all lead? And how dangerous they are?

Eakins went on to condemn the attempts of some students to draw a line "between the living and the dead body, and getting with the young women on the foolish side of the foolish line," to discuss obscenity in that regard.[122] Eakins may have offended many of his female students and their parents, but he never patronized them by assuming that they were not equally capable of training for employment as professional artists.[123]

It is likely that some of Amelia Van Buren's gray hairs were won during Eakins' troubles. In July 1887, he wrote to her of his "crimes":

> Being the only figure painter in ... Philadelphia habitually using the naked model, I have whenever not too inconvenient to me, allowed my most promising pupils to work from my models. I have also encouraged my advanced pupils to work from each other when the state of their purses precluded the employment of regular models at home, and I have corrected much of such work. I have also made photographs of the naked figure including my own. I have spoken of medical things with the freedom of a physician....
>
> My life has been very simple and honorable, and singularly free from complications and is all of it open to any friend.
>
> Hence if anything you may have heard may need explanation or refutation, I trust you will write to me as I count upon your good sense and refinement.[124]

Whether or not we choose to believe Eakins' defense, it is

important to distinguish between the actions and statements the artist readily admitted and those accusations he bitterly denied. Because so much of the language of this period was coded, particularly in written communications, it is difficult to determine precisely the offense that lost Eakins his job—his final straw. But one thing is certain, given the relative unpopularity of many of the artist's pedagogical beliefs—it is not surprising that his reign came to an end in 1886. Ultimately, as we have seen, many factors were responsible for the demise of Eakins' anatomy program.

Even William Williams Keen, Eakins' intellectual companion at the academy, was nowhere to be found when his colleague needed supportive defense. Keen proved his lack of affection for his colleague's painting style in 1902, when he chose William Merritt Chase to paint his portrait for Jefferson Medical College (fig. 37). As his grandson writes: "More acceptable to Keen (and probably more acceptable to his daughters as well) was to commission William Merritt Chase, a *respectable*, professional portraitist, whose 1902 portrait of Keen made the doctor appear taller. Eakins never would have indulged in such flattery."[125] Although Keen undoubtedly would have agreed with Eakins that "distortion" in the medical realm was unacceptable, his taste in art was more conventional. Clearly, Eakins did not see beauty in art in the same way as Beaux, Inness, or even Keen.

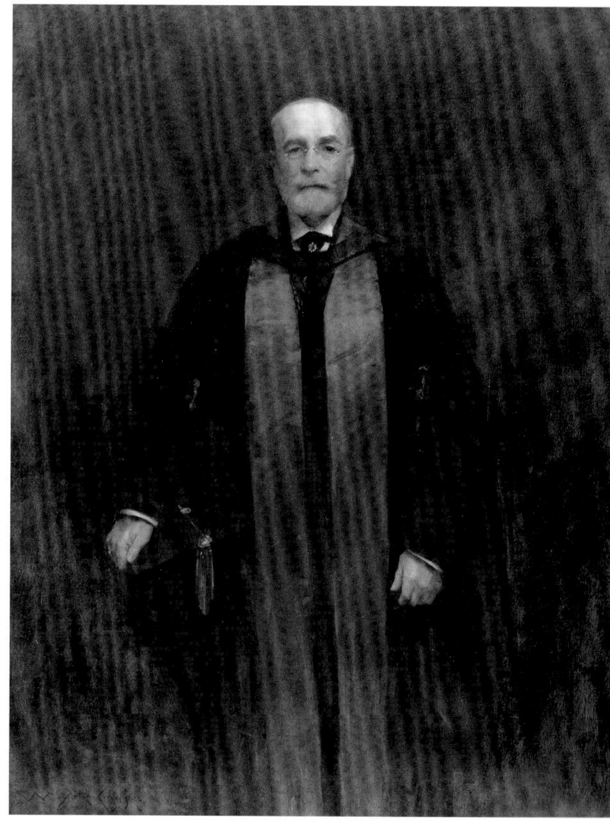

Fig. 37. William Merritt Chase, *William Williams Keen, Jr., M.D.*, c. 1901. Oil on canvas, 67 × 52½ in. © Courtesy Thomas Jefferson University, Philadelphia. All rights reserved.

I would like to conclude this chapter by returning to its opening thread with a short account of the American Anthropometric Society, which was established exactly forty years after the Mütter Museum in Philadelphia, in 1889. Edward Anthony Spitzka, Eakins' later portrait subject, wrote an essay in 1902 that described the research the society had enabled him to conduct.[126] The essay was titled "A Study of the Brains of Six Eminent Scientists and Scholars Belonging to the American Anthropometric Society." Spitzka had news both good and bad to report: "The chief object of the society was the preservation of the brains of its members.... The brain of Walt Whitman, together with the jar in which it had been placed, was said to have been dropped on the floor by a careless assistant. Unfortunately, not even the pieces were saved. The brain of Dr. [J. William] White is in good condition." Spitzka went on to compare the brains of great men with "normal brains of men executed by electricity." In somewhat grievous news for art historians, Spitzka found the following averages: "The brain weights of those in the Exact Sciences average 1542g ... and in the Fine Arts 1479g." Whitman's brain, presumably weighed before its demise, was near the bottom of a list of 115 eminent brains organized by weight.[127]

My point in recalling this bit of history is to remind modern readers that stepping into (or onto) the minds of nineteenth-century scientists is a necessarily disorienting experience. Privileges we now take for granted were then hard-fought, and attitudes toward the body were both more prudish—and more ghoulish—than those to which we are accustomed. But this point of view was the filter through which Eakins understood his world, his art, and his personal relations. It is not necessarily a filter we can easily recreate for the purpose of our own examinations, and it is clearly not an optical arrangement welcomed by many in Eakins' world—although they identified and understood it better than we do today.

There is no doubt that Eakins' study of anatomy bordered on the compulsive, but placed in the context of his medical colleagues, including Keen and Spitzka, it was hardly unique. Celebrating every part of the body, for Eakins, and for Whitman—albeit with his relatively light brain—after decades of repressed knowledge of structures and feelings, was a great adventure in the second half of the nineteenth century. And it is possible that Eakins might have escaped his troubles had he stuck with his program of drawing, painting, and modeling the nude.

The case has been made that finances, or loincloths, or (here) the perils of co-education were chiefly responsible for Eakins' fall from grace at the Pennsylvania Academy, but another factor is surely to blame: the artist's use of photography in documenting and furthering his intellectual passion for the study of the nude. Once Eakins progressed from the production of paintings and sculpture, which were considered acceptable creative media, into photography, which was considered a documentary medium, there was little to protect him from the censure of his fellow Victorians. Although Eakins lost several teaching positions as the result of his emphatic and egalitarian program of anatomical study, this loss was minimal in comparison to the personal difficulties he and his students faced when he transformed his camera lenses into "anatomist's eyes."

CHAPTER FOUR

Art, Pornography, Freak Shows, Medical Pictures, and the Guilty Pleasures of Photography in Nineteenth-Century Philadelphia

Thomas Eakins' artistic methods never have been the subject of much debate. The artist created preparatory drawings, photographic studies, oil sketches, and modellos that survive in preparation for finished works, and he wrote a lengthy manuscript on perspective that carefully explains his approach to the formulation of pictorial space. The surfaces of his finished works rarely hide the marks of brushes, palette knives, carving tools, pencil, or wash. In addition to the self-evident process in Eakins' own creations, a number of students, colleagues, and portrait subjects recorded his methods themselves or recounted them to art historians.

Given everything we thought we knew, it came as something of a surprise when conservators preparing for the 2001 exhibition of the artist's work at the Philadelphia Museum of Art discovered underdrawings and small incised lines in some of Eakins' paintings. These marks prove that the artist transferred forms directly from photographic images projected onto his canvases. Eakins' efforts to scrub his finished surfaces of evidence by covering or filling in the transfer marks with paint also were revealed. The practice was confined to just a few paintings between 1879 and 1885, from *A May Morning in the Park* to *Swimming*. Nevertheless, for an artist so disposed to exhibiting his (usually) laborious methods, his unwillingness to mention the trick is notable.

The artist's silence about his experiments with projector (probably a "magic lantern") and canvas can only lead us to conclude that he perceived the practice as disreputable and not in keeping with the persona he crafted for public view. Even Susan Eakins claimed not to have known of the trick. She reported that her husband "only used a photograph when impossible to get information in the way he preferred, painting from the living and moving model. He disliked working from a photograph—and absolutely refused to do so in a portrait."[1] The artist's cover was not blown until "technical examinations" using infrared reflectography found him out.[2]

Photography posed philosophical problems for artists from its inception. While many painters in Europe and America hailed the fabrications of chemistry and light revealed to the public by Joseph-Nicéphore Niépce, Louis Daguerre, and Henry Fox Talbot in 1839, others foresaw in the new medium an inevitable decline in business for more traditional image makers. An acerbic *New Yorker* critic quipped upon news of the invention: "The Dagueroscope [*sic*] and the Photogenic revolution are to keep you all down, ye painters, engravers, and, alas! the harmless race, the sketchers."[3] As this quick study noticed, photography called into question the fundamental utility of the skills artists possessed. A scientist writing in the same precipitous year boasted that the daguerreotype required "no knowledge of drawing."[4] Some artists must have wondered whether the painful months they spent copying dusty plaster casts suddenly had been rendered a waste of time.

More troubling was the worry that artists no longer would play a unique and central cultural role; for millennia it was the

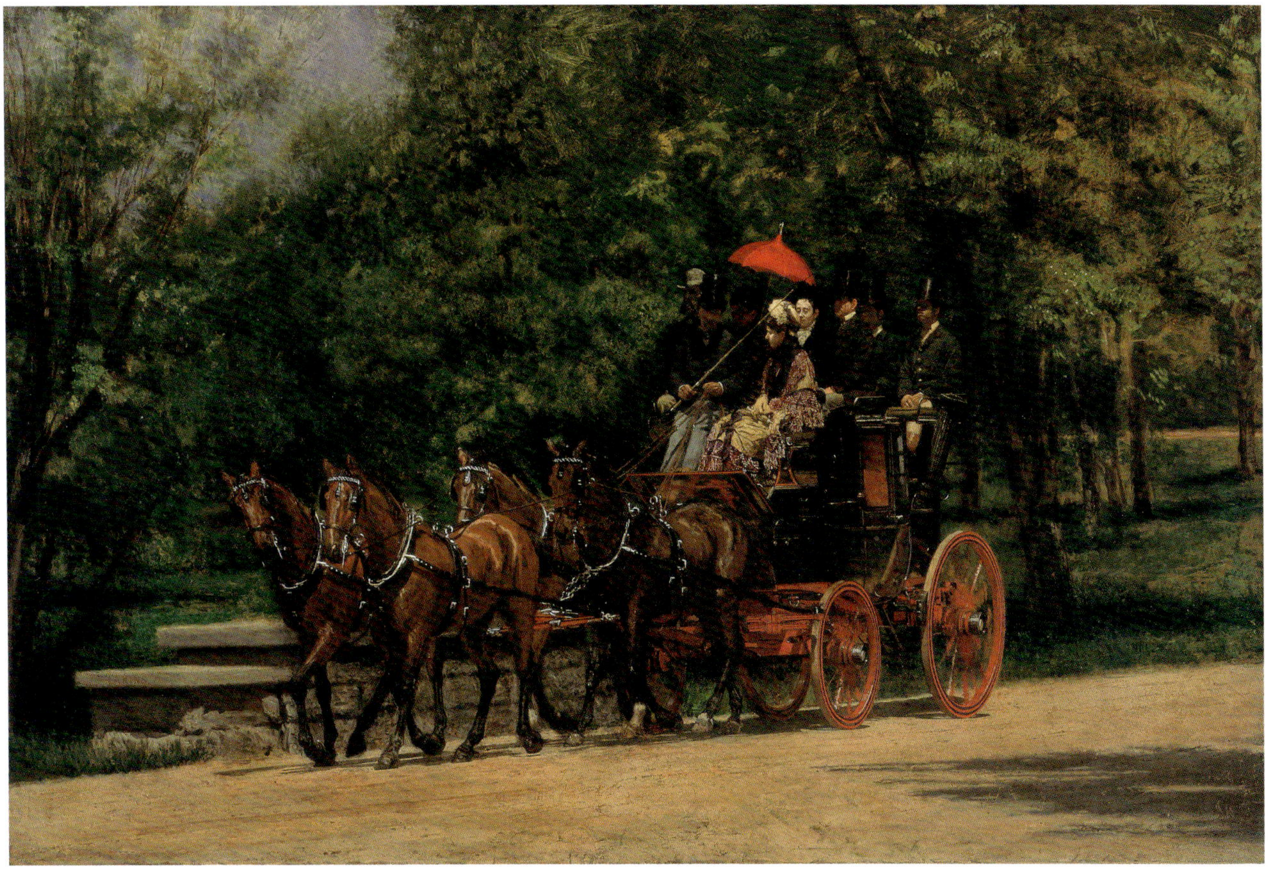

Fig. 38. Thomas Eakins, *A May Morning in the Park (The Fairman Rogers Four-in-Hand)*, 1879–80. Oil on canvas, 23 ¾ × 36 in. Philadelphia Museum of Art. Gift of William Alexander Dick, 1930.

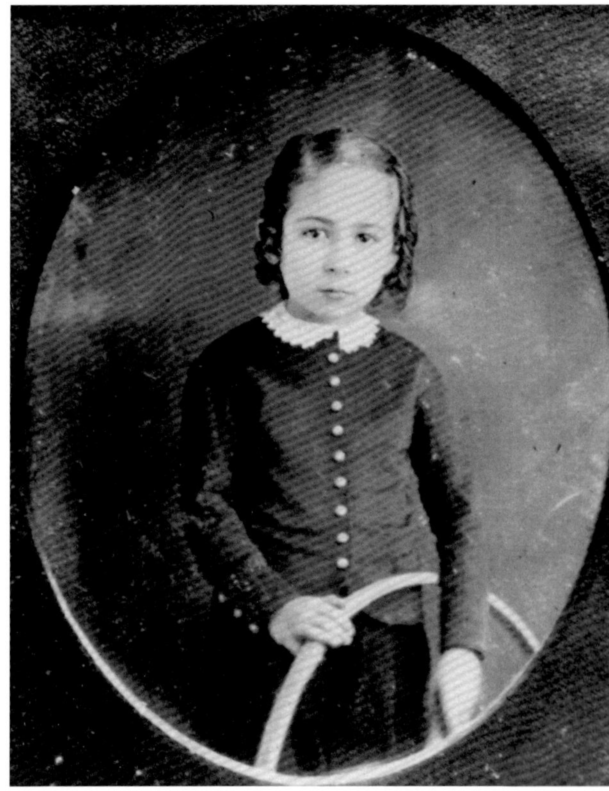

Fig. 39. Unknown photographer, *Eakins at about age six*, c. 1850. Daguerreotype, 3 ½ × 2 11⁄16 in. Courtesy of the Pennsylvania Academy of the Fine Arts, Philadelphia, Charles Bregler's Thomas Eakins Collection. Purchased with the partial support of the Pew Memorial Trust.

work of artists to record and document the world, and to fabricate its visual fantasies. As Arthur C. Danto notes, "Eakins's use of techniques influenced by photography as a means to further artistic fidelity ironically contributed to the progress of a technology that would undermine the idea of verisimilitude in painting."[5] Realism always had its detractors, but when photography could do the same documentary job better, it seemed even more open to question as an artistic credo.

Despite the various threats posed to nineteenth-century artists by the invention of photography, Thomas Eakins always seemed a blithe spirit regarding use of the camera. He certainly never vocalized any of the concerns about photography that other observers and critics of the nineteenth-century art scene took pains to address. To the contrary, Eakins wholeheartedly endorsed photography for artists and art students. He made photographs for both personal and professional study purposes, and he spent a good deal of time working on improvements to the cameras he bought and built. He also drafted an essay on his efforts that Kathleen Foster describes as "a snapshot of a heady moment when amateur experimentation was pressing forward the frontiers of photographic technology."[6]

At the Pennsylvania Academy in 1879, students hardly could have missed seeing their professor's extraordinary preparations for a painting commissioned by Fairman Rogers, the chairman of the committee on instruction. For *A May Morning in the Park*, Eakins learned about equine physiology using studies by Etienne-Jules Marey and photographs by Eadweard Muybridge, as well as his own early (and now lost) efforts with a camera. Eakins also created perspective studies, oil sketches, and wax modellos.[7] The finished painting demonstrated how an artist might integrate photography with more traditional preparatory techniques (fig. 38). Before the discovery of Eakins' methods in the early 1880s, one could hardly have read into this artistic production, his teaching methods, or his written statements any ambivalence about the role of photography in the training and work of a fine artist.

Yet there is no doubt now that Eakins did have some ambivalent feelings about the medium that were difficult to reconcile with his public views—that he found a use for photography so subversive he could not quite own up to it. In that regard, Eakins employed the relatively new medium in a furtive manner similar to the many nineteenth-century Americans who traded photographs in saloons and the back rooms of book shops. The subversive underbelly of photography in the nineteenth century was its ability to capture and record things that should not be seen, and to challenge the fundamental ground rules for who could do the looking. Eakins' photographic indiscretions may have been of a tonier sort, but they still amounted to a private—and guilty—pleasure.

Like most middle-class Philadelphians, before 1880 Thomas Eakins and his family primarily were consumers of photographs, rather than producers of them. Formal studio portraits of Eakins as a boy are typical of the photos families paid for in the antebellum period (fig. 39). The poses were stiff, and clothes and grooming reflected the relative rarity and expense of the event. This mode of photographic production was significantly challenged after 1879, when "the advent of dry-plate negatives ... opened photography to ready experimentation by all." Now, exposure times were faster, and cameras were smaller and more portable.[8]

No longer limited to indoor poses held uncomfortably in a photographer's studio, families like the Eakinses now could record more informal scenes, such as Margaret Eakins and companions on the beach in New Jersey in 1880 (fig. 40), or Tom at thirty-five in that same year, in an overgrown yard, scowling in his trademark worn and unfashionable clothing (fig. 41). Many of the photographs that may be attributable to Eakins over the course of his lifetime fall into this category of publicly acceptable production typical of the era.[9] The Pennsylvania's Academy's large collection of almost 550 images by Eakins and his circle, for example, includes 182 portraits (33 percent), 71 clothed figure studies (13 percent), 61 animal subjects (11 percent), and 8 landscapes (2 percent).[10]

It is not surprising that Eakins used a camera on so many occasions. Philadelphia in particular boasted a vibrant and inventive community of photographers in the second half of the nineteenth century, and one of the most prominent of these was Coleman Sellers. Sellers was a grandson of Charles Willson Peale who organized amateur camera clubs and lived next door to Eakins during the artist's youth. In the tradition of his grandfather, Sellers experimented with optical devices, and he invented the kinematoscope. Eakins' proximity to Sellers in his childhood is a good reminder that he was among the first generation of artists raised in an era in which photography was never a novelty.[11]

During his three years of study in Paris, from 1866 to 1869, Eakins used photography in two modes typical of his generation as well: both as a polite tool of social exchange, and for professional purposes. In several letters sent home to Philadelphia between 1866 and 1868, Eakins thanked family and friends for the photographs he received from them and indicated his hope that they had received the photographs of himself and his professors that he had sent in return. In the early, homesick days of his overseas training, photographs were tangible proof of the existence and well-being of loved

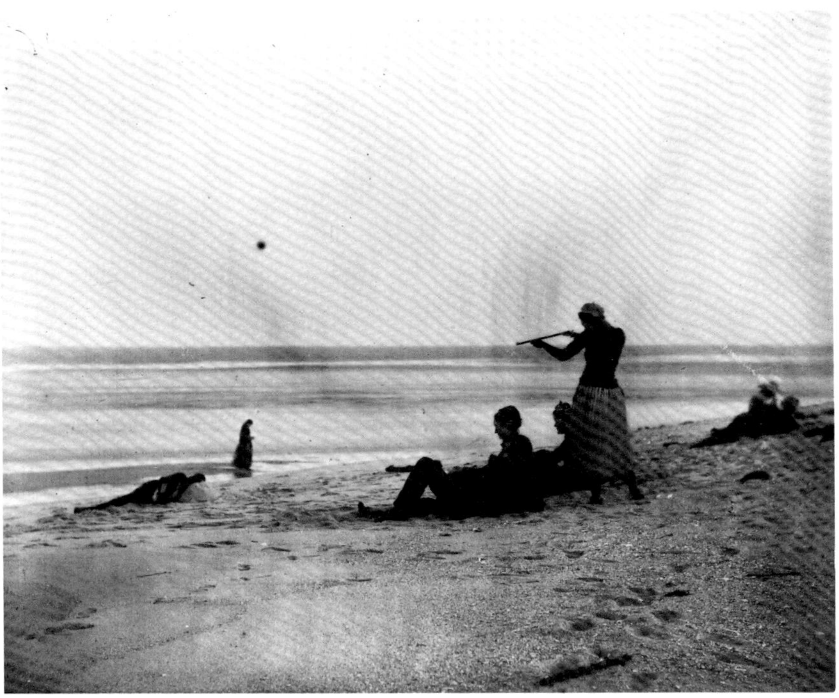

Fig. 40. Thomas Eakins, *Margaret Eakins and other figures on beach at Manasquan, New Jersey (?)*, c. 1880. Dry-plate negative, 4 × 5 in. Courtesy of the Pennsylvania Academy of the Fine Arts, Philadelphia, Charles Bregler's Thomas Eakins Collection. Purchased with the partial support of the Pew Memorial Trust.

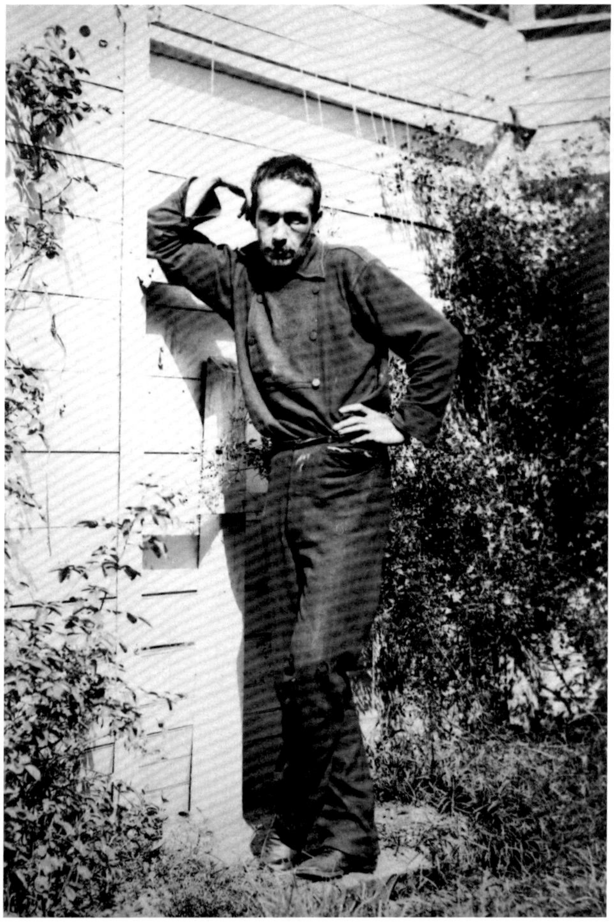

Fig. 41. Susan Macdowell Eakins, *Thomas Eakins at about age thirty-five, leaning against fence*, 1880. Gelatin silver print, $6\frac{7}{16} \times 4\frac{1}{2}$ in. Courtesy of the Pennsylvania Academy of the Fine Arts, Philadelphia, Charles Bregler's Thomas Eakins Collection. Purchased with the partial support of the Pew Memorial Trust.

ones, and then served as memory aids as his stay in Europe grew to several years.

Eakins' use of photographs for professional purposes also grew with the length of his stay abroad. In letters to his parents, Eakins accounted for purchases of photographs of his professors, "stereoscopes," and "life studies."[12] In the latter instance in particular, the artist was following the example of the Parisian painters around him, who patronized a large industry devoted to the production of photographs of the nude also called *academies.*

The most famous photographer of academic nudes in France during the time Eakins was there was Gaudenzio Marconi, the "self-styled king of the genre" who boasted of his official role as "Photographe de l'Ecole des Beaux-Arts" (although such a position seems never to have existed).[13] To emphasize his virtuous appeal to artists, Marconi posed nude men, women, and children in modes that advertised their artfulness, mostly featuring the types of poses seen in academic life study classes. Especially popular were poses reminiscent of classical Greek and Roman statues, and poses designed to show major muscle groups and shifts in weight. Beginning in the 1850s, important French artists including Ingres, Courbet, Gérôme, and Delacroix all collected these life studies.

Like other purveyors of photographic academies in the nineteenth century, Marconi frequently promised that the artist would save on modeling fees.[14] Eakins certainly bears out this promise—he recorded buying photographs in Paris more often than paying models' fees. Among the expenses Eakins listed in the scrupulous accounts he sent home, he included a portrait of Gérôme that cost 1 franc, a landscape for .80, and four photographic life studies that cost 8 francs.[15] The higher price of the life studies reflected the more ample profit margin their subject matter could demand from desiring audiences—it never was necessary to show a paint box to buy the photographs.

Although many of the academies purchased by Ingres, Gérôme, and presumably Eakins had the official sanction of the French government for use specifically by artists, they circulated far more broadly than intended. As Thomas Waugh writes, in short order even "the most functional of anatomical studies became fodder for leering wankers as well ... in postcard format on urban streets, mass-produced for tourists in France and other Mediterranean countries, and circulated freely though the sexual underworld, even as ads for brothels." It is hard to imagine that the other audiences for academies were unknown to Eakins along with their relatively chaste function as drawing aids.[16] Chasteness, of course, was hard to come by in a medium so devoted to the precedent set by painting.

Although France did have and enforce anti-obscenity laws regulating nude photographs more than a decade before Anthony Comstock came on the scene in America, these laws had little effect on the circulation of photographic nudes. If a photographer went to the trouble of registering his images with the Bibliothèque Nationale de France (and presumably if he paid a fee to the attending bureaucrat), he could then legally market and sell them as "studies for painters."[17]

The problem, of course, is that even the most venerated Greek and Roman statuary often are erotically charged, sometimes with sexual relations at the heart of the scene. Some of Marconi's government-registered photos, including one example presumably imitating *The Rape of the Sabines*, required that the models act out a scene involving physical contact between naked bodies and presumably on the verge of intimate relations (fig. 42). Like *The Roman Daughter*, a man's mouth here is quite close to a woman's breast, but now his hand also gropes her naked buttocks, the scene involves full and frontal nudity, and of course, they are real individuals seen through the camera lens, not badly painted inventions with an attendant exculpatory pamphlet.

Fig. 42. Gaudenzio Marconi, *Nude couple posed in the classical idiom (probably imitating "The Rape of the Sabines")*, c. 1856. Photograph. Bibliothèque Nationale de France.

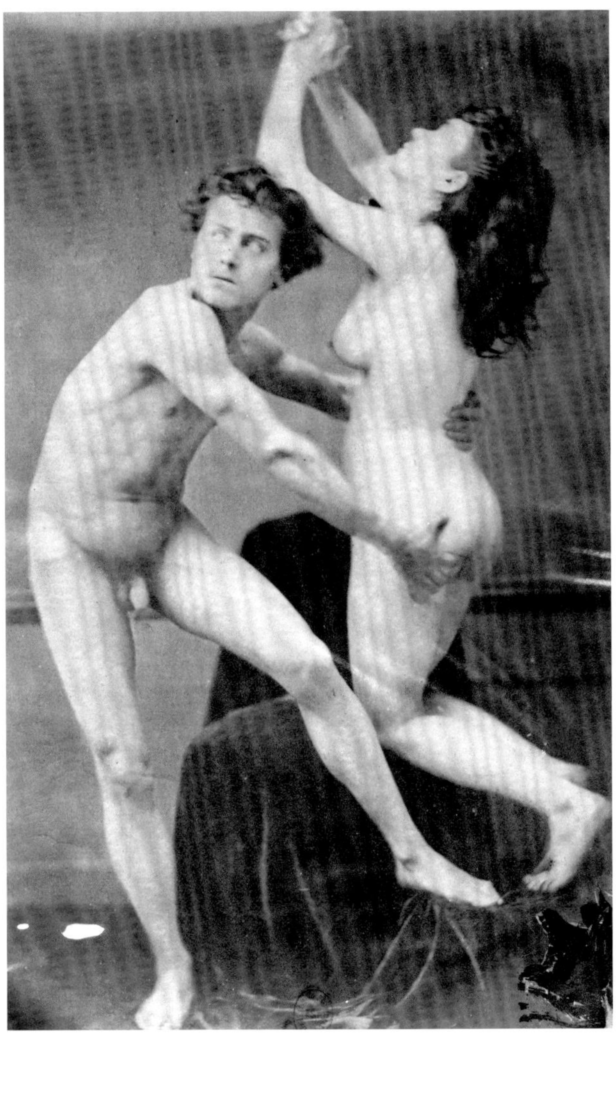

Only slightly more subtle were Marconi's many photographs of women posed in the mode of the domestic and exotic genre scenes so popular in the French Salon at the time, including the coy scene *Nude with a bonnet* (fig. 43). Although Marconi might have liked to advertise that he worked for artists at the prestigious Ecole des Beaux-Arts, in fact this image demonstrates how he already had tweaked his repertoire to compete with other photographers for the vast audience of paying voyeurs who had no intention of painting or drawing from the scenes. Waugh notes that "before the end of the 1850s, some photographers of the female nude had already abandoned the cold studio look of the early figure studies and were using explicitly erotic codes of gesture (a slightly opened thigh), gaze (a coy look at the camera), and decor (the draped and tasseled alcove instead of the drafty studio pedestal)."[18]

Eakins almost certainly was aware of the thin line between life study and pornography when he wrote to his father in 1867 regarding a potential purchase of photos for Benjamin's friend George Holmes: "on receiving your [letter] about finding out about the models of which Mr. Holmes spoke to you ... I send you the list of the subjects already issued. They are photographs from the—finest models & statuary of the Greeks, paintings & drawings of the Italians, a few French and Hollanders.... The list I send will hint very well at the average selection. The statuary heads would be the most appropriate to buy for Mr. Holmes & maybe—one or two whole statues."[19]

Eakins displayed some delicacy in mentioning the quality of the models in the photos but then suggesting the more "appropriate" choice of statue heads for Mr. Holmes. He probably was not so "appropriate" in his own purchases. For an artist struggling to learn to paint the nude, the opportunity to save money on models would have been a much more

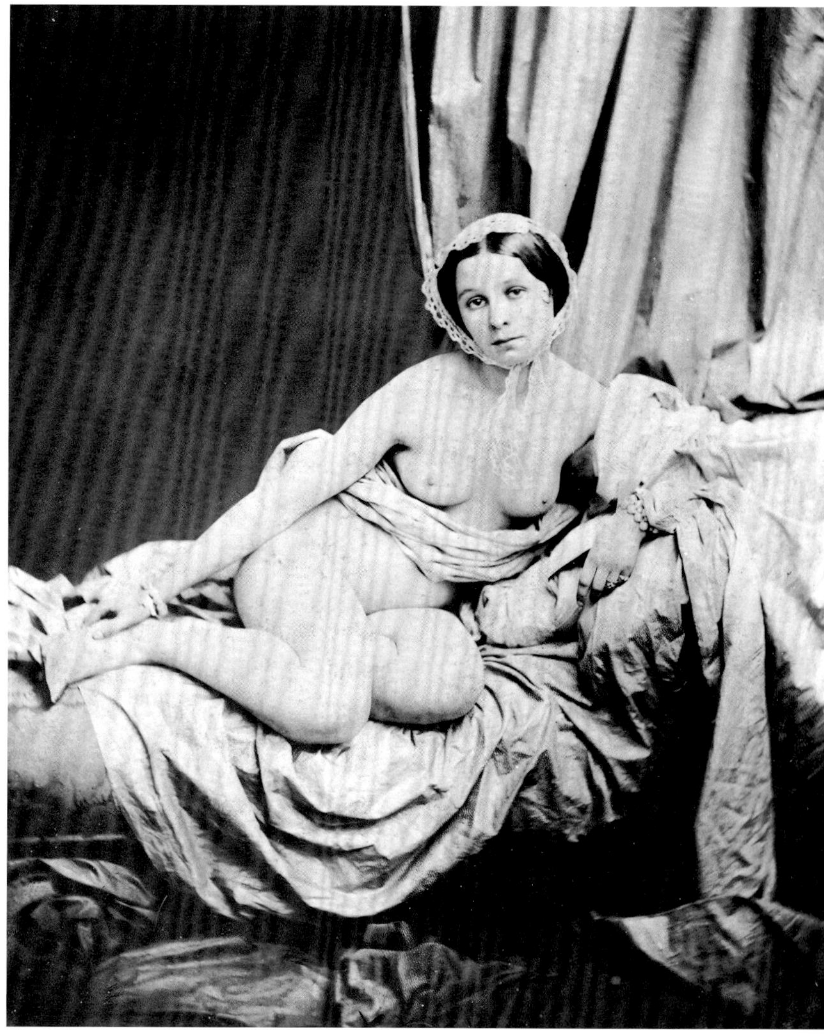

Fig. 43. Gaudenzio Marconi, *Nude with a bonnet,* 1856. Photograph. Bibliothèque Nationale de France.

pressing concern. Whether or not Eakins used life studies as autoerotic aids—and whether he chose male and female models, together or separately—would have been entirely his own decision to make in the lonely studio apartments he inhabited by himself while studying abroad.

In Paris on his own, Eakins certainly did not have to worry about the type of criticism George Holmes might have received for the display of nude photographs in his living quarters. Here also, Eakins was far from the lectures of the moral reformers of his youth. In November 1868, he wrote exuberantly to his sister Frances (Fanny) of his impending visit home for Christmas, looking forward in particular to eating oysters. "By eating oysters you improve your mind provided they contain phosphoric properties and other mirific substances of which the human brain is made, the which has already been noted and expounded by Reddy Vogdes, who had the experience along with Francis Wayland, doctor in mental, moral and idiotic sciences."[20]

Vogdes was Central High School's professor of moral hygiene who assigned students a textbook written by Francis Wayland. Wayland was a president of Brown University and author of the tome called *The Elements of Moral Science,* which included such chapter headings as "The General Duty of Chastity." His moral principles required chastity for all except "individuals who are exclusively united to each other for life." Wayland stressed: "Inasmuch as unchaste desire is strongly excited by the imagination, the law of chastity forbids all impure thoughts and actions; all unchaste conversation, looks, or gestures; the reading of obscene or lascivious books, and every thing which would naturally produce in us a disposition of mind to violate this precept."[21] Wayland certainly was not a Frenchman, and he undoubtedly would have complained that government-registered stereoscopic artist's "life studies" like Bruno Braquehais' image of a model seen from a low angle scarcely could fail to create "a disposition of mind to violate this precept," at least if the viewer was prone to enjoy such views (fig. 44). The broad array of life study photographs available for sale in Paris assured that a range of other tastes was accommodated as well. Eakins' assumption that Holmes would not have wanted to purchase images of models (at least through a well-respected friend) indicated his awareness that the climate in America was different.

But while it certainly is true that Philadelphia was no Paris, it was a matter of degrees rather than constitution; Americans also enjoyed the opportunity to purchase photographs of nudes in large numbers. Both new printing technologies and the social impact of the Civil War caused the American pornography industry to expand in the 1860s. Large numbers of American men fighting both in the North and the South were removed from their homes and families for long stretches of time. In this environment, obscene materials routinely circulated among both soldiers and officers. One Captain Tousley was so disturbed by the traffic, and the army's failure to stop it, that he "wrote directly to Commander in Chief Abraham Lincoln, enclosing as evidence a circular advertising 'New Pictures for Bachelors.' ... For twelve cents a piece or $1.20 a dozen, men could purchase twelve-by-fifteen-inch pictures, suitable for framing. Most of the advertised pictures placed the man in the role of voyeur observing groups of young women in various states of

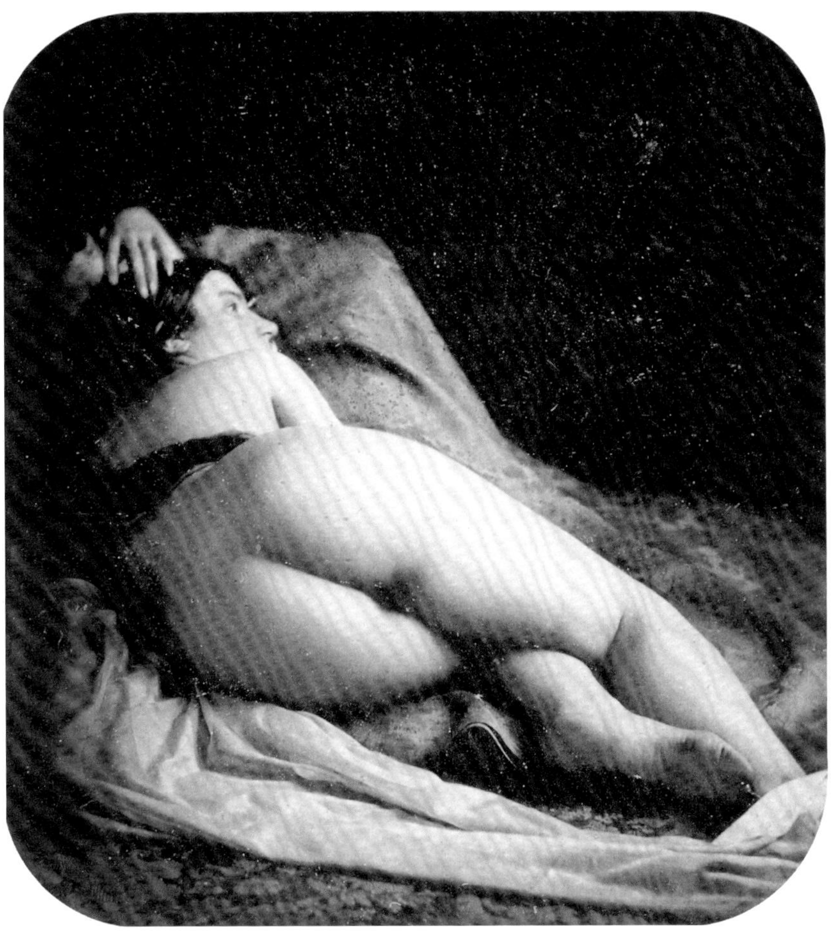

Fig. 44. Bruno Braquehais, *Nude female, reclining, from rear*, 1858 or later. Right side of colored stereoscopic daguerreotype. Collection, Budapest Museum.

undress. In 'Wood Nymphs' Frolic,' for example, girls 'engaged in a rustic dance ... in all the consciousness of innocence, caring little whether or not they are seen in their nude and interesting frolic.'"[22]

In spite of the captain's complaint, obscene materials continued to circulate in large numbers throughout the war. In 1863, the widely available catalogue of H. G. Hoskins and Company of New York City listed erotic books, including "Prostitution in Paris" and "Venus in Cloister," in addition to dildos, condoms, and stereoscopic pictures at nine dollars per dozen. For three dollars a dozen, one could order carte-de-visite photographs of subjects that included "two or more figures photographed from life, engaged in sexual enjoyment."[23]

For thousands of years, of course, art had served the function of depicting erotic fantasies—the difference in the second half of the nineteenth century according to William Gerdts was simply that in "pool halls, saloons and hotel bars, photographic nudes now mingled on the walls with copies of French paintings like Adolphe William Bouguereau's *Nymphs and Satyr* (1877)," and individuals from all social strata could own images they found erotic.[24]

Thomas Eakins may never have entered a pool hall or purchased a lurid view of a derriere, but it is impossible to imagine that such images were unknown to him. Three years in Paris, consorting with a large circle of French and American men, ensures that he understood the format, conventions, and style of the photographs called "life studies" or even "bachelor's pictures." Both categories of images shared an emphasis on images of nude females and sometimes males in sexually charged scenarios, and were sold, censored, regulated, and politely not discussed by proper women and men in similar manners at home and abroad. And although it never has been suggested that Eakins set out to make photographic pornography, the comparison of his works with the more commercial genre nevertheless is useful in establishing the taboos and protocols surrounding his images and their reception in the nineteenth century.

In spite of the delicate legal and social issues regarding the sale, ownership, and display of photographic nudes, Eakins began producing them as soon as dry-plate technology made

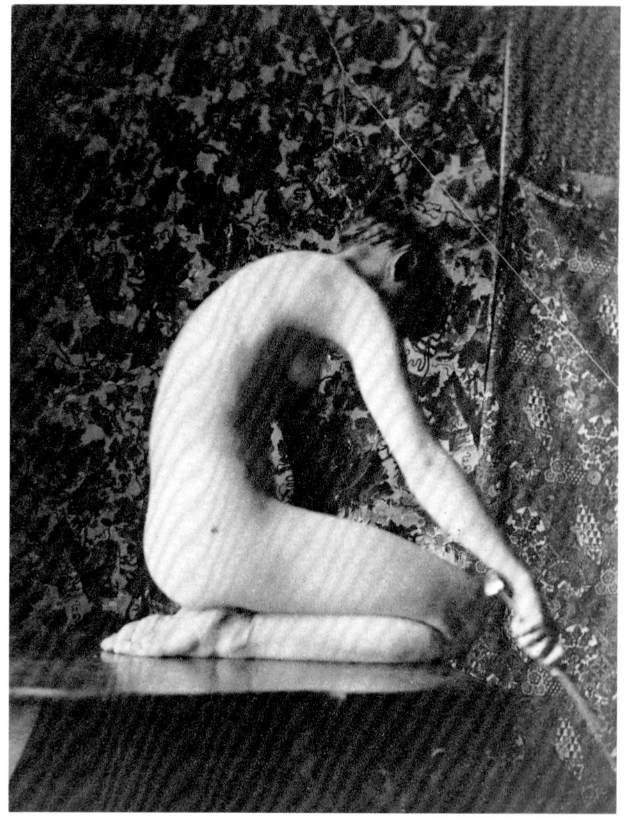

Fig. 45. Thomas Eakins, *Female nude kneeling on table*, c. 1884. Albumen print, 3 13/16 × 3 1/16 in. Courtesy of the Pennsylvania Academy of the Fine Arts, Philadelphia, Charles Bregler's Thomas Eakins Collection. Purchased with the partial support of the Pew Memorial Trust.

it possible and affordable for him to do so. The Pennsylvania Academy collection contains 218 photographic prints from Eakins' circle devoted to study of the nude, making up the largest single group in the collection (39 percent), plus another 86 negatives of this genre.[25]

Eakins' photographs of the nude have inspired a great deal of writing by historians, in part because the experience of looking at them often requires some processing in modern minds. There are numerous photographs of the artist himself. Writers singing the praises of *The Gross Clinic* also know what its brilliant creator looked like stark naked—standing, running, jumping, and often staring back at us. We also share an intimate view of his wife, Susan, and many of their close friends. More disconcerting are a few photos of nude children, sometimes looking shy, women with masks over their heads, signifying a sense of shame, and then of course the series of three photos of Eakins holding a nude female model. What was he thinking? Should we really be seeing this?

Located precisely in these questions lie the great challenges and opportunities of Eakins' nude photographs. Whatever his motives may have included, nevertheless what he and his colleagues accomplished is a compendium of images that comprehensively survey, and challenge, the conventions of nudity and voyeurism in the nineteenth century.

Historians at the Pennsylvania Academy chose the following categories to organize their collection of Eakins' photographs of nudes: women indoors, children indoors, men indoors, men outdoors, men in sports, nudes with horses, and scientific photographs including the standing "naked series" and nudes in motion. Although attribution and dating are often imprecise in the case of photographs, the studies all date between 1883 and 1892, and appear to have been produced by Eakins and a small circle of friends and students. All told, the size and breadth of the group is impressive.

On their surface, the nude photographs by and of Eakins and his circle bear great similarity to the life studies the artist was familiar with in Paris. In the indoor photos made at the Pennsylvania Academy in the mid-1880s and later at the Philadelphia Art Students' League, we see props similar to French equivalents, including drapery, an oriental carpet, a sword, a plant, and some assorted furniture. The poses range from overtly artful—a woman curled in a beautiful kneeling pose (fig. 45) and Eakins reclining, seen from the rear in the mode of Braquehais (fig. 46)—to plainly straightforward (fig. 47). Some of the photos reveal their classroom setting—we see artists sketching, model platforms, easels casually included in the frame. In many ways, Eakins followed French conventions he already was familiar with in composing these images, and the only truly innovative aspects of the photos were their more amateurish casualness and the fact that they were made on American soil.[26]

If it occurred to Eakins as a professional art instructor to make sure his educational photos did not look like the kinds of images that circulated in France both as life studies and as pornography, his attempts were only partly successful in this group. Some of the reclining poses echo Braquehais' better-lit and framed photos, and certainly the series of Eakins with a naked model is redolent with the titillating narrative of

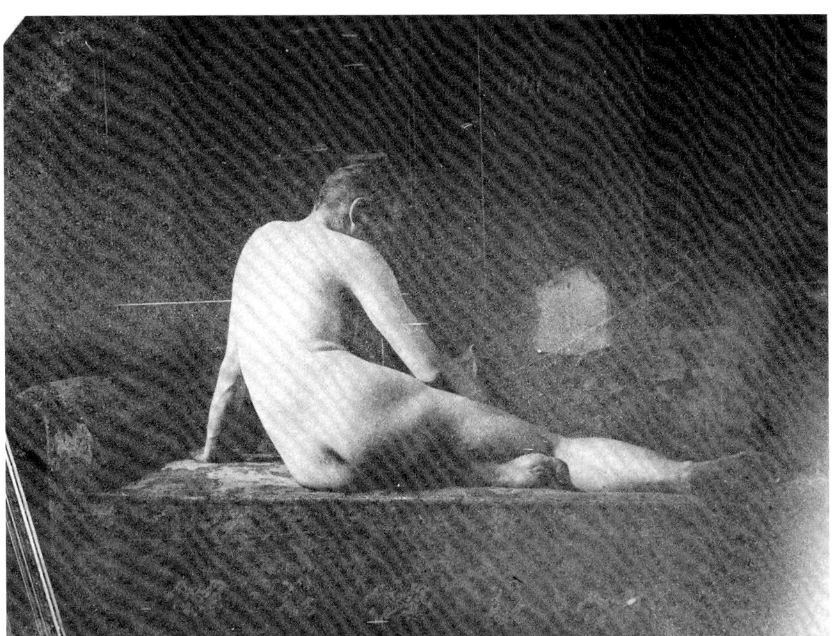

Fig. 46. Circle of Thomas Eakins, *Thomas Eakins nude, semireclining on couch, from rear,* c. 1883. Platinum print, 5⅜ × 7¼ in. Courtesy of the Pennsylvania Academy of the Fine Arts, Philadelphia, Charles Bregler's Thomas Eakins Collection. Purchased with the partial support of the Pew Memorial Trust.

abduction also capitalized on by Marconi and his following of "leering wankers" in the *Rape of the Sabines*. A variety of less charged classical poses by both Marconi and Eakins demonstrates the vibrancy of the Greco-Roman tradition as it crossed from the realm of fine art to the new medium of photography.[27] These examples all demonstrate that the most obvious influences on Eakins' photos of indoor nudes were French and classical examples. Other images were more unprecedented.

Although the Greeks and Romans often incorporated public nudity into their festivals and daily life and portrayed that nudity in works of art, the nineteenth-century adoration of all things classical did not often extend to outdoor disrobing. Eakins was quite unusual in photographing nudes outdoors, although the practice resulted in especially useful studies of the body in natural light.[28] The insights from these photos certainly helped Eakins as he worked on *Arcadia* and *Swimming*.

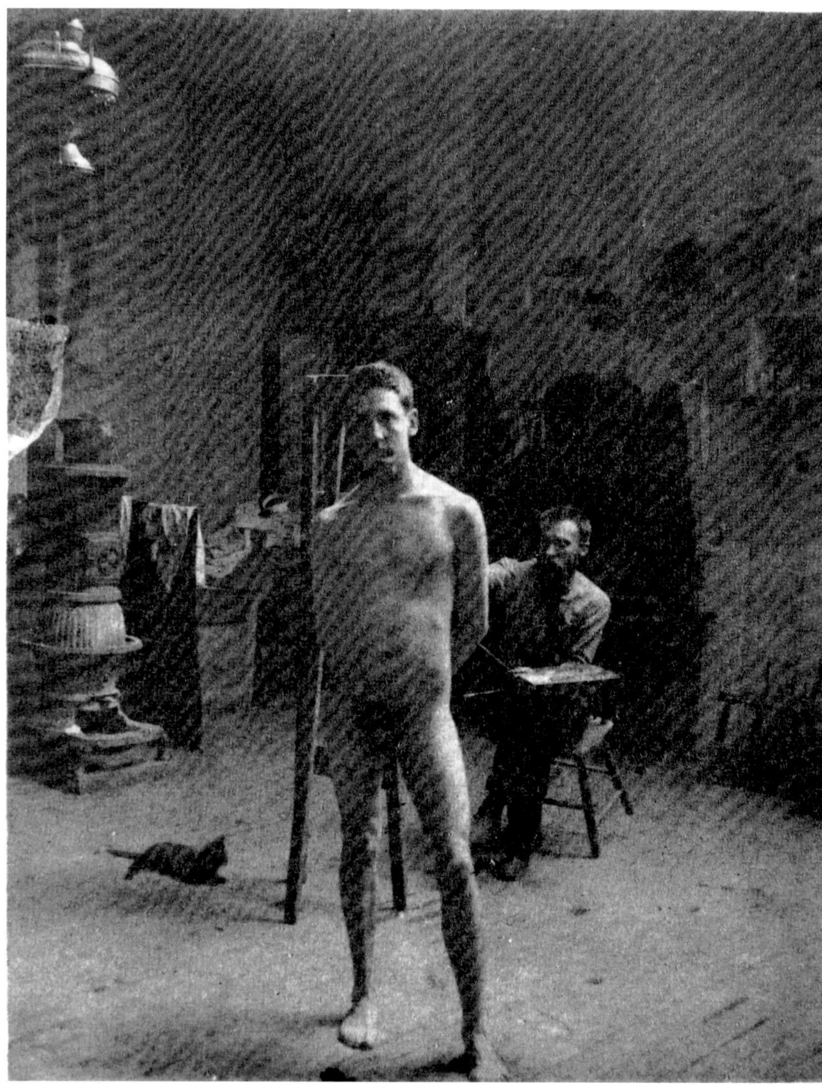

Fig. 47. Thomas Eakins, *John Wright nude, posing for George Reynolds at easel*, c. 1889. Cyanotype, 4½ × 3 9/16 in. Courtesy of the Pennsylvania Academy of the Fine Arts, Philadelphia, Charles Bregler's Thomas Eakins Collection. Purchased with the partial support of the Pew Memorial Trust.

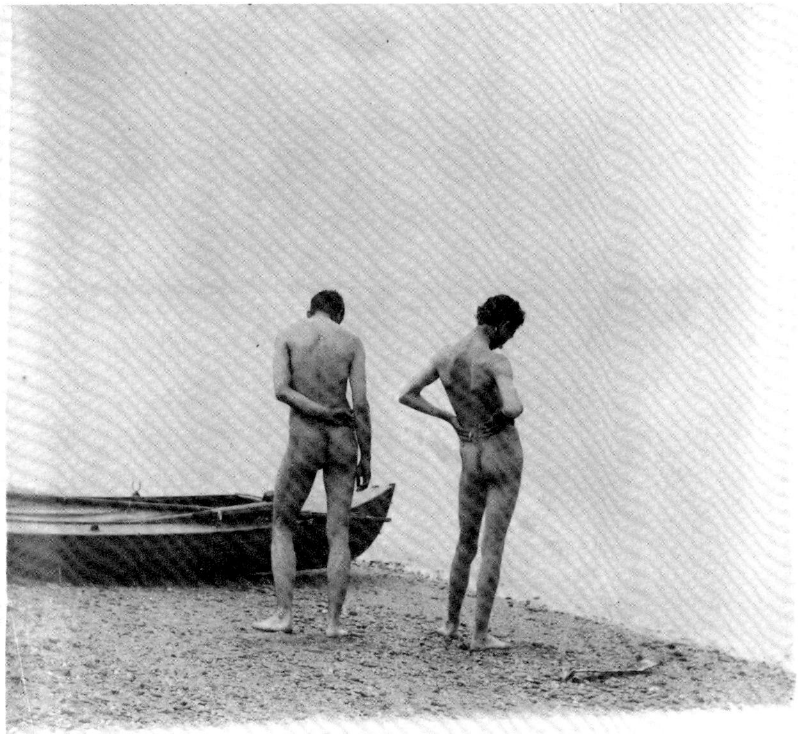

Fig. 48. Circle of Thomas Eakins, *Thomas Eakins nude and J. Laurie Wallace nude, from rear, in front of boat at shoreline*, c. 1883. Albumen print, 3 ½ × 4 in. Courtesy of the Pennsylvania Academy of the Fine Arts, Philadelphia, Charles Bregler's Thomas Eakins Collection. Purchased with the partial support of the Pew Memorial Trust.

In spite of the novelty of the outdoor setting, however, the change of scenery did not amount to much else. Outside the classroom setting, models struck similar poses as indoors, often standing casually or in athletic stances requiring flexion of a number of important muscle groups, as in a photograph of a male nude in a wide stance prepared to throw a rock, or from the rear sitting or lying down and propped on an elbow. The chief changes from indoors to fresh air were more space for groups of figures, scenic backdrops, natural lighting, and the gender of the models. Women do not appear as nude figures outdoors in Eakins' photographs, with the exception of a small number of images of Susan.

This gender difference is entirely in keeping with conventions for same-sex nudity at the time. Although there certainly were isolated radical groups like the "free love" advocates who indulged in mixed public nudity, there is no evidence that Eakins advocated their views or practiced them outside his smallest inner circle. Even Walt Whitman consistently disavowed any support for free love advocates.[29]

Putting aside the few pictures of Eakins' most devoted female student—his eventual wife—the much larger number of images of men seen individually and together in wooded and seaside settings includes preparatory photos for *Swimming*, and less staged scenes such as *Thomas Eakins nude and J. Laurie Wallace nude, from rear, in front of boat at shoreline* (fig. 48). The resemblance of the poses in these photos to indoor versions demonstrates the convergence of Eakins' inexhaustible desire to study the nude with the invention of affordable equipment enabling him to extend his terrain. With dry-plate negatives, strong-minded purpose, and presumably isolated settings, Eakins forged a new category of photographic production—the outdoor male nude.

One of the reasons Eakins' photographs so often have been analyzed for their Grecophilic attributes is their unusual emphasis on male nudes. Elizabeth Johns, for example, describes the series of photographs of naked men and boys in a wooded landscape preparatory to painting *Arcadia* as a celebration of "the male physique" in "an era in which male friendship and beauty were celebrated throughout the Mediterranean." She goes on to demonstrate the ways the poses each are inspired by well-known Greek and Roman sculptures.[30] And Jonathan Weinberg writes: "Eakins's goal in *Swimming* could be said not only to re-imagine the classical body in a modern setting but also to restore the earlier prestige of the male nude. One exalted precedent for the theme of men swimming is Michelangelo's *Battle of Cascina*,

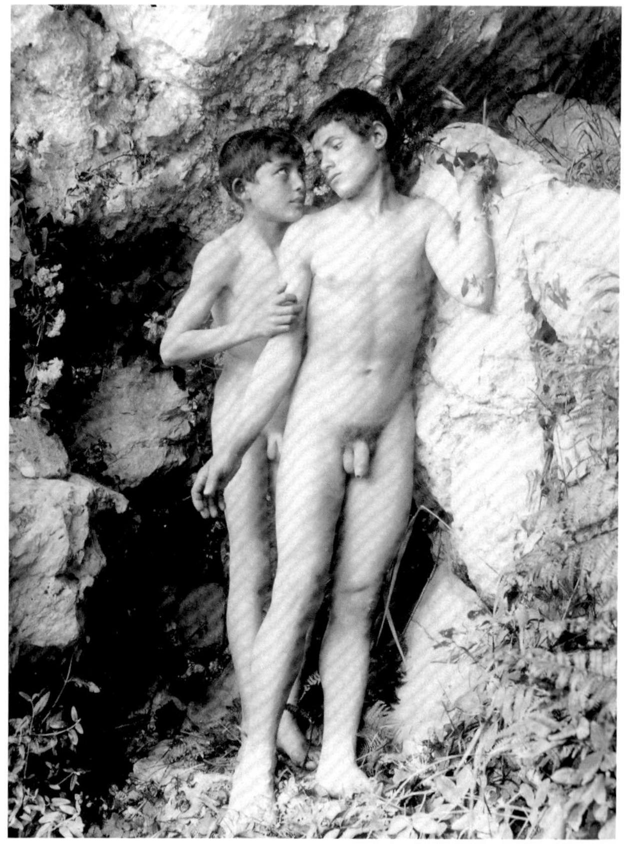

Fig. 49. Baron Wilhelm von Gloeden, *Youths in grotto*, c. 1885–1905. Gelatin print. The J. Paul Getty Museum, Los Angeles.

whereas the young man at the apex of Eakins's pyramidal composition, his buttocks thrust out and his arms akimbo, evokes the heroic pose of Donatello's *David* (albeit in reverse and seen from the behind), the first great Renaissance nude."[31] Given the relative rarity of the male nude in American visual culture before the twentieth century, it is not surprising that Weinberg's study titled *Male Desire: The Homoerotic in American Art* begins with Eakins.

It is unlikely that Eakins consciously thought about ways to heighten the eroticism of his photographs of male nudes, but he was quickly followed by other artists who certainly did. Sometime around the 1890s, Baron Wilhelm von Gloeden began photographing Sicilian boys and young men in seductive poses at his Mediterranean villa, thus inaugurating the profitable industry of gay male photographic pornography. A turn of fortune in his illustrious family prompted him to sell postcards of his images to tourists. In America, Fred Holland Day followed suit around the turn of the century.[32]

One of the innovations Eakins introduced that these later artists emulated was his presentation of male models in traditional female poses. In his photo with Wallace at the beach, for example, Eakins lifts his arms above his head in a convention more usually popular for women because it helped display their breasts. This simple gender twist became the norm in purposefully homoerotic photography, such as von Gloeden's languorous *Youths in grotto* (fig. 49), modeled on images of women in similar embrace. Eakins' indoor photos as well capture men and women in the same seated and standing poses.

Other elements of Eakins' and von Gloeden's work are less comparable. One immediately apparent difference between von Gloeden's *Youths* and *Eakins and Wallace* is the dramatic and romantic narrative suggested by the touching and gazing in the later photo—an obvious contrast with the earlier scene in which the men look simply like they are displaying their bodies for the camera. In Eakins' scenes with more narrative content, including men wrestling or swimming, the storyline supplied by the artist still remains markedly slight in contrast to von Gloeden's boys, surrounded as they often are by props and backdrops.

Another distinction is clear as well between Eakins and von Gloeden. In his broad survey of gay male eroticism, Thomas Waugh also notes a typical emphasis on "the centrality of the genitals" and their "coy aestheticization, with light, shadow, scale, props, or gesture."[33] Although the inclusion of the penis is similar in the work by von Gloeden and Eakins, the style in which it is rendered is substantively different. In contrast to many of the images intentionally produced as homoerotic pornography a decade later, Eakins and his circle never made an effort to adjust lighting, scale, or composition to highlight the "centrality" of genitals.[34]

Although Eakins' male nudes did break with conventional precedent in their outdoor settings and typically female poses on occasion, at the same time he adopted quite different conventions in the paintings he intended for public display. Eakins chose not to depict the penis in his paintings of male nudes, including *Arcadia* and *Swimming*. This bow to contemporary norms demonstrates that he understood and abided at least this aspect of the taboo against the display of the male nude in fine art. The artist also only once displayed a female using full frontal nudity in a painting—his last version of *Wil-*

liam Rush (fig. 50), now in Hawaii. The phrase "anatomically correct" still signifies a level of detail in rendering that even Eakins did not necessarily think appropriate for fine art audiences. The artist identified far fewer rules for his photographs, perhaps because of the obviously liberal precedents set by life studies and pornography, but also because he intended them for professional use rather than public display.

Four significant points are important in positioning Eakins' photographs of nudes in the context of their time. Photographers like Marconi and von Gloeden of course were businessmen seeking profit, gauging the interests of artists, "bachelors," and tourists. Commercial photographers manipulated lighting, hired attractive models, and chose poses that were staged in a manner that often suggested a theatrical or sexual narrative. Eakins in contrast never created a photograph for the purpose of sale. He deemed all of his photographic nudes to be preparatory or instructive, and most were created under the aegis of the curriculum at the Pennsylvania Academy and later the Art Students' League. The photographs seem not to have circulated beyond limited circles of students and professional artists.

A second important point is that Eakins never concealed the fact that he was producing the photographs. In fact, the Pennsylvania Academy circular of the committee on instruction for 1883–84 recorded that photographs of models had been made that year in cases in which "the model was unusually good, or had any peculiarity of form or action which would be instructive."[35] Eakins later followed Gérôme's example by filling the walls of the Art Students' League with prints of his nude studies.[36] Whereas photographs intended for commerce as sexual materials were viewed, and traded, in furtive circumstances, Eakins never treated his images in a similar manner.

Another important difference between Marconi, von Gloeden, and Eakins lies in their visual styles. Photographers of commercial life studies justified the cost of their products in part through their superior quality compared with the images amateurs could create. These photographers therefore balanced their compositions and adjusted lighting to convey deep contrast in rendering forms. Overall, the photographs appear studied, formal, and professional. In contrast, the lighting in all of Eakins' indoor and outdoor nudes is haphazard—at times revealing a pictorialist sensibility, but more often suggesting a lack of attention.

Finally, Anne McCauley notes that the commercial French academies "differ from Eakins's more amateurish efforts in their melodrama and the introduction of appropriately passionate facial expressions to correspond with the poses."[37] Again in contrast to Marconi and von Gloeden, there are no emotional stories in Eakins' photographs—these are bodies before a camera lens. The contrast between the professional performance of the models in Marconi's *Rape of the Sabines* and the emotionless visage of Eakins as he holds up the female model is striking. The difference between the two abduction scenes is similar to the contrast seen between John Rubens Smith's art anatomy tome, filled with its overt expressions of "orderly" and "disorderly" moods, and William Williams Keen's text, in which the appearance of emotion never was addressed.

Just as Eakins made his own body casts from cadavers, dismissing French versions as "prettified," he also made his own less prettified photographs of human anatomy. In this sense, his approach to the body without adornment via flattering lighting or angles—or neutering via fig leaf or gesture—was a logical extension of his approach to the body in other aspects of his teaching methods. In all these ways, Eakins' photographs bear the hallmarks of medical, in addition to French and classical, influences.

Nineteenth-century Americans photographed naked bodies for two primary purposes—erotic franchise and medical-scientific documentation. In the former category, they imported many more French examples than they produced, but in the latter category, Americans were themselves prolific. Daniel Fox and Christopher Lawrence note that "in Britain, France and the United States after about 1850, professional journals regularly reported attempts to apply photography to every area of medical interest, including anatomy, physiology, histology, and pathology."[38] Medical use of the camera was only one example of an expanding list of devices doctors used in making their practices more rigorous and specialized.

Jacob Mendez DaCosta, whom Eakins painted in 1893, for example, delivered regular exegeses on the benefits of

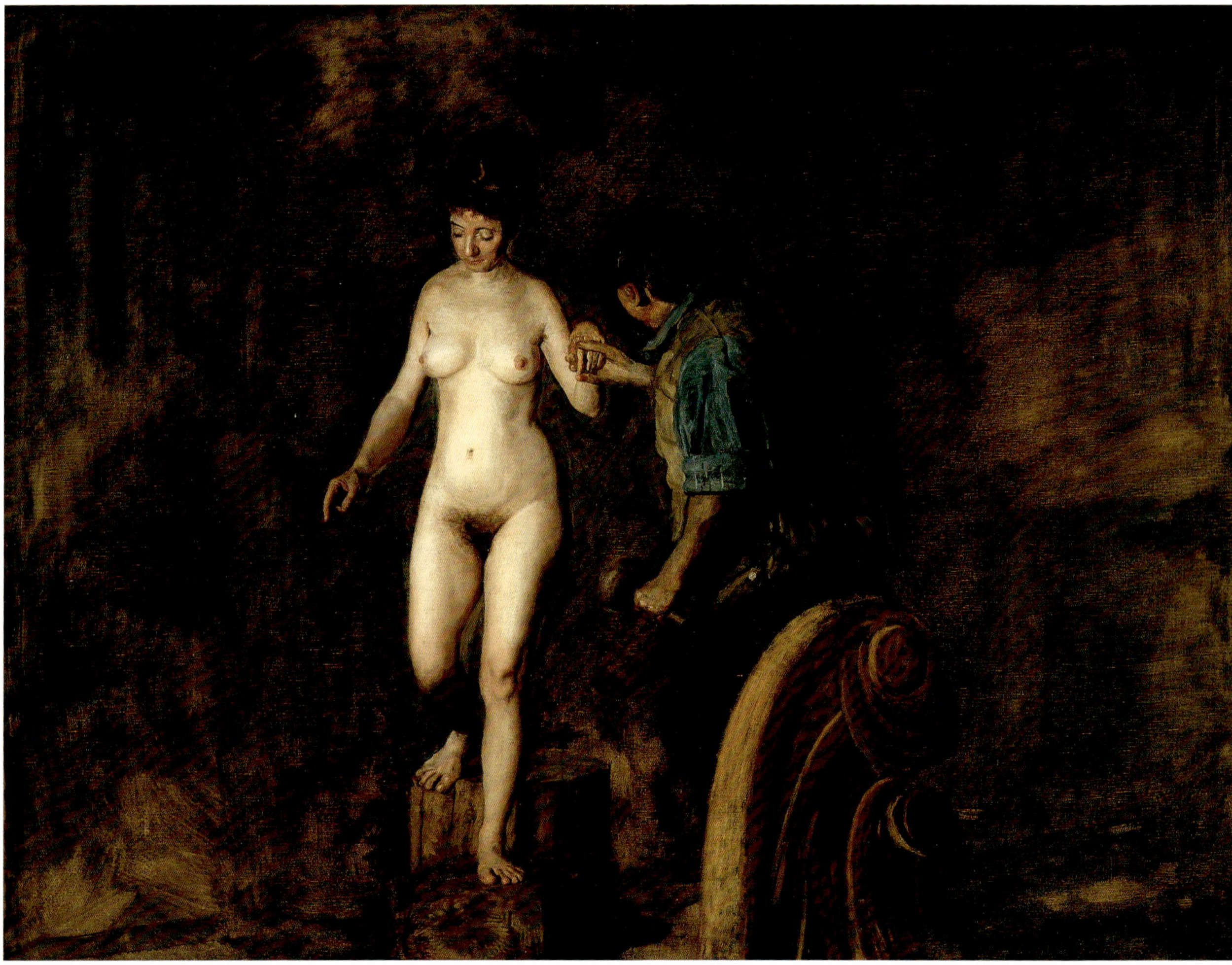

Fig. 50. Thomas Eakins, *William Rush and His Model,* c. 1907-8. Oil on canvas, 35 ½ × 47 ½ in. Honolulu Academy of Arts. Gift of the Friends of the Academy, 1947.

mechanical devices in medicine, including the camera. In 1872, he (presumably) humorously addressed incoming students at the Jefferson Medical College with the following "glimpse into [the] future":

> Madam is in her boudoir, reclining on the sofa, in expectation of her medical attendants. A drag drives up, from which alight two servants with heavy bags, who assist four doctors to descend. The fraternity is announced, and, followed by the servants, enters the room. The bags are deposited; the servitors withdraw, and after the exchange of a few remarks the examination begins. Dr. Ready, the junior practitioner, conducts the first inquiries, makes the (18) ordinary investigations of the different organs, and before finishing pulls out of his pocket a tablet containing the volumetric examination of every fluid in the body, completed since his last visit. This is looked at by all. Dr. Reckoner then takes traces of the movements of the heart, of the pulse, of the action of the muscles, records the velocity of their contraction, and estimates the amount of nerve-supply, showing the diagrams and figures to the patient, who inspects them with the look of a connoisseur. Dr Eyeman now applies the ophthalmoscope, which photographs as well as is used to see by.
>
> Later in the examination, Dr. Magnet, the physicist on the team, steps forward with a "modified, portable Ruhmkorff coil" and after analysis and consultation by "the fraternity" the patient is advised to take "a few glasses of soda-water, and a daily ride on horseback."[39]

DaCosta's whimsical vision of the future revolved around his certain expectation of both disciplinary specificity and the abundant use of new diagnostic devices, including the camera. Both of these predictions were born out, though in quite different style, in the decades that followed.

The most common subjects of early medical photography were people suffering from "extraordinary deformity of unusual interest." A good example is "Plate VII. Venous Tumor" (fig. 51), in which the photographer posed the subject so that both the unaffected and the cancerous cheeks were displayed—an interestingly similar approach to display of the breasts in Eakins' *The Agnew Clinic*. Other images of surgery from this era reveal the artist's relative restraint in

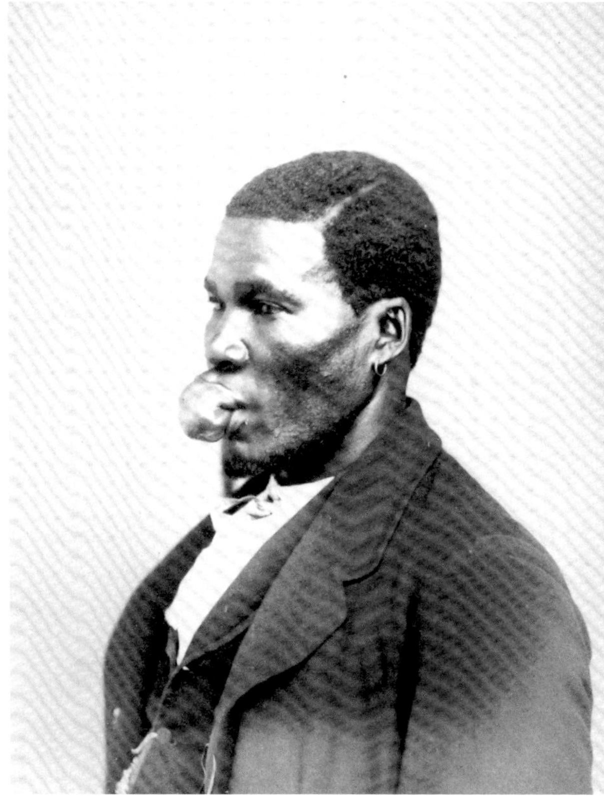

Fig. 51. Unknown photographer, "Plate VII. Venous Tumor," c. 1870, published in Louis A. Duhring and Francis Fontaine Maury, eds., *Photographic Review of Medicine and Surgery* (Philadelphia: J. B. Lippincott, 1871–72). Collection, Boston Medical Library in the Francis A. Countway Library of Medicine.

depicting the blood and gore of nineteenth-century surgery as compared with the real thing.[40]

Just as a large number of photos vacillated between categories of "life studies" and "bachelor pictures," many medical photographs also crossed boundaries into the realm of low amusement. Throughout the second half of the nineteenth century, some doctors weighed in about Amazons, or pygmies, who had been found and brought to American concert halls, fairgrounds, and museums. "To the joy (and often at the instigation) of showmen, debates raged among scientists and laypersons alike as to whether a particular exhibit actually represented a new species or was simply a *lusus naturae* or 'freak of nature.'"[41]

Despite their seemingly noble purpose of documenting disfiguring genetic and pathological conditions, early medical photographers of such subjects as the man with a tumor on his cheek had difficulty signifying how their products were different from the freak show souvenir postcards that circulated widely in the public. Exhibits at the Mütter Museum, including the livers of the popular circus stars Chang and Eng, demonstrate the particular mix of medicine and circus that emerged in the nineteenth century. Tom Thumb, the hairy lady, and other "freaks" all served as profitable subjects for promoters and photographers during Eakins' era. According to Robert Bogdan, by the 1860s, Americans bought upward of four hundred million photographs of "human curiosities" annually.[42]

Even in the circus arena, a mix of art, science, and even Grecophilia influenced the subjects and style used by photographers. In retrospect, there seems to be little difference between "teratologists"—physicians studying "monsters" and

Fig. 52. Mathew Brady, *General Tom. Thumb, wife & child*, 1863. Photograph. Collection of Robert Bogdan.

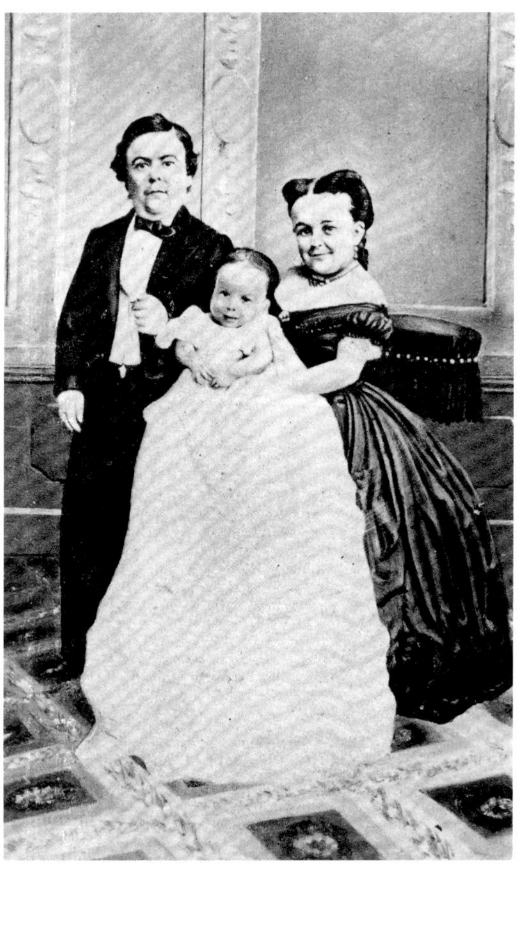

often searching for the modern equivalents of ancient mythological creatures—and freak show promoters like P. T. Barnum. Prominent portrait photographers of the day, including Mathew Brady, used their portrait-making skills and equipment to earn considerable profits in both medical and freak show genres.

General Tom. Thumb, wife & child (fig. 52) is a good example of how circus performers were photographed. Tom Thumb and his wife, Lavinia—"the most photographed woman of the century"—are evenly lit in a photograph with deep contrast, tight grain, and balanced composition. They are dressed in fancy clothes and surrounded by emblems of wealth. While stylistic elements make them appear more attractive for paying customers, the costumes and props help remind audiences of the storyline behind the pair. The "lovers in miniature" famously celebrated their marriage in 1863 at the Metropolitan Hotel. In attendance were the elite of New York society, including the Astors, Vanderbilts, and Belmonts. President and Mrs. Lincoln could not attend but sent a "spectacular set of Chinese fire screens."[43]

To keep the story interesting, Barnum decided that Tom and Lavinia should be a happy "miniature" family, so he had them appear with a baby, which Lavinia later admitted was not their own. In fact, Lavinia's similarly diminutive sister died in childbirth due to complications from giving birth to a five-pound child.[44] In other examples of freak photographs as well, Bogdan notes that subjects were "posed in front of ... painted backdrops depicting scenes that ranged from jungle terrain to Victorian parlors. Props were selected, costumes worn, and the pose struck—all to reflect the image that the manager and the subject wanted to promote.... In addition, negatives were doctored, with, for example, additional hair added to exhibits whose abundance of hair was their oddity."[45] Whether the storyline was abduction, or the happy family, photographers in the nineteenth century followed the lead of genre painters in using style and props to tell a story likely to sell.

At a time when the most sober physicians—including Gross, Agnew, and Keen—were struggling to standardize and improve medical education, accredit their members in professional organizations, and distinguish themselves from

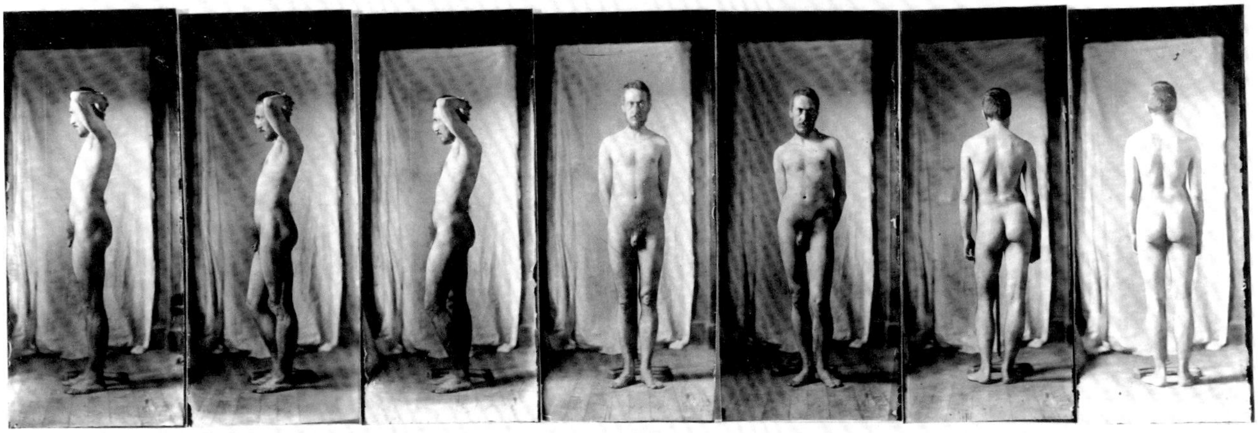

Fig. 53. Circle of Thomas Eakins, *Naked Series: Thomas Eakins in front of cloth backdrop, poses 1–7*, c. 1883. Dry-plate glass negative, 4 × 1 11/16 in., composite photo from seven negatives. Courtesy of the Pennsylvania Academy of the Fine Arts, Philadelphia, Charles Bregler's Thomas Eakins Collection. Purchased with the partial support of the Pew Memorial Trust.

"eclectic" practitioners, the association between human pathology and freak show fare was unwelcome to say the least. With medical photography growing in importance, it became increasingly clear that careful distinction—and professional policing—were needed.[46] The British medical journal *The Lancet* came under particular attack in 1865 when it published an engraving made from the photograph of a doubled set of male genitalia. The picture was condemned as a "mere mask for obscenity."[47] The goal in following years became the production of medical journals that clearly were not amusing to popular audiences.

During the next decades, medical photography evolved into a more discrete discipline that signified its unique seriousness of purpose by presenting the body in an identifiably different manner—chiefly by using stark lighting and neutral backgrounds. The resulting "non-style" in medical photography formed an obvious contrast with more commercial examples.[48] Martin Kemp notes that the pictorial conventions of Gray's *Anatomy*, whose first edition was issued in 1858, also incorporated a "non-style … designed to preach the objective values of a professional class dedicated to a high scientific understanding of the mechanisms of the human body."[49] "The apparent neutrality of the 'non-style' was itself a very special mode of rhetoric, the rhetoric of disinterested objectivity."[50] Medical photography in short evolved a style most notable for what it didn't have—namely aesthetic lighting, props, and narrative content.

This medical non-style is clearly embodied in almost all of Eakins' images of nudes, but especially in his last categories of nude photographic production—his "naked series." These images were markedly different in both style and format from the indoor and outdoor nudes that bore the influence of French and classical models. In the naked series, as Douglass Paschall points out, Eakins used the camera to professionalize art education in the same spirit in which medical schools and universities were standardizing and raising the reputations of their own curricula—creating, in short, a "professional class."[51]

In the case of the naked series, this meant photographing a series of models each in the same seven standing poses, so that bodies could be compared. The seven images were printed and mounted on cardboard strips, in the following sequence:

> Profile, heels together, hips straight
> Profile, right leg bent
> Profile, left leg bent
> Front, arms behind head or back, legs straight
> Front, with leg bent
> Rear, knees together, legs straight
> Rear, left leg bent.[52]

The finished product resembled a pack of anatomical flash cards that measured roughly three and one-half inches high by ten inches wide. The models range from a young boy to an elderly man, and they include Eakins himself (fig. 53) and his future wife, Susan Macdowell; almost all seem to have been made in 1883.[53]

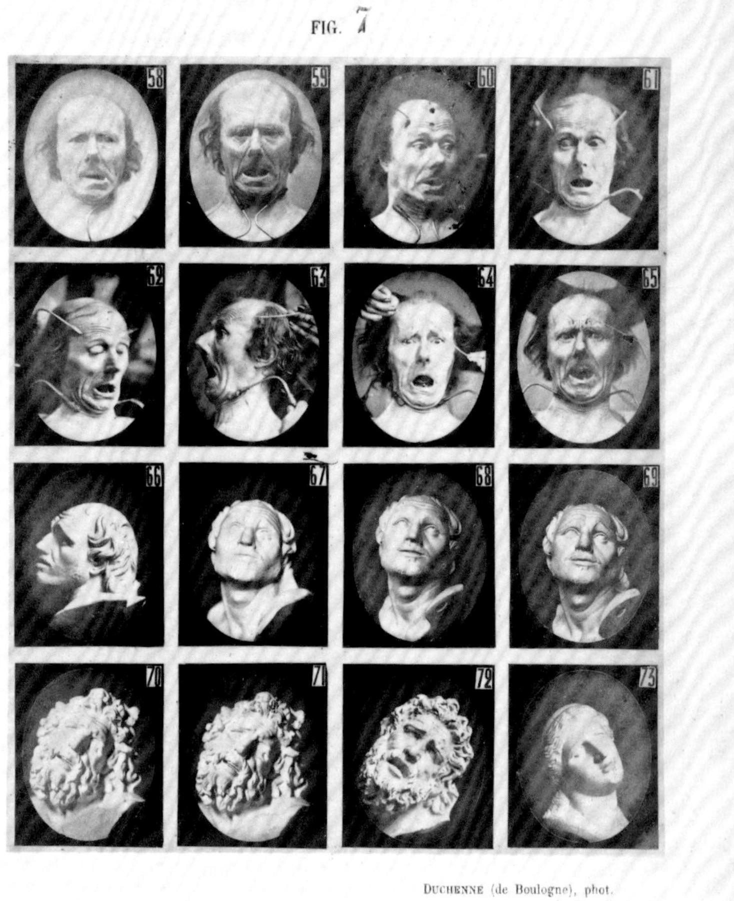

Fig. 54. G. B. Duchenne de Boulogne, "Fig. 7," from "*Mécanisme de la physionomie humaine, ou, Analyse électro-physiologique de l'expression des passions,* 1876 (originally published 1862). Collection, Boston Medical Library in the Francis A. Countway Library of Medicine.

Here the medical "non-style" was applied to artist's studies as never before—the figures stand in raking light, with no storytelling props or attributes—the only narrative is that they stand in the sequence of simple poses choreographed by the photographer. Although certainly the Greeks posed kouros and kourai figures in similar manner, it hardly is likely that classical themes were uppermost in Eakins' mind.

In comparison, G. B. Duchenne de Boulogne also toyed with the new non-style of medical photography for the use of artists, while maintaining an interest in ancient art. Duchenne recorded the facial expressions of a man stimulated by electrical currents in his book *Mécanisme de la physionomie humaine, ou, Analyse électro-physiologique de l'expression des passions,* first published in 1862. Beneath those frightening images, he compared the heads of famous Hellenistic and Roman sculptures to demonstrate that photography was more true to reality than art (fig. 54).[54] This was medicine as tragic comedy and entirely in keeping with the art anatomy tomes of men like John Rubens Smith. There is no question that Duchenne's appeal also extended to the types of audiences intrigued by freak shows. Keen acquired *Mécanisme de la physionomie humaine* for the Pennsylvania Academy library soon after its publication, but Eakins obviously avoided this sort of theatricality in his own mix of art and science.[55]

In contrast, Eakins' naked series aptly is seen by Maria Chamberlin-Hellman as a "photographic anatomy archive" that complemented Keen's efforts to assemble "a collection of published books and periodicals to provide the academy students with a wealth of anatomical studies and illustrations."[56] Indeed, the naked series was entirely in keeping with Keen's idea that the spine (rather than any emotional state) was the most important element for understanding and depicting the body. In his unpublished artistic anatomy manual, Keen wrote: "[The spine] … both in man and all the lower vertebrates is the basis on which their bodies are constructed. All other parts are but modifications or appendages grouped about the spine; thus the Head and the pelvis are modified vertebrae and the limbs are only appendages."[57]

Eakins not only photographed his subjects with particular emphasis on the centerline of the body, but he also then traced this central axis of the spine in line drawings, for example comparing his own body with those of J. Laurie Wallace and Jesse Godley (fig. 55). In both photos and line drawing, there is a distinctive absence of any contextualizing props, aesthetic lighting effects, or material objects that might suggest the social status or any other narrative context for the models. This was quite a different type of nude than the indoor and outdoor series with its easels, Arcadian references, and sporting activities—here was the body even further deconstructed of its social assignations, existing only as an example of biological engineering. While a Freudian analyst might see in the line drawing a repressed desire for homoerotic layering, it also simply is true that Eakins had stopped looking at French life studies, and started aiming his camera with "anatomist's eyes."

Fig. 55. Thomas Eakins, *Comparative Analysis of Anatomical Photographs*, c. 1883. Black, blue, and red ink and graphite on thin tan wove paper, 3 5/8 × 2 1/4 in. and 3 5/16 × 8 1/2 in. Philadelphia Museum of Art. Purchased with the SmithKline Beckman (now SmithKline Beecham) Fund for the Ars Medica Collection.

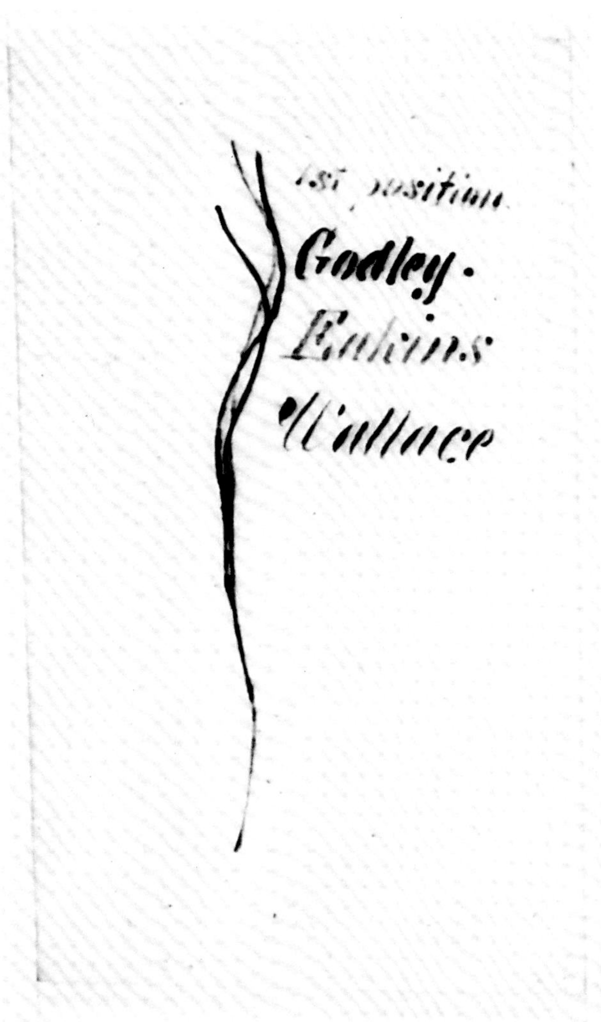

Eakins differed from most medical photographers of his day in that the subjects under his gaze were not examples of lusus naturae or pathological anatomy, but rather models who were "unusually good, or had any peculiarity of form or action which would be instructive," as he stated in the academy circular. We may recall that Keen differentiated between medical and artistic anatomy in two chief respects—compared with the comprehensive Gray's *Anatomy* he contributed to for medical students, in his artistic treatise Keen avoided discussion of interior structures not relevant to understanding the surface of the body. Keen also studiously avoided discussion of any pathological anatomy in his lectures to artists.

What Eakins meant by "good models" were those with no evidence of deformities and little fat that would hide important anatomical structures. Keen certainly was in agreement in his own curricular choices for artists. It is interesting that Charles Willson Peale made a similar distinction decades earlier. In his Philadelphia museum, Peale for a short time "exhibited albinos and other 'human curiousities' but believed they attracted too much frivolous attention. He thought that the proper subject of science should be regularly occurring specimens, not the unusual," as Bogdan writes.[58] Victorian preference for the macabre unfortunately superseded Peale's elegant Enlightenment model of public museum exhibition.

All the displays of human misfortune seen in freak shows of Eakins' era are troubling and sad, but particularly so is their frequent inclusion of Native Americans and other eth-

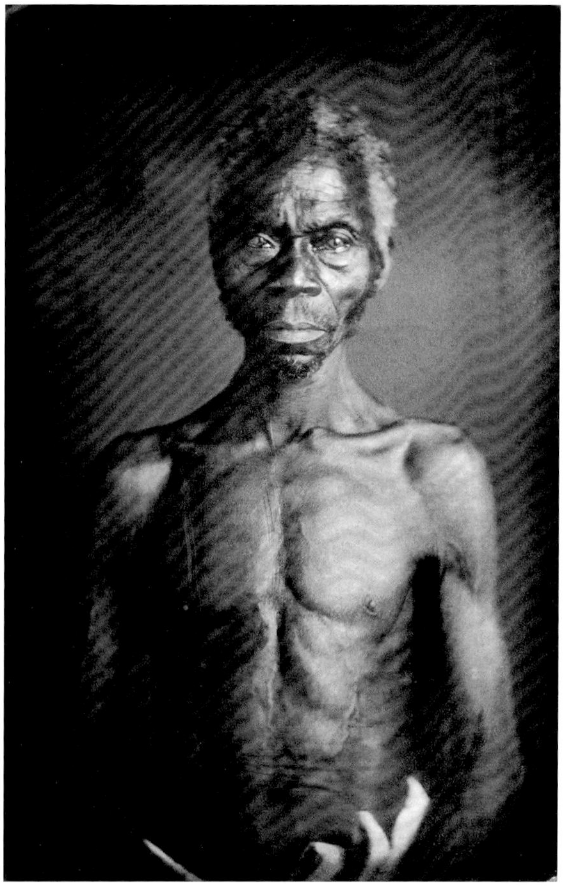

Fig. 56. J. T. Zealy, *Renty, Frontal*, 1850. Daguerreotype. Peabody Museum of Archaeology and Ethnology, Harvard University.

nic groups, who often were presented along with "albinos, dwarfs, joined twins, etc" as "human oddities."[59] Anthropological photographers cashed in on the interest in a similarly messy mix of art, science, and hucksterism as the freak show genre. Men like the Harvard natural scientist Louis Agassiz, for example, documented Native American life by photographing individuals with costumes, props, and backdrops that codified them as exemplars of static classifications. Here, the attributes of the portrait subjects were even more important than in pornography, which simply suggested a subject's availability. These photographs were meant to serve a serious purpose of documenting vanishing traditions—What do they wear? What do they hold? Where do they live?

In 1850, Agassiz began another kind of anthropological project. He hired J. T. Zealy, a South Carolina daguerreotypist, to photograph Africans working on local plantations, and to record the region of Africa they had come from. Among these now famous images is *Renty, Frontal* (fig. 56). The goal of such photographs was to chart the change in anatomical types across a geographic map. Such a project stripped its subjects even of social referents.

As Alan Trachtenberg writes, "Zealy's [photographs] convert individuals to tokens of a type—a different order of humanness. Both groups of images represent their subjects through what Foucault calls the 'eye of power.'"[60] Trachtenberg goes on to compare the anthropometric images of Agassiz and Zealy with the phrenological pictures of Mathew Brady, who documented the appearance of the mentally ill and criminally insane in addition to freaks. According to Trachtenberg's analysis, all of these can be seen to "refer to a code of rectitude presumed to make distinct the line between right and wrong, crime and obedience and, by extension to the racial hierarchy, black and white."[61]

One of the favorite techniques of anthropological photographers, who developed their own stylistic conventions in similar manner to medical colleagues, was to use a grid as backdrop for their subjects. As Trachtenberg notes, with the grid anthropologists could pretend to quantify "degrees of humanness" based on racial profiles.[62] Stylistically, there could be no better signification of the medical—here pseudoscientific—"non-style" than the grid. In place of the backdrops and props typical of life studies, pornography, and freak show acts, anthropological photographers supplied instead the preeminent symbol of the modern, scientific quest for quantifiable knowledge.

Eakins may consciously have avoided including models of color in his group of forty-one individuals (only one African-American man was photographed) because doing so inevitably would have signified an anthropological rather than an artistic or anatomical project—it is certainly true that, in the context of the time, comparing bodies across racial lines would have been an entirely different endeavor.[63] Even today, we have a difficult time seeing the body of the African-American model in the naked series without considering the implications of his racial status, rather than the center of gravity in his spine (fig.

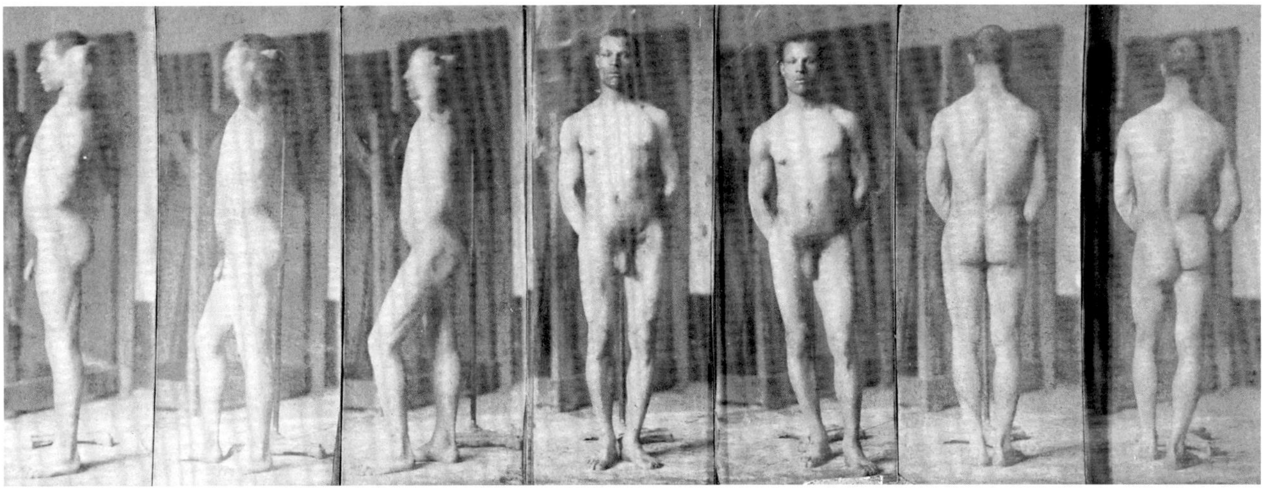

Fig. 57. Thomas Eakins, *Naked Series: African-American male, poses 1–7*, c. 1883. Seven albumen prints mounted on blue board, 3 1⁄16 × 8 3⁄8 in. Courtesy of the Pennsylvania Academy of the Fine Arts, Philadelphia, Charles Bregler's Thomas Eakins Collection. Purchased with the partial support of the Pew Memorial Trust.

57). Eakins had dissected enough black bodies to know that structurally they were no different from white bodies, but he still may have not wanted to distract from the goal of the project, which at its core was about artistic anatomy.[64]

There is another charged category of human subject that Eakins photographed—children. On a few occasions, Eakins photographed his nieces and nephews nude on their Avondale farm (fig. 58) and used unnamed child models in academic indoor and outdoor posing sessions, including the one boy seen in the naked series. For their own time, these images are largely unremarkable. Children frequently appeared nude in photographs and paintings in the nineteenth century without much discussion of the merits or potential dangers involved in such display. It may seem obvious today that photographs of nude children suggest their vulnerability, but their signification in the artist's own era was radically different.

Several gifted historians have studied the frequency with which Victorian artists depicted nude children. Among those, David Lubin stands out as an author who has attempted to help readers recapture the paradigms of another age. In *Picturing a Nation*, Lubin notes that Victorian culture believed in the innate goodness of children, and their lack of sexuality, yet it "seems to have put blinders on adults who could look at photographically realistic representations of nude or seminude *middle-class* children—representations that in earlier or later eras would have been deemed lewd—and yet not consider them as such."[65]

Rev. Charles Lutwidge Dodgson, better known as Lewis Carroll, is the leading example of a photographer whose life and work have been reevaluated with anxious care. He bought his first camera in 1856, and he stopped photographing in 1880, just as Eakins was beginning his own experiments. His photographs today are renowned for their technical and aesthetic virtuosity—but also for their suggestive subject matter. Carroll made no effort to hide his love for prepubescent girls. He spent a great deal of time with them, corresponded with them in passionate letters, and drew and photographed them nude when circumstances permitted. Vladimir Nabokov was a somewhat ambivalent fan of Carroll. He translated *Alice in Wonderland* into Russian but then created his canonical anti-hero Humbert Humbert, a pedophile, with Carroll in mind.

Nabokov's literary choice is indicative of the treatment Carroll has received by twentieth-century authors. As Douglas R. Nickel writes, "Seen through the filter of the modern age, Carroll's life and activities—his writings, his photography, his social relationships—all appear suspect, distorted by a postmortem diagnosis that reduces his biography to deviancy and his creative works to symptoms."[66] There is no doubt that Carroll's "diagnosis" is more difficult to accept when we also recall with fondness the joy of reading the author's marvelous children's stories, written in large part for the same girls he photographed.

In the past century, a number of biographers have attempted to contextualize Carroll's provocative images with different strategies. Carroll was particularly in love with Alice Liddell (fig. 59), the middle daughter of the dean of Christ Church, who served as the inspiration for *Alice's Adventures in Wonderland* and *Through the Looking-Glass.* Carroll befriended the Liddell sisters in the early 1860s, and in 1862, on a hot day in July, he made up the story of Alice on a boating party down the Thames with the three girls as avid listeners. In following years, he extolled his love for Alice and other girls in letters, signing them with kisses and protestations of love. After 1867, several of these girls posed in the nude for Carroll to photograph or draw, and he recorded all their sittings in a diary. He zealously guarded the pictures while he was alive, collected more images of nude girls from the photographer Gertrude Thomson, and then destroyed most of them before his death. Today only four prints and a few drawings of nudes survive from his large collection.[67]

There is no evidence that Carroll sexually molested any of the girls he spent time alone with and photographed in his famous studio at Oxford, where he worked as a mathematics professor. Nevertheless, in modern times such passionate and attentive behavior generates more than just the "current of whispers" that spread in the 1870s and 1880s.[68] Today, as Nickel points out, it "seems necessary somehow to pass a sentence on the Oxford don before considering a verdict."[69] Scholarly debate over the meaning of Carroll's photographs and the extent of his relations with his girl subjects has blossomed into a cottage industry of apologists and detractors. In his 1995 biography of Carroll, for example, Morton Cohen carefully documents his subject's relationships with girls, and demonstrates the pains Carroll took to gain approval from parents and acquiescence from subjects. Mocking other modern essays on Carroll, Cohen writes: "These analysts seem to be engaged in a contest to win a prize for the most outlandish reading of the texts.... One ... tells us that *Alice* represents Carroll's own birth trauma ... and some Freudians suggest that the book is about a woman in labor, that falling down the rabbit hole is an expression of Carroll's wish for coitus, that the heroine is variously a father, a mother, a fetus, or that Alice is a phallus (a theory that, at least, provides us with a rhyme). We can see her as a transvestite Christ if we

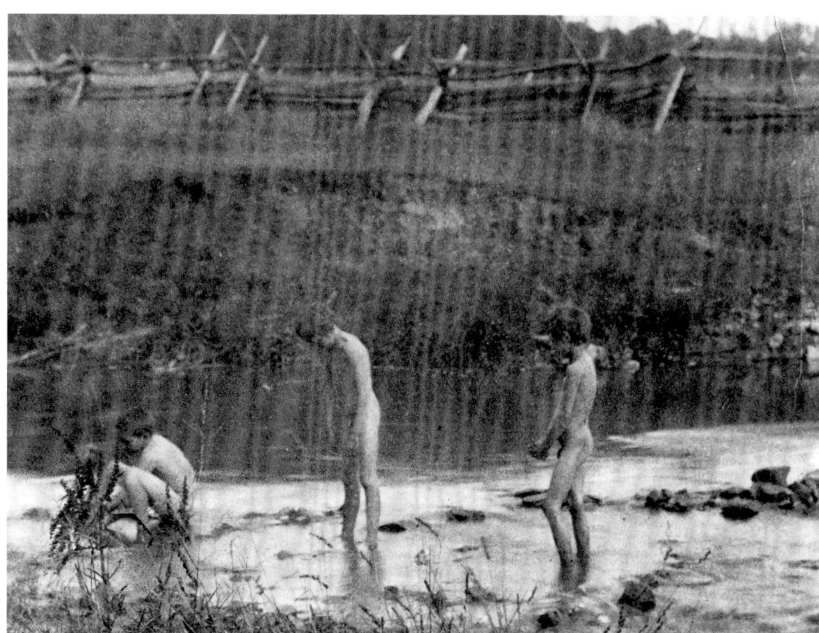

Fig. 58. Thomas Eakins, *Three Crowell boys nude, in creek at Avondale, Pennsylvania*, c. 1885. Platinum print, 3 1/8 × 4 1/16 in. Courtesy of the Pennsylvania Academy of the Fine Arts, Philadelphia, Charles Bregler's Thomas Eakins Collection. Purchased with the partial support of the Pew Memorial Trust.

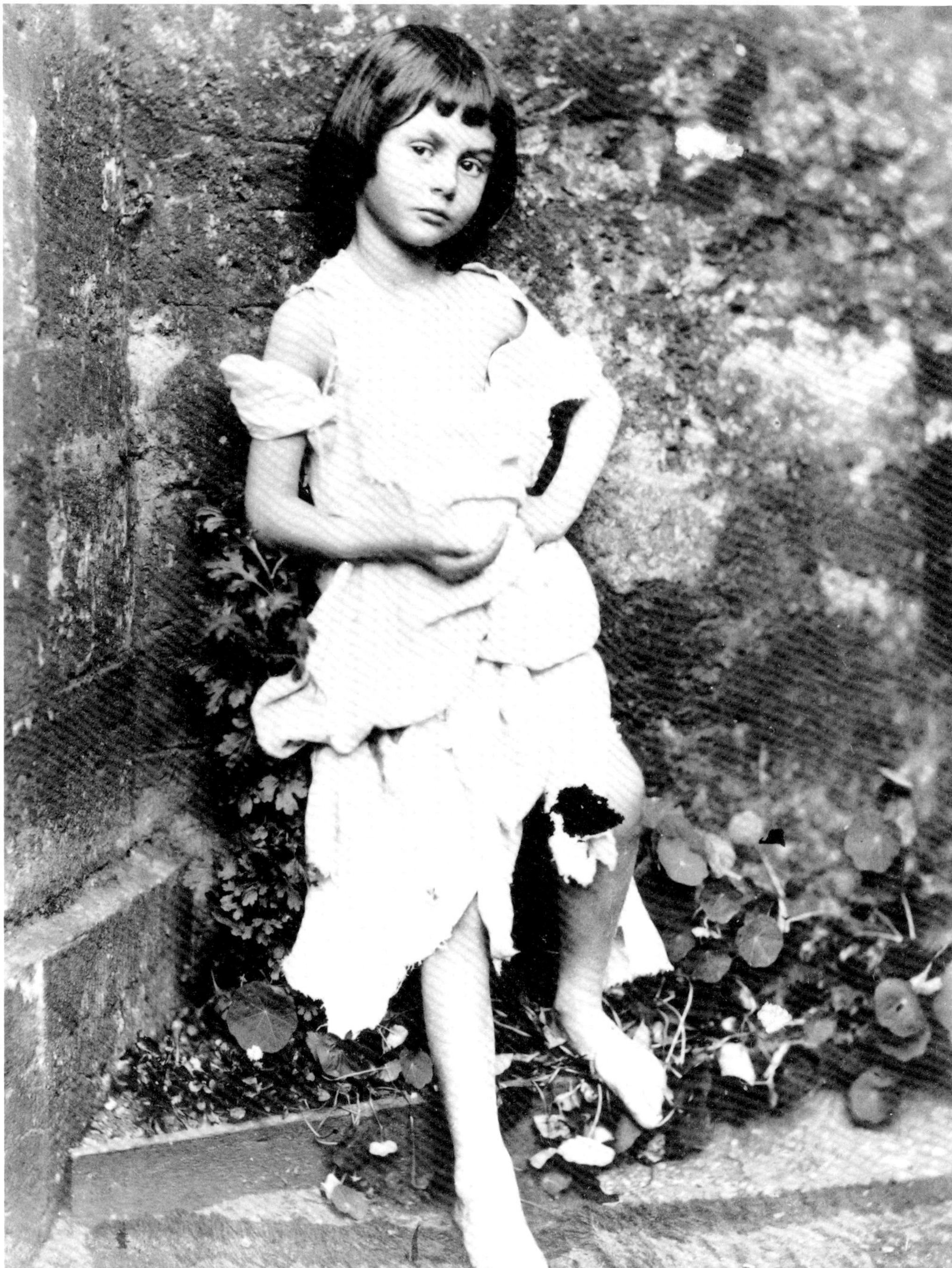

Fig. 59. Charles L. Dodgson, *Alice Liddell as a beggar child*, c. 1860. Photograph. Morris L. Parrish Collection, Department of Rare Books and Special Collections, Princeton University Library.

choose or, if we follow the tortured reasoning of a more modern writer, we can consider Carroll himself as the first 'acidhead.'"[70] Rather than accepting any of the claims he caricatures, Cohen chooses instead to read Carroll as a straightforward denizen of Victorian repression—sexless, if not without passion.

This type of interpretation presents its own pitfalls. Carol Mavor complains that such readings of "innocence" are generated not by historical perceptions, but by our own inability to discuss the issues: "Cohen is interested in presenting Carroll as 'repressed' by Victorian culture, and therefore innocent.... What Cohen fails to see is how he in turn is repressed by our own society, and how this repression governs his reading of Carroll. Confronted by the taboo combination of child and sexuality, such critics refuse to 'see.'"[71] Repression is, by its very nature, a difficult thing to document, and the same issues face biographers of Eakins as they do biographers of Carroll.[72] Nickel's summation of the problem of interpreting Carroll applies in equally apt manner to Eakins: "The burden falls on us to determine to what degree his photographs signify a real pathology, a Victorian cultural norm that has since shifted, or simply a blank screen upon which we project our own anxieties about the welfare of children."[73]

One of the most surprising aspects of Carroll's story for modern readers is that parents of the girls he photographed continued to deliver them up to his studio, often unaccompanied, for nude posing sessions even after "rumors" were widespread. Clearly, as Lubin notes, an ideology of innocence allowed these parents to dissociate their children's nudity from the possibilities of sexuality. Undoubtedly, the ubiquitous prevalence of images of nude children—even on postcards and advertisements—helped create a climate in which such display seemed benign.

The conventions defining acceptable public representation simply were different for children than for adults in the Victorian era—children's nudity was not deemed a problematic invitation to abuse, as it surely is today. Judging by Eakins' own letters and the art work that surrounded him during his life, this description certainly held true in France as well. In 1866, he wrote to his father from Paris about the new model in Gérôme's atelier:

> Our model is a little girl ten years and four months old. a most beautiful little creature. She has posed ever since she was three years old, her little brother nine years old poses too. and the money that the children & parents who belong to a theatre, earn, enables them to give their children an education and good feeding. She can write very well and has very sweet manners. She is very modest & timid, certainly not about her nakedness because she is the same naked as dressed.
>
> The past few days she did not speak at all, but now she knows the most of us by name and when the time of repose comes, she runs around the room to see the studies. We have had her now two weeks she knows us pretty well, we can see her character, and I don't think I ever saw a nicer little girl.[74]

It is unclear why Eakins wrote to his father about the girl who modeled at the école, but it may well have been because he was surprised by the experience and used the opportunity to report the child's exposure for the sake of art, and its direct benefit to herself and her family. Certainly in Philadelphia it was hard enough to get an adult to pose naked.

Although is it likely that child models were far more common in Paris than in Philadelphia, in Eakins' time it was useful to know how to paint children nude due to the popularity of "girl paintings" by artists like Seymour Guy. Mary Cassatt was relatively unusual in depicting naked children of both sexes, but even so such images hardly were rare, and they were not considered provocative.

In his essay on Guy's *Making a Train* (fig. 60), David Lubin argues that the artist's girl paintings reflect the post–Civil War emphasis on the innocence of children and their vulnerability to forces outside rather than within themselves—in particular immigrants, the poor, and the technological world. This was a welcome change from Sylvester Graham's emphasis on the innate evil of children that needed to be carefully doused with cold showers and fed wheat biscuits. As Lubin points out, images of innocence and vulnerability like *Making a Train* "constituted ... a popular discourse that in reconfirming gender stereotypes helped perpetuate the hierarchy of the sexes and ward off from a white, middle-class, male-dominated social order threats arising from militant feminists and other agents for social

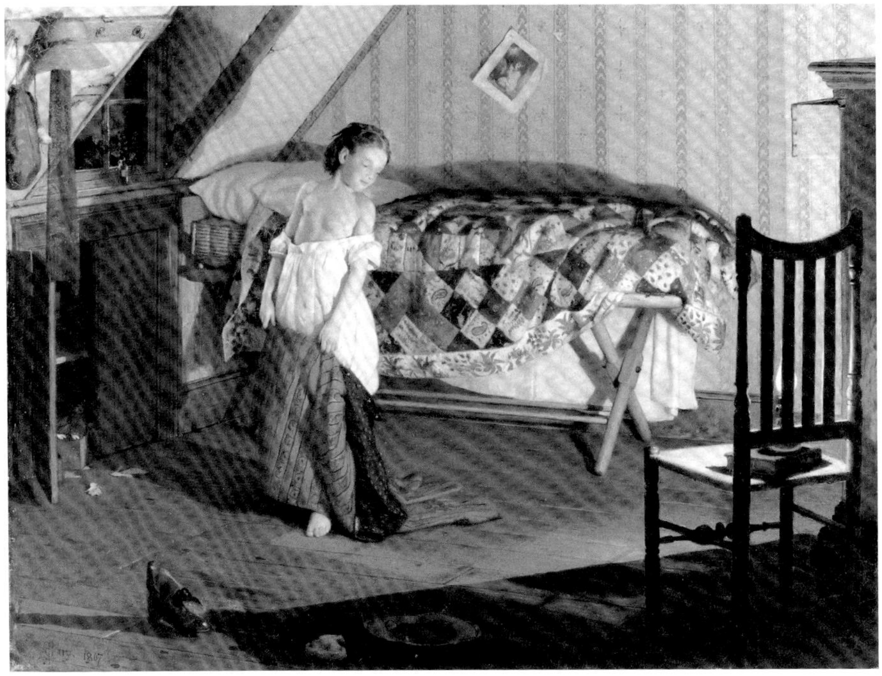

Fig. 60. Seymour Guy, *Making a Train*, 1867. Oil on canvas, 18⅛ × 24⅛ in. Philadelphia Museum of Art, The George W. Elkins Collection, 1924.

change."[75] Certainly, with her nightgown lowered to imitate a wedding dress, Guy's half-naked girl subject looks unlikely to storm any barricades.

Eakins rarely painted children, but when he did, as in *Baby at Play* and *Arcadia*, his images hardly fit Lubin's characterization of Guy's appeal. In *Baby at Play*, the young Ella Crowell, who is clothed, looks intently at her blocks, focused on learning both physics and the alphabet (fig. 61). Jules Prown sees the painting as an extension of Eakins' commentary on teaching and learning in *The Gross Clinic*; Eakins painted his young niece in the backyard of the family home "in the wake of the rejection" of the artist's infamous surgical portrait. Juxtaposing both learners—Ella Crowell the toddler and Gross the professor—Prown observes, "*The Gross Clinic* represents the culmination of a creative life; *Baby at Play* explores its beginnings."[76] In the case of the latter painting, there is little to suggest that Eakins was thinking in any way about the female qualities of his subject. Rather, he depicts the child in an activity, and a pose that transcends or rather predates gender.

In *Arcadia*, Eakins painted children clearly old enough to self-identify their own gender (fig. 62). As in *Baby at Play*, however, Eakins performed his usual twist on a popular theme by making the sex of his subjects ambiguous, or at least obscure. As Martin Berger writes:

> Despite his interest in physiology, not to mention the efficiency with which the depiction of genitals would demonstrate the model's sex, Eakins chose not to rely on such obvious signs. In the Metropolitan Museum of Art's version of *Arcadia*, Eakins represented three nude figures lounging in a pastoral setting. At first glance it is easy to interpret all three bodies as male, but close inspection reveals that the model lying with her back to the viewer is actually a woman. What announces the woman's sex is the small bun in which her hair is tied at the nape of her neck rather than any uniquely female bodily features. Although all the models are naked, what alerts us to the woman's sex is a cultural construction of "femaleness" (namely, her hairstyle), rather than the picturing of any biological differences. In the end Eakins's constructions of gender were rarely as straightforward as the mere essentialization of anatomical parts.[77]

Because Eakins (presumably) mixed the sex of the subjects in his painting, but provided few articulations of culturally constructed gender, his audience is not permitted to ruminate here on the innocence and benign vulnerability of girls, without also considering boys in this passive role as well.

Although Mary Cassatt often displayed the genitals of her baby subjects, she also managed to subvert gender norms compared with Guy by presenting both genders in the same poses and contexts. Because her subjects are so young, they

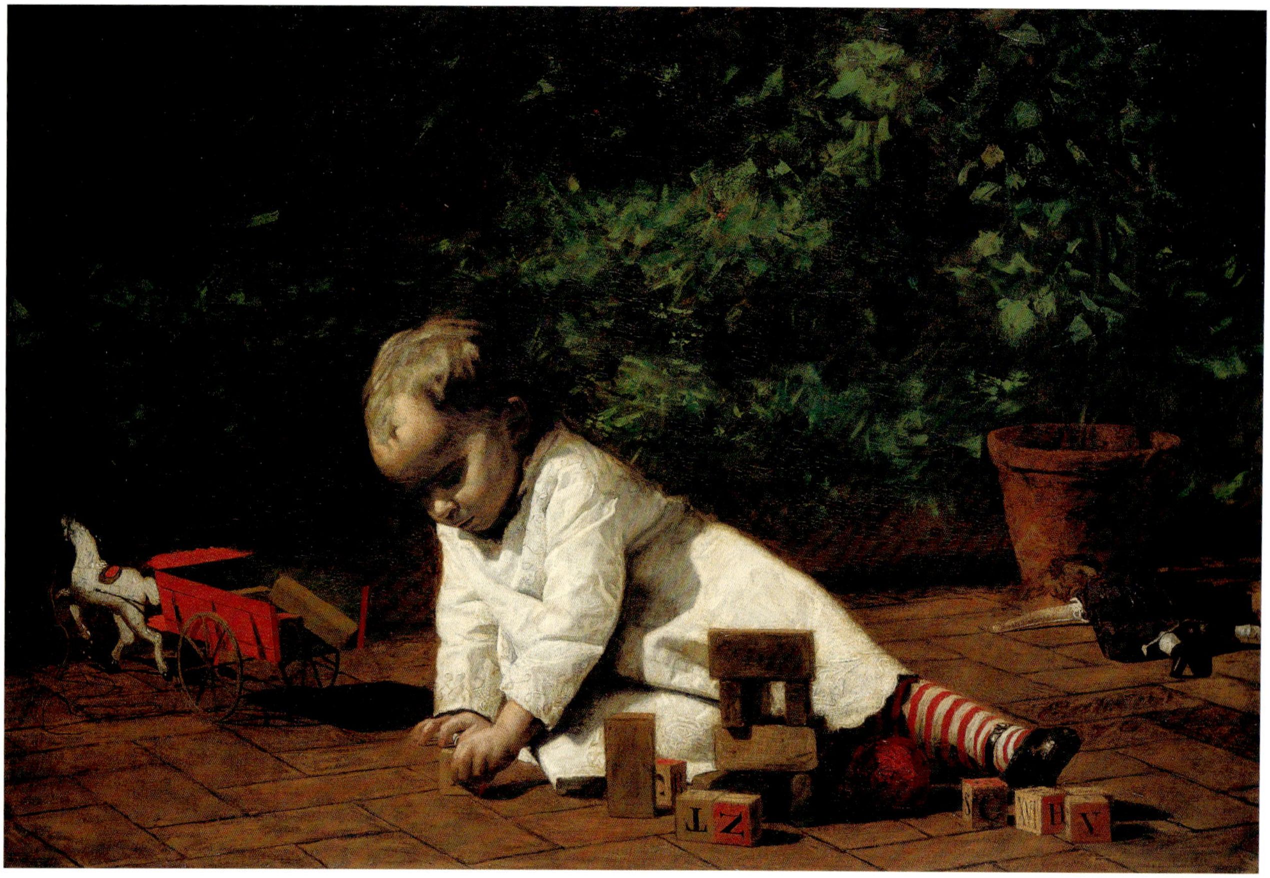

Fig. 61. Thomas Eakins, *Baby at Play*, 1876. Oil on canvas, 32 ¼ × 48 ¾ in. National Gallery of Art, Washington, D.C., John Hay Whitney Collection.

don't have a conscious awareness of whether they are boys or girls. In this world, babies are the ultimate proof of equality between the sexes—male and female babies are cuddled, bathed, fed by their mothers in the same nurturing manner, and painted with the same lush surfaces. When children developed the ability to distinguish their gender, Cassatt was no longer interested in painting them naked.

In Eakins' photographs of his nieces and nephews, he similarly pictured them at an age in which any gender awareness on the part of audience or subjects is at best only partial. These children may have been old enough to feel shy and thus turn from the camera, or Eakins may have asked them to turn simply because the view of the spine from the rear perfectly illustrated Keen's lecture on the growth of the body:

> One other joint and I am through with the Spine. Contrast the upper neck of the model or that of the Venus Callipeye and the Skeleton. See what a great hollow there is just below the head by the muscles attached to the back of the head. Something of the same sort is seen in a young child's neck, especially a baby's. The muscles are not yet developed. The erect posture not being at first a possibility there is no need of these muscles. But gradually they develop and fill out the neck. Where they reach an unusual development as in Heracles the head neck and back become almost a continuous vertical line.[78]

Seen through "anatomist's eyes," particularly in the Victorian era, there wasn't an age before which it was unethical to look at a body.

In her study of Eakins and Cassatt together, Linda Nochlin warns against reading too much into any of these images given the difficulty of recovering their original meanings.

> One might almost speak of Cassatt's lust for baby flesh.... The psychoanalytic terms "displacement," "repression," and "sublimation" inevitably creep into the discourse when the subject of sexuality is broached in relation to the works of both Cassatt and Eakins. Yet we must be wary of anachronistic readings of the

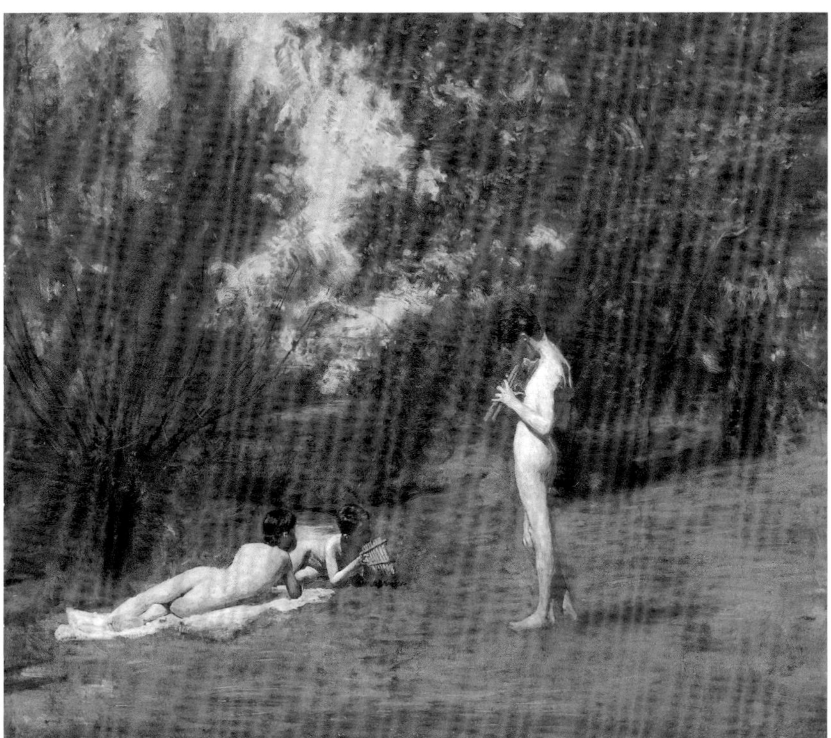

Fig. 62. Thomas Eakins, *Arcadia*, c. 1883. Oil on canvas, 38⅝ × 45 in. The Metropolitan Museum of Art, New York. Bequest of Miss Adelaide Milton de Groot (1876–1967), 1967.

> mobility of desire and its objects. For the nineteenth century, the naked bodies of children were often envisioned as simultaneously pure and desirable.... Although it is tempting to see Cassatt's lusciously nude babies as examples of Freudian "displacement"—to assert that in the absence, in the representational codes of the time, of socially acceptable mature objects of female desire she simply displaced that desire onto immature ones—this may not be the case at all. Desire takes many forms at different historical moments and in different situations and we decide what is "normal," what "displaced" or "repressed" at our peril. What Eakins and his contemporaries might have envisioned simply as healthy male bonding in the out-of-doors, in his various representations of naked men, boys, and adolescents, may well be read as homosocial or even repressed homosexual desire today.[79]

Nochlin makes a case here not for viewing Cassatt or Eakins as repressed, lustful, or innocent but rather for not making a case at all, given the difficulty of reading the sexual clues of another era. It certainly is true that what we assume to be erotic or even obscene today often was not discussed as such in the nineteenth century, and in general the qualities that made a work acceptable or unacceptable for public display seem curious today.

One of the most prolific critics of the day was Edward Strahan, who wrote a series of reviews of American collections for the *Art Amateur* in 1880, including in his discussion paintings of nudes recently purchased in Paris. In assessing D. O. Mills' collection, his most important category of concern was not lewdness but lifelikeness. In agreement with Inness, Strahan felt that if a nude was too close to the real, rather than the ideal, it was simply unacceptable. So, for example, Gérôme's *Cleopatra Before Caesar* was "realistic rather than ideal—I have happened to draw from the same hired model in Paris, and know certainly the extreme accuracy of the master's study." That accuracy was deemed a problem. The artist's *Snake Charmer,* on the other hand, today a disturbingly erotic image of a young boy, found great favor. The figure of the nude boy holding the serpent was described as "statue-like ... modeled with the clean precision used by the old carvers of ivory crucifix."[80] The centrality of the boy's exposed buttocks, and the large number of grown men enjoying the entertainment, did not cause Strahan to bat so much as a single eyelash.

So did Eakins think he was doing something bad when he photographed children? It is quite likely that this was not among the guilty pleasures of the medium for the artist. Children's bodies do not appear to have been contested terrain in images of the nineteenth century, despite their firm standing in that category today.

All the photographic projects examined thus far—formal and casual portraits, life studies, pornography, images of circus performers, medical, anthropological, and child subjects—help position Eakins' own images among the corpus of his day. From this diverse body of work, Eakins made choices to incorporate elements of style and subject matter from many of the categories, while also sticking close to the idea of artistic utility, defined in his own particular manner. Another photographer of his era and place also wove together strands of these diverse projects in his own work. In a final effort to tease out the threads of art, science, and sexuality that wound together around the question of what was acceptable in nineteenth-century nude photography, no example is more instructive than that of Eadweard Muybridge, whom Eakins admired, worked with, and later dismissed. The progress of their work together not only charts the ethos of the time especially well, but it also spans the decade of Eakins' interest in photography. After he abandoned Muybridge, Eakins put down his camera and returned to more traditional artistic methods.

There is little question why Thomas Eakins originally was drawn to the work of Muybridge. Since childhood, Eakins had loved mathematics, and he created perspective drawings particularly in the 1870s that allowed him to quantify his compositions to an extraordinary degree. In the late 1870s, this interest was expanded to incorporate the idea of graphing forms in motion, rather than the static objects typically painted by artists. Muybridge's experiments with photographic sequences of horses and people in motion were at the cutting edge of photographic technology, chronicled in sensationalist articles in the nation's most important journal devoted to the subject, the *Philadelphia Photographer.*

In the 1870s, Eakins' interest in this work also was encouraged and supported by his employer and patron Fairman Rogers, an important figure in the course of Eakins' life and the life of Philadelphia more broadly. Rogers was not only the chairman of the committee on instruction that hired Eakins at the academy but also a man with highly compatible interests and temperament. Trained as a civil engineer, Rogers lectured on physics at Harvard and then the University of Pennsylvania. In 1871, he resigned from teaching to pursue his own interests and serve on the board of trustees of the university, a position he held until 1881. "Rogers's two passions, outside his engineering work, were photography and horsemanship."[81]

These two passions came together in the work of Eadweard Muybridge at Stanford University, where the photographer attempted to create accurate successive photographs of horses in motion in the 1870s. The legend has since been refuted that instigation for the project arose from a $25,000 bet made by the former governor of California, Leland Stanford, with a wealthy friend over the arrangement of horse hooves during a gallop. Stanford indeed did hire Muybridge to use photography to determine whether all four hooves left the ground at once. And in response, Muybridge did set up "a battery of twenty-four cameras" on a track on the campus of Stanford University and accomplished the goal. The project seems now only to have satisfied a gentlemen's debate, however, rather than a bet. Whatever the impetus for them, the photographs Muybridge produced did prove with certainty that Stanford's most famous, scientifically bred horse, Occident, was fully airborne for a moment in its stride.[82]

Back in Philadelphia, Rogers and Eakins together reviewed Muybridge's published images in 1878 and were impressed with the work. However, they found inaccuracies resulting from the twenty-four points of view; Eakins set out to correct and "improve" the results. In 1879, Eakins drafted a letter to Muybridge, asking him to "dispense with your lines back of the horse in future experiments.... Have one perpendicular centre line only behind the horse marked on your photographic plate.... Do you not find that in your old way the perspective [is] very troublesome? The lines being further off than the horse a calculation was necessary to establish the size of your measure."[83] After making his own corrected drawings based on the photographs, Eakins was able to produce an acceptable view of a trotting horse as seen in a zoetrope—a device that spun a strip of sequential photographs (or drawings). The viewer looked at the strip through an eyehole as the device spun and enjoyed an experience quite close to early movies.

Proud of what Eakins had accomplished, Rogers wrote an article for the *Art Interchange* in 1879 describing the artist's success at correcting and adapting Muybridge's photographs:

> Mr. Eakins plotted carefully, with due attention to all the conditions of the problem, the successive positions of the photographs and constructed, most ingeniously, the trajectories, or paths, of a number of points of the animal, such as each foot, the elbow, hock, centre of gravity, cantle of the saddle, point of cap of the rider, &c.... The value of these investigations to the artist is very great. It is certain that nearly all the attempts to represent the gaits of either animals, or men, in painting, are extremely unsatisfactory, and it is only by thoroughly understanding the mechanism of the motion, that the artist will be able to portray it in a satisfactory manner.... There are many interesting speculations as to how this new information may be utilized by the painter, for which we have not the space at present.[84]

At the time of this essay, Eakins was hard at work trying to invent an artistic style that proved the worth of these studies—and Rogers was eager to help. In 1878, he commissioned Eakins to paint his four-in-hand carriage based on the research they had conducted together. To help establish the usefulness of the work for art education, Eakins made a zoetrope for the academy and placed it in the library. A student recalled, "when you turned the Zoetrope rapidly you could see the horse galloping and the man's shirt and sleeves fluttering in the wind."[85]

Although Rogers undoubtedly helped Eakins at the time, the long-term benefits of the connection are questionable. Rogers convinced Eakins that his idiosyncratic and unpopular methods were in the right—and then retired from the academy board of trustees in 1883, leaving Eakins there alone to support the unpleasant results of their agenda. Also, despite Rogers' promise of interesting ways the photographic experiments might be used, it isn't clear that Eakins benefited from photographic influences in any personal or professional way. When the painting Rogers commissioned, *A May Morning in the Park*, was exhibited in 1879, it met with harsh criticism for its odd mix of painterly and photographic effects. A reviewer of Muybridge's work in the *New York Times* went so far as to use the painting as a demonstration of the ill results of the photographer's project: "Like many other discoveries, the truths revealed by the camera were misinterpreted by some men and applied in such a fashion as to excite ridicule.... A painter in Philadelphia, for instance, made a picture of a four-in-hand in which the four horses were drawn according to positions which have been revealed as really those of a trotting horse, yet in effect completely absurd."[86] Rogers' departure from the board of the academy meant that Eakins no longer benefited from a supervisor who shared his narrow interests—and disagreed strongly with his critics.

Although *May Morning* ultimately failed to impress art critics as an example of how Muybridge's work could help the cause of art, Rogers, Eakins, and others in Philadelphia's scientific community were no less enthralled when it was announced in 1883 that Muybridge would come to Philadelphia to continue his work. The race for improved photographic technology was a compelling drama in the 1880s, covered in newspapers and magazines on a frequent basis.

Dr. William Pepper, provost of the University of Pennsylvania, can be credited with bringing Muybridge to conduct experiments on campus. The cost of the research—ultimately totaling more than $40,000—was contributed by a group of wealthy university scientists, including Pepper himself. Pepper supervised other necessary arrangements as well. Muybridge's research laboratory on the grounds of the veterinary hospital included:

1. Shed containing 24 cameras
2. Cameras for taking for-shortened things
3. Shed covered all over inside with black cloth for background
4. track about 4½ ft wide[87]

Despite all the expense involved, there is no doubt that Muybridge's arrival at the University of Pennsylvania was a proud accomplishment for Pepper—and a signature moment in his career as provost.

In 1887, at the time Muybridge published the culmination of his Philadelphia work, *Animal Locomotion: The Muybridge Work at the University of Pennsylvania—The Method and Its Result*, Pepper wrote an essay to introduce the photographs that explained his agenda:

> It is fitting that a few words should be said here in regard to the connection of the University with this work, and the motives which led its authorities to assume the supervision of it.
>
> The function of a university is not limited to the mere instruction of students. Researches and original investigations conducted by the mature scholars composing its faculties are an important part of its work, and in a larger conception of its duty should be included the aid which it can extend to investigators engaged in researches too costly or elaborate to be accomplished by private means.
>
> When ample provision is made in these several directions we shall have the university adequately equipped and prepared to exert fully her great function as a discoverer and teacher of truth.[88]

Pepper's justification for the expense of Muybridge's work is extremely telling.

Pepper was a medical school professor when medical schools were moving toward the Johns Hopkins model, requiring more hours of laboratory work and disciplinary study toward the goal of "discovering new truth," rather than the more practically focused clinical training of previous years. The ticket for good universities as a whole seemed to be to move in the same direction—placing more emphasis on scholarship and research than teaching. Eakins of course implicitly understood this goal as he adopted the same motive in formulating the curriculum of the Pennsylvania Academy. The academy and the university were to be places that generated new knowledge rather than just professing what already was known. To Pepper, Muybridge seemed an excellent candidate to add luster to the university's reputation as a prominent and distinguished research institution. Others, however, needed convincing.

Although Muybridge had achieved fame as a photographer, his work did not fall neatly into any of the new disciplinary categories. It was not necessarily medical, or artistic, or even uniquely a feat of engineering. Pepper used this to his advantage in raising funds for the work by creating an oversight committee designed to draw the maximum practical benefit from the work—and funds for its support. Formed to ensure the "thoroughly scientific character" of the work, as Pepper wrote, his committee consisted of (and they were listed in this order): two medical doctors, one physicist, one veterinarian, two engineers, Thomas Eakins, Edward H. Coates, as the new chairman of the committee on instruction at the Pennsylvania Academy, and Harrison Allen, medical doctor and professor of physiology, who served as secretary of the committee.[89] The committee included at least three Central High School graduates—Eakins, Allen, and Dr. Francis Dercum, a specialist in nervous diseases. The order of the specialties listed was carefully drafted to reflect the priorities and preferences of university administrators.

The original intention of the scientists from the committee was to obtain photographs demonstrating the movements and gait of patients with nervous disorders for the edification of medical students.[90] It is not surprising that the concept of photography for the purpose of medical education at this point seemed the most saleable to university supporters. The idea that Muybridge's work might lead to better treatments for nervous diseases was simple and direct, and it seemed to convey indisputable rationalization for the nudity in the works.

It also is not surprising that "diseased" people were the first to be photographed. Medical photography in the 1880s still focused on pathological (bordering on freak show) anatomy—at the university, the medical "non-style" was meant to be taken to new levels of quantifiable professionalism and seriousness. Muybridge, for example, included the image of a naked "woman weighing 340 pounds" in his series; he studied animals as well so that the work promised to be of additional use to the department of comparative anatomy and zoology, where Harrison Allen taught.

Although engineers were listed after physicians as likely beneficiaries of the work, in fact Muybridge mostly fell into this category. His experiments with camera shutters were complex and progressive, and ultimately the most obvious contribution of the work. Artists came last in Pepper's estimation. Clearly they would benefit from photographs that could save the time and expense of model's fees (as life studies always had), but the desirability of the end result still was an unclear and somewhat contested question.

Ultimately, the photographs Muybridge made reflected the interests of the committee Pepper drew together. In 1887, Muybridge prepared 782 series of photographs for publication, including 562 of humans, 100 of horses, and another 120 of various animals. The resulting massive publication was a relatively small sample of the photographs Muybridge had taken while working at the University of Pennsylvania, a total estimated at 30,000.[91] Eakins was on the scene for much of this time, assisting Muybridge, and also using the facilities to make his own photographs.

The details of the collaboration between Eakins and Muybridge on the mechanical devices used to photograph continuous motion have been well studied. In general, while Eakins is not given credit for changing the course of photographic technology, he is recognized for "making valuable technical improvements in already known devices."[92] What is more noteworthy for art historians interested in the development of photography at this point perhaps is not the mechanics of how it was done, but rather how conventions of style and subject matter were constituted or subverted in the process.

Muybridge of course needed to work especially hard to satisfy the first goal of the project, the documentation of pathological nervous disorders. Dr. Pepper was a specialist in such mental "deficiencies," as they were termed, as was Dr. Francis X. Dercum, P.D., Ph.D., instructor in nervous diseases, and another member of the committee. Dercum wrote of a case Muybridge photographed on his behalf in the preface to *Animal Locomotion:* "Mr. Muybridge having at his command a 'Marey' wheel, the writer resolved to test the possibility of photographing tremors.... The first case selected was one of typical *paralysis agitans.* It was a woman, fifty-six years of age.... In making the experiment, the patient, as in Marey's experiments on the normal walk, was dressed in a suit of dark-blue tights. On these a white stripe ran along the outside of the arm from the shoulder to the wrist and hand, upon which a bright metallic button was sewed. The legs were similarly striped.... The patient was then seated on a chair, and at a given signal she raised both the arm and leg of one side." Dercum was able to gather some data from this experiment, although one may question the usefulness of knowing that "the arm sweeps over thirteen intervals before the stripe touches the nose and chin." The "diagnostic value" seemed to lie in the professor's proof that the clearly paralytic subject could move only *very* slowly.[93]

Nevertheless, as a matter of record, Muybridge's photographs of this woman had succeeded in documenting pathological anatomy using the medical non-style in a manner more credible than it had been done before. Measurement was the project of the day, and Muybridge was in that sense somewhat successful. As for the medical value of the work, modern viewers may feel less confirmed in their support. In a letter to a colleague in 1929, Dercum recorded more of the historic work:

> He also photographed for me a woman in convulsions. The subject that I selected was an artist's model.... She was unusually intelligent and complied with the necessary details of the experiment. The convulsions were induced artificially by means which have been already described elsewhere. Both the beginning of the convulsion as she sat at a table, later in a chair and finally when she was placed while in convulsion on the mattress before the camera, are illustrated in Mr. Muybridge's plates. I may say that this was the first time that convulsions of any kind were ever photographed.... I need hardly add that the artificial induction of convulsions came soon to be regarded by myself and friends as of such a nature that they were early discontinued.[94]

By 1929, it undoubtedly must have been clear to Dercum that having a record of the appearance of artificially induced convulsions served no beneficial purpose and certainly did not justify the pain inflicted.

Harrison Allen didn't wait four decades to voice skepticism about the project. In the preface to *Animal Locomotion*, Allen was spare in his description of the impact Muybridge's work had on his own. Referring to himself in the third person, Allen wrote of his own essay:

> Many of the statements could have been deduced from data already accessible to the writer, but since he wrote the paper immediately after the inspection of the photographs his conclusions may be said to be based upon them. At the same time he has not hesitated to include materials not embraced by the photographs. Whenever practicable the study of a given series was carried on at the same time that the animal itself lay dissected before him. For example, when studying the photographs of the elephant, he had the good fortune ... to dissect the limbs of an elephant. He has also dissected the horse, the ox, the raccoon, the sloth, the skunk, the Virginian deer, and the domestic cat.[95]

Rather than praising Muybridge's work, Allen asserted here the supremacy of the real thing—dead and dismembered—over the photographic evidence.

In his prefatory essay, Allen further expressed doubts in general about the value of photography to the field of comparative anatomy, terming conclusions based on the photographs "not in all respects satisfactory." He nevertheless completed his essay in the preface to *Animal Locomotion* by pointing out examples of "flexion, extension, abduction, adduction, pronation, and supination" in the plates.[96] He then went on at length to analyze the photographs of the nervous patients, including one man "under the care of Dr. William Pepper."

> H.S., aged twenty-eight years, single, is an engineer by occupation, and had been working on a railroad in Wyoming Territory until three or four months ago, when he came to this city. When a child he had diphtheria, which was followed by dropsy and paralysis. Later he was thrown on a hot stove and severely burned, the scar being visible on the epigastrium. When twenty-two years of age he had typhoid fever. He denies having had gonnorrhoea or syphilis, although intercourse with loose women is acknowledged. Careful investigation fails to reveal any trace of specific infection. He has used alcohol in considerable quantities, but he has never been intoxicated. He uses tobacco in great excess, smoking as many as fifteen cigars on some days, and chewing a large plug of tobacco every twenty-four hours.[97]

Clearly, H.S. was not a follower of Sylvester Graham, "Reddy" Vogdes, or Francis Wayland. It is doubtful nonetheless that charting the patient's sins and graphing his spastic condition as photographed by Muybridge helped him recover from the inexplicable condition.

By 1884, it was clear that Allen was not alone in questioning the value of Muybridge's work. A series of letters written by Eakins' student and successor at the academy, Thomas Anshutz, to J. Laurie Wallace is telling of the mood on campus.

> You want to be kept posted on the Maybridge [*sic*] business. Well he is making some very nice photographs of men and women doing things. Such as throwing, jumping, stepping down and up, etc.
>
> These are all made as I crudely explained on one plate. So that it shows the figure at intervals of a few inches as it goes through the movement. These images, of course frequently overlap but do not seem to confuse on that account. The work is, of course, done with one lense.
>
> He has not yet done any work with his series of lenses and I hear they do not work. The shutters are too clumsy and slow. The university people are dissatisfied with the affair as he cannot give them the result they expected. Which was to photograph the walks of diseased people paralytics etc. so that by means of the zoopraxiscope they could show their peculiarities to the medical student. This it seems however cannot be done even with the best known contrivances So they would like to fire the whole concern but they have gone too far to back out.[98]

Perhaps simply because Pepper had taken so much money from important donors, the university did see the project through to completion, and the committee and Muybridge together negotiated a deal with Lippincott to publish the series, with introductory essays by Allen, Dercum, and Pepper.

Eakins was also supposed to write an essay for the book in which he finally would explain the value of photographic studies for artists. But it was not to be. Only months before the launch date, Edward Coates requested, and then accepted, Eakins' resignation from the academy. The essay never materialized. Perhaps because of the firing at the academy, Coates was the member of the committee to raise a rather obvious question: "The human figure series should I think be carefully examined and considered. If the work is to be published at all the usual question as to the study of the nude in Art & Science must be answered Yes. Otherwise the greater number of the 562 series [of human figures] would be excluded. At the same time there are *probably* some lines to be drawn with regard to some of the plates. That there will be objection in some quarter to the publication would seem to be most likely if not inevitable. Dr. Keen may be quite right as to the undesirability of conciliating one enemy but I am inclined to believe this point worthy of consideration at least."[99] The invocation of Keen's name is interesting, since he was not technically involved with the project, but there is no doubt that the academy and the university were intertwined as overseers of Muybridge's work thanks to the makeup of the oversight committee.

Given that Eakins' firing over issues of nudity had occurred so recently, it comes as no surprise that Coates should have raised "the question of nudity" before members of the committee as they looked forward to publication of the project. Indeed, Muybridge had gone far beyond even Eakins' liberal use of the nude at the academy in photographing subjects for his series. Children, disabled people, pathological types, professional models, all had stripped down for Muybridge's cameras on the campus of the university. Most famously, many of the university's premier student-athletes had been drafted for the project, demonstrating—in the buff—such sports as pole vaulting that were staples of collegiate athletics.

The university magazine reported the photography sessions with unreserved enthusiasm: "Some of our athletes have been photographed while performing feats of strength and agility. Twenty-four photographs are taken of a man in the simple act of turning a hand-spring.... It is hoped that athletes of other colleges may be interested in this work."[100] The daughter of Mr. J. Liberty Tadd, the first principal of Philadelphia's School of Industrial Art, modeled in the nude, and his widow was so unembarrassed by the work that she later proudly identified her as "the child seen in most of the photos."[101]

In 1888, a *New York Times* writer reported on the work, again with nonchalant appraisal of its many nudes: "The Series of nude and partially draped infants, children, women, and men teach us to analyze the bend, the sway, the oscillation, the muscular changes in human figures. In creeping up a stair an infant raises arms and legs in the same way, the same order, as a horse or dog walks. In walking a woman swings her feet very differently than a man."[102] What today is surprising about such neutral commentary is the sheer buffoonery of so many of the series. Can the reporter be speaking with seriousness about the women who pour water on each other (fig. 63)? Or the "woman chasing another with a broom"? The "mother spanking a child"? Naked boys and girls not only make an appearance in the photos—two carefree boys play leapfrog. As Marta Braun insightfully writes: "The scientific purpose served by a study of one woman chasing another with a broom or a girl falling into a pile of hay is impossible to fathom without directions. Are we to understand that there are … numerically expressed laws that can be derived from 'Chickens Being Scared by a Torpedo,' the final plate in *Animal Locomotion*?"[103] It truly is hard to believe that Muybridge, the enterprising photographer born near London in 1830 as Edward James Muggeridge, was not also in some ways a con man, posing as a scientist to get paid to visualize his scandalously silly, subversive, and often erotic whims.[104]

As Braun further points out, the manner in which the photographs were made held no hope of being rigorous enough to provide verifiable data: "In spite of the anonymity of the gridlike background in these pictures, the seeming objectivity of the camera and authenticity of results, and even the evident seriousness of the direction under which the work was carried out, these pictures are inconsistent with what we understand to be a scientific analysis of locomotion. The unsystematic and incongruous aspects of Muybridge's photographs effectively obscure any knowledge of the underlying laws governing the mechanics of movement. In many cases the moving limbs are hidden by drapery."[105] Muybridge's ruse—his guilty pleasure—was far more wasteful of time and resources than Eakins' hidden experiments with a projector carried out around the same time.

Fig. 63. Eadweard Muybridge, "Plate 406. Woman pouring a bucket of water over another woman," c. 1884, originally published in *Animal Locomotion: An Electro-Photographic Investigation of Consecutive Phases of Animal Movements, 1872–1885* (Philadelphia: University of Pennsylvania, 1887). From the Collections of the University of Pennsylvania Archives.

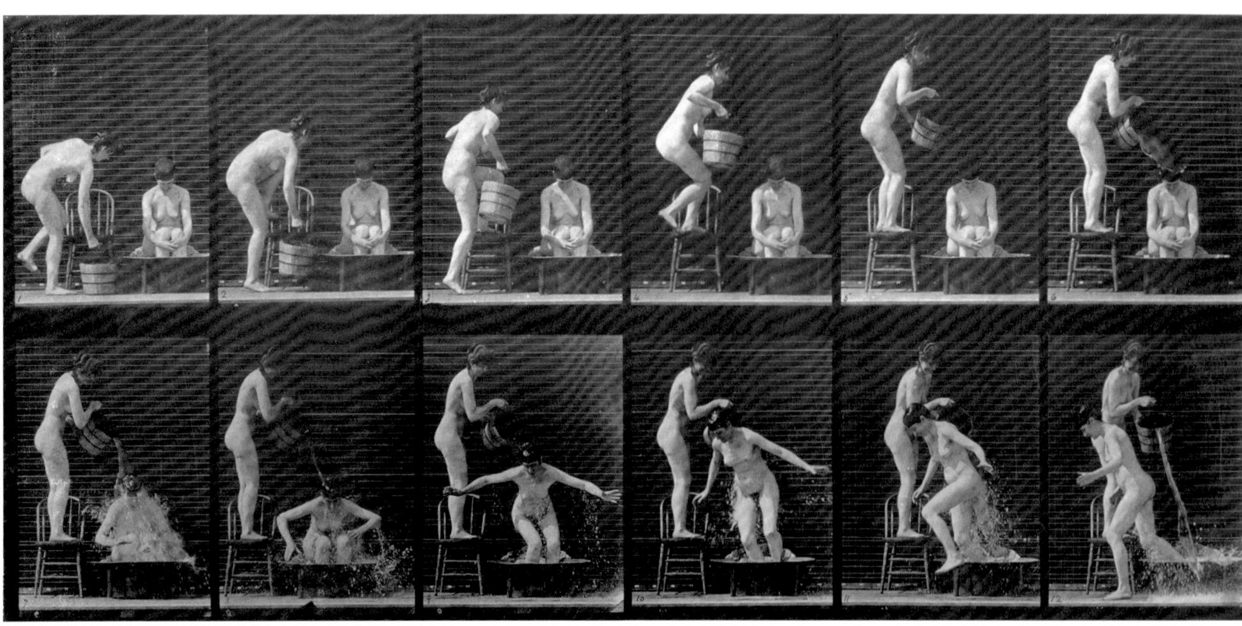

In retrospect, it is baffling why others besides Coates failed to raise the "question of nudity." In a climate in which even photographs of Salon paintings respectable in Paris were subject to seizure under Comstock's campaign to enforce censorship laws, how is it possible that "the question of nudity" could occur to so few as a potential difficulty?[106] As Braun notes, Muybridge's images in many cases were so close to pornography as to constitute a distinction without a difference: "The photographs objectify erotic impulses and extend voyeuristic curiousity in a language we now recognize as taken from the standard pornographic vocabulary. Naked women kneel in supplication and crawl around on their hands and knees or on all fours. They meet and kiss, disrobe each other, pour water down each other's throats, and dump buckets of it over each other's heads. They also smoke—a practice confined at that time to actresses or other 'loose' women."[107]

Coates' point, that the committee perhaps should be prudent though not prudish, resulted in an intelligent compromise. The entirety of the series would be published, but in order to limit the clientele for the photographs, Lippincott required a minimum purchase of one hundred plates, which could be selected from the larger group described in a prospectus that indicated whether the subjects were animal or human, clothed, partially draped, or nude. One hundred plates cost $100, or subscribers purchasing six series would receive all 781 plates in a portfolio.[108] Today, Muybridge's original *Animal Locomotion* survives in different configurations in libraries depending on the preferences of the original buyer.

Although his work received uneven reviews in Philadelphia, Eadweard Muybridge left the city a success, in contrast to Eakins' treatment around the same time. One might imagine that this difference owed to varying degrees of social connection and acceptability, but in fact Muybridge and Eakins shared similar reputations for their unconventional dress and behavior, and Muybridge in fact sounds like much more of a boor. Dr. Dercum politely recalled: "He was so busy that he did not have much time to go to a barber and therefore his hair and beard were at times unduly long."[109] Another colleague "remembered that a lunch specialty was cheese—for which he shopped way down on South Street—with live maggots in the holes. The maggots, Muybridge explained, were simply large 'cheese germs.'"[110] Muybridge's erratic behavior was so infamous in California that a modern neurologist suspects he may have suffered orbitofrontal cortex injuries as the result of a stagecoach accident in 1860. After that time, "friends and colleagues ... called him impatient, nervous, irritable, untidy, easily excited, and eccentric."[111]

A much more important issue than scandalous lunch fare and ragged appearance—but remarkably not as much commented on—was Muybridge's sordid past. In California in 1874, Muybridge had killed a man named Harry Larkyns, whom he accused of adultery with his wife, resulting in the birth of a son Muybridge never accepted.[112] At the trial, Muybridge's plea of insanity was not accepted by the jury members, but they acquitted him nonetheless. "Afterward it was said that they were all married men, and the jury foremen convinced them that they would have done the same if they found their wives had lovers."[113] Gordon Hendricks describes the silence of the committee members on the subject: "Surely everyone knew about [the Larkyns murder] but went out of their way to avoid mentioning anything embarrassing to their distinguished visitor."[114] Again, the unequal treatment of Eakins and Muybridge is quite surprising.

Even in perhaps the key trait that led to Eakins' demise, Muybridge set the precedent. Both men were entirely willing to "disrobe readily," but here again Eakins was outdone in his dangerous habit. In the spring of 1885, when Muybridge projected his first successful images for the trustees of the university, the distinguished gentlemen in attendance may have been surprised when they realized that the series captured Muybridge himself walking up a stepladder naked.[115] Eakins never went so far in his own institution—yet the reaction of University of Pennsylvania administrators was to grumble privately—and continue funding the venture.

It is clear that Muybridge and Eakins were in some senses kindred spirits as bohemian outsiders among patrician trustees. In this way, they encouraged and influenced each other, and it is not hard to imagine that the university's continuing support of Muybridge may well have led Eakins not to take seriously the complaints that were growing at the Pennsylvania Academy at the same time. Ultimately, Eakins' break with Muybridge had nothing to do with any of the photographer's peculiarities or scandals. Eakins' complaint was that Muybridge "was trying to popularize the experiments and Eakins wanted to go at them in a more scientific manner."[116] In retrospect, the naked series is at least as credible a scientific project as *Animal Locomotion.* But while Muybridge dined on his Philadelphia work for years to come, Eakins' naked series ended with quite a different result.

Nearly a century after the publication of *Animal Locomotion,* in 1978, Olympia Galleries in Philadelphia exhibited forty-one sets of multiple photographs of standing male and female nudes photographed in identical sequences of seven poses—the lost "naked series." The photographs had been found by descendants of Edward Coates, wrapped in brown paper and tucked away in a safe deposit box. The address on the package that directed it to Coates was penned in the hand of H. C. Whipple, curator and librarian of the academy who kept the minutes for the committee on instruction in the 1880s.[117] While Muybridge and his photographs toured Europe and America following their publication in 1887, Eakins' images lay in a brown paper shroud after 1886, entombed in a private safe.

Edward Hornor Coates was a Quaker, educated at Haverford. He went on to become a financier, but like Eakins he was intensely interested in scientific study of the body. He served on the board of trustees at the Pennsylvania Academy from 1877, as treasurer from 1878 to 1886, and as chairman of the committee on instruction from 1884 to 1890. Along with Eakins, Coates was collegial with Muybridge and in fact pledged $5,000 to fund the excess expenses of his work at the University of Pennsylvania.

As Kathleen Foster notes, Coates obviously received the naked series as chairman of the instruction committee during discussion of the scandals that forced Eakins out. Although he might have destroyed the group, instead he kept it hidden away, showing both his concern and his admiration for Eakins. Part of Coates' decision to abandon Eakins may have been at the prompting of his wife, an upper-crust classicist and aesthetic poet. Her mentor, Matthew Arnold, was anathema to Whitman. Mrs. Coates and Arnold spent their time talking and writing about beauty—it is highly unlikely that they enjoyed Eakins' work.

Coates' feelings about Eakins undoubtedly were more ambivalent. There is no question that he essentially fired the artist. A year later though, when James Scott rejected Eakins' commissioned sculptures *Spinning* and *Knitting,* Coates bought them from him and presented them to the academy, thus saving face—and fees—for the artist.[118] Coates of course is also the patron who diplomatically returned *Swimming* and took instead the *Pathetic Song* in 1885.

Because Coates ultimately had the background and training to appreciate Eakins' projects and pedagogy, he is an interesting focus for discussion of why it was that Eakins, and not Muybridge, lost his position. When Coates posed the inevitable "question about nudity" at the University of Pennsylvania, he insisted that it must be answered yes—but at the academy his answer was instead a resounding no. Given the example of Muybridge across town, it cannot be that the difference lay in the poses, or the lighting, or the gender or ages of models or their pathology or health. In fact, Eakins' photographic nudes all fit perfectly within their various contexts—the tradition of French academies, the popularity of classical example, the peculiar bent of medical research, and the depiction of the nude child as unremarkable. Eakins like Muybridge also refused to treat his photographs in a furtive commercial manner. The difference lay instead in Eakins' subversion of the most elemental rules of nineteenth-century voyeurism. It wasn't the subject being gazed upon that was so contested in the nineteenth century, but rather who got to do the looking, and in what context.

Although the style and subject matter of Thomas Eakins' photographs all fell into categories that were acceptable at various strata of society, he broke many of the basic rules of voyeurism operative in the age. Picturing working-class, poor, or "freakish" women, including the insane, as Muybridge did, was never questioned or considered an ethical infraction. Photographing naked middle-class Philadelphians, and then making those images available for consumption by other middle-class Philadelphians, including women, transgressed rules about class and gender distinction that Eakins should have known were immutable. When Muybridge photographed students from the University of Pennsylvania, they were male students, whereas Eakins used both male and female students from the academy as models. This choice simply wasn't available to Muybridge because the University of Pennsylvania was still an all-male institution.

Part of this also had to do with how males were presented to the women who might view them. "The proliferation of girl paintings in the decade after the Civil War can be explained in part by the prevalent notion that girls—as opposed to women—were still soft and malleable in nature as well as in physique."[119] Eakins' depiction of boys and men with the same conventions as women destroyed operative illusions about power, distinction, and privilege. Muybridge, in contrast, photographed men performing athletic feats while women performed domestic chores or mirrored the poses seen in pornography. The distinction of active male and soft, "malleable" benign female was preserved.

An excellent comparison with Eakins' subversion of the nude is Howard Roberts' *La Première pose* (fig. 64)—an award-winner at the Philadelphia Centennial at a time when Eakins' *Gross Clinic* was displayed only behind medical equipment in the hospital exhibition hall. Here was a sculpture of a fully nude woman presumably cowering at the shame of posing naked for the first time. In contrast, the models in Eakins' photographs almost always exhibit freedom and not shame. *La Première pose* may well have been so popular because it allowed its viewers to gaze at an ideal naked female body while being assured that she was not the kind of person who would enjoy it. Our sense of power in the face of her humiliation is complete.

David Lubin writes that "voyeurism, by any definition, suggests detachment, estrangement, viewing from a distance. It is the perceptual difference embodied by the voyeur—literally, his standing back from the scene he gazes upon—that allows him to take measure of his sexual difference, his so-called masculinity."[120] But what if the voyeur submits to the gaze equally as the subjects of his own? Kathleen Foster assumes that Eakins' eagerness to pose in the nude, and to display his own body, is the result of "latent narcissism and exhibitionism," and this may well be true.[121] But it is at least an equally compelling idea that Eakins disrobed in an earnest effort to demonstrate his point that posing for the sake of art was not debasing.

In this sense, Eakins might again be said to have invented a paradigm that would be adopted by later generations of photographers of homoerotic images. As Thomas Waugh writes: "In straight eroticism, gender-determined positions within a power hierarchy exactly echo identical positions in real society outside the frame, and thus tend to validate, if not reinforce, gender hierarchy. In gay eroticism, no such exact echoing is present. Here power roles are not pre-assigned and thus have the potential to be in flux—interchangeable, ambiguous, spontaneous, multivalent, and egalitarian."[122]

Fig. 64. Howard Roberts, *La Première pose,* 1873–76. Marble, h. 51¼ in. Philadelphia Museum of Art. Gift of Mrs. Howard Roberts, 1929.

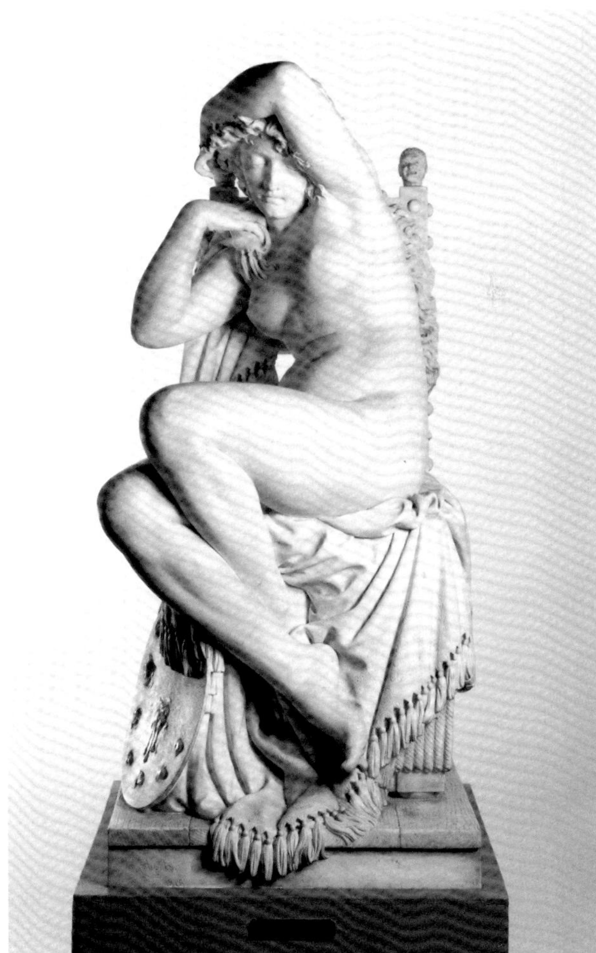

This list of adjectives is extraordinarily precise in defining the aspects of Eakins' photographs that were so revolutionary. The models—men, women, and children—strike the same poses in the same settings. Sometimes, poses seem asynchronous with gender stereotypes—Eakins with his hands over his head, for example, or Susan outdoors. None of the studio sessions seem carefully planned—sometimes a model's poses are as stiff and formal as the stances commonly struck in a portrait studio, many other times the shutter has snapped on a scene of utter informality. In all of this there is an easy exchange of power—sometimes the photographer snaps the shutter, at other times he is the model. Women lie down, men lie down. Students are models, and teachers are models. The obliteration of all these hierarchies layered a veneer of sameness onto all the bodies displayed. Muybridge never went that far, even though he did pose as well.

The fundamental taboo broken by Eakins was about who could look at whom. Women were traditionally meant to be looked at—they were not supposed to look back at men with the same "eye of power." This of course is precisely what Eakins did in his own institution. Elizabeth Johns describes the nude posing sessions at the Pennsylvania Academy as an "avowal of artistic community" that "set himself and his followers apart not only from ordinary laymen but also from less thorough artists.... He made students' acceptance of his attitude a carrying card for membership in his circle."[123] By including women in this fraternal "circle," Eakins gave them the power to be voyeurs as well as certified art professionals.

The Muybridge oversight commission in contrast found a way both to release the images of those muscular male student-athletes—but also to preserve control of the gaze. *Animal Locomotion* could be purchased only by wealthy buyers and institutional patrons—assuring an overwhelmingly male audience. In some ways, this model followed on Rabelais' (and Krafft-Ebing's) habit of writing the punchline to the dirty joke in Latin.

When Eakins displayed the naked bodies of his students in *Swimming*, and in the photographs circulated as life studies at the academy, he set those images free, and set women free to view them, with their own mix of artistic, scientific, and sexual responses. Jonathan Weinberg writes that although Eakins "did not include a woman in *Swimming*, he knew that when it was publicly exhibited, women would see it. They would be able to look closely at naked men, some of whom take the passive roles usually assigned women in art. In general, the modern male nude troubles the postmodernist concept of the gaze as being always male, and the object of the gaze as being always female. I think it is likely that Coates was disturbed by *Swimming* not just because of its homoeroticism per se but because such homoeroticism made the male body open to both male *and* female fantasies."[124]

All of Eakins' nude photographs, and his painting on view at the academy, multiplied the opportunities for fantasy, and extended those opportunities equitably. The images were too erotic for some, erotic to the wrong people for others, and for yet another group it is possible as well that the unerotic response they felt when they looked at Eakins' skinny nudes was sometimes part of the problem. Eakins' images of the body seen through anatomist's eyes can be viewed as denying the essential sexiness of the body. Sometimes, we rather want art, and in particular images of the nude, to offer us "pleasurable visions" that inspire our fantasies.

Muybridge, in contrast a slicker navigator of public morals, as Janine Mileaf writes, managed "a strategic positioning of his research between science and art [that] fostered work that otherwise would have been deemed scandalous."[125] Starting in the realm of science, and working toward the look of art and pornography, Muybridge's footing was in a field that already enjoyed less compromised access to the body. Eakins operated in reverse.

If we look not at what people espoused, but at what they paid for, a different picture emerges of Victorian attitudes toward the body, just as it would today if surveys of professed taste were compared with actual visual consumption. In the post–Civil War United States, Americans bought images that promoted sexual titillation through a choice of attractive subjects and aesthetic presentation styles (in the manner of the day). They also paid to see "freaks of nature" either as amusements or scientific studies, and ethnic and racial types that made them feel comparatively normative. Americans also bought self-aggrandizing and memorializing portrait photos in large numbers.

The type of photos Eakins made crossed so many of these categories that they tripped nearly every social guide wire. But we also must remember that each of these categories was so ill-defined—life studies doubled as pornography, freak show promoters and accredited teratologists shared interests, and artists and scientists including Duchenne, Muybridge, and Eakins all had difficulty staying within a singular disciplinary genre—that any inventive photographer of the nude was courting disaster. Although the nineteenth-century world was well on its way to specialization, with photography following, the rules for the medium were as yet even more uncodified than those established for painting, and all the terrain was contested—and filled with land mines.

For nineteenth-century photographers, the categories of image production fluctuated so widely that their boundaries were almost imperceptible. For us today, the subjects of our biographies—like the photographs—also sometimes fluctuate unstoppably between conventional and unconventional, sacred and profane. It isn't possible now to fix the image, and it wasn't then either. In the final analysis, all we can say of men like Marconi, Eakins, Carroll, and Muybridge is that they each used creativity and skill to find a new way for photography to serve as the century's most tantalizing guilty pleasure.

CHAPTER FIVE

Scandalous Exposures The Trials of Thomas Eakins, William Smith Forbes, and Oscar Wilde

Thomas Eakins, Dr. William Smith Forbes, and Oscar Wilde all endured scandalous trials in the late nineteenth century as a result of their infractions of rules governing human bodies. For Eakins, the bodies were nude and female, for Forbes they were dead and black, and for Wilde, young and male. Although Wilde's trial took place in London's Old Bailey, Forbes' in the courts of Philadelphia, and Eakins' in the less litigious arenas of workplace and home, all three men were front-page news in Philadelphia in the 1880s and 1890s.

The scandals Thomas Eakins instigated and then endured fall into two major periods: 1885–86, and then 1895–97. The first round of scandals was far more public, and demonstrates how vital and loud discussions were about art, art education, and nudity in the late nineteenth century. The second round of scandals, centering on accusations that Eakins destabilized his niece "in the style of Oscar Wilde," demonstrates the opposite—a conversation that took place in private homes. Both of Eakins' rounds of major controversies were informed by the scandals of other men—Forbes in 1882, and Wilde in 1895.

It is rare that disputes about art education ascend to the pages of major city newspapers today, but in 1886 the resignation of Thomas Eakins from the Pennsylvania Academy of the Fine Arts was clearly newsworthy. On February 15, page one of the *Philadelphia Evening Item* led with the headline "The End of Eakins," and the *Philadelphia Evening Bulletin* featured an article titled "Professor Eakins Resigns" on page six.

These early notices blamed "trouble in the life class" that had been "brewing for some time" as the cause of Eakins' ouster. The *Bulletin* reporter secured a statement from an unnamed board member (or "director") who attributed the issue to a "difference of opinion" about methods of instruction that amounted to a "tempest in a teapot." The informant expressed his confidence in Eakins as a teacher and a student of Gérôme, but also noted that the artist "had a number of enemies who made trouble for him and the committee thought it best for the interests of the class that he should resign."[1]

The *Evening Item* was far less generous in its treatment of Eakins. Terming the artist "eccentric," the paper went on to complain that he always had been "a mistake." The reporter continued: "Very few of the scholars who graduated from the Academy have amounted to anything.... The majority of the directors have been in favor of Mr. Eakins. And why? Principally because they know very little about Art, and because they were being constantly informed by Mr. Eakins' friends that he was a pupil of Gérôme. And so he was. But who would ever have known it? Mr. Eakins cannot paint a good picture. His latest work, 'The Bathers,' which was in the December exhibition of the Academy, was more than usually bad."[2] The reference here to the style of *Swimming*, which had been exhibited at the academy in the fall, is a good indication either that the public cared little about the display of nude men as subject matter in paintings, or that they were not willing to discuss the matter. Even in the midst of recounting the artist's sins, the morality of the display never made it to the long list of the *Item*'s complaints.

The reality of the situation inside the academy was far different from these accounts. In contrast to newspaper reports, which only hinted at "trouble" in the life class, it is clear that nude posing by female students was the chief impetus for the directors' actions. Board minutes between 1882 and 1885 reveal a fair amount of friction between Eakins and his supervisors: several people wrote to complain about the exposure of female students to male nude models, female students complained about the impropriety of having male students pose in their life classes, Eakins demanded a substantial pay raise in April 1885, and then in the fall of that year he removed the loincloth from a male model in front of female students when such uncovering expressly had been forbidden by the board. Although we might imagine any one of these incidents resulting in Eakins' censure, in fact none of them rose to the level of board action—the artist was undeniably a difficult employee, but not yet indefensible.

What finally moved academy directors to ask for Eakins' resignation were complaints by the artist's "enemies" that female students had posed for each other, for their professor, and before the camera. Following a board meeting at which grievances were aired, Edward Coates, chairman of the committee on instruction, informed Eakins by note on February 8, 1886, "a change in the management of the Schools is deemed to be necessary." It may have been at this time that Coates came into possession of the "naked series." As Kathleen Foster and Cheryl Leibold amply demonstrate in their comprehensive review of the "trouble" at the academy, Coates' phraseology in this brief note summarized a much larger discussion.[3] Eakins tendered his resignation the next day.

At the beginning of his ordeal, Eakins had little understanding of the depth of the accusations against him. His first letter to Coates after his resignation explained the circumstances in which he had displayed his pelvis to Amelia Van Buren (who remained an ally throughout his life, whether or not she approved of the display). After providing his version of the incident, Eakins wrote: "If the Academy Directors wished to enquire into my personal or professional affairs in order to act upon what it seems to me did not concern them, I think they should have at least investigated them, and if any thing suspicious appeared to them, they should have told me just what it was, and have asked of me the explanation. The whole conspiracy against me was so secret that I could only guess at my accusers and of what they might have accused me, nor would any one enlighten me. The subsequent action of the Directors was to my mind cowardly cruel and dishonorable."[4] Eakins was only beginning to understand the "trouble" his enemies had made for him. He should have known that his photographs of and with nude students were potentially far more damaging than the exposure of one part of his body, on one occasion, to a single collegial woman. Yet at this point he seemed to think he had found out the whole truth of the matter.

Of course, the photos were not a secret at all, and in March, Eakins wrote back to Coates with a letter that reveals the infilling of many more gaps in understanding on his part. Eakins' tone in this letter, filled with crossed-out passages, is furious. He starts by rejecting Coates' suggestion in a February 18 letter (now lost) that the artist's own friends were the most to blame for his "unpleasant consequences" (presumably because they had agreed to pose in the nude). Eakins goes on to contest Coates' statement that the "facts in the case" had remained within the committee: "No sooner was I out of the school than your same informers repeated even to new scholars in the school, and to outsiders that I had made photographs of my female pupils naked. And that I was a libertine, which is a lie." Eakins then indicated his understanding that his brother-in-law, Frank Stephens, was at the center of the rumor mill. Stephens was married to Eakins' youngest sister, Caroline, and living in the family home on Mount Vernon Street at the time. Frank Stephens' cousin Charley was engaged to Alice Barber, who appears in many of the nude photographs.

Next, Eakins laid out a series of justifications for his photographic project, all conveyed in an emotional tirade: "My figures at least are not a bunch of clothes with a head & hands sticking out but more nearly resemble strong living body's [*sic*] than most pictures show, & my subjects have always been decent.... And in the latter end of a life so spent in study, you at least can imagine that painting is with me a very *serious* study, that I have but little patience with the false modesty which is the greatest enemy to all figure painting." Eakins concluded his passionate letter to Coates by noting, "I myself see many things clearer now than I did when in my first surprise I was stabbed from I knew not where."[5] Eakins gradually was coming to understand the actions and motives of his "enemies," but so were the readers who understood the academy trouble only through public newspaper accounts.

On February 15, newspaper readers in Philadelphia knew only vaguely that life class study, aesthetics, and enemies were involved in the trouble at the academy. The nature of the news story quickly shifted, however. Just a day after the *Philadelphia Press* and the *Item* reported Eakins' dismissal, they turned to coverage of the aftermath of this event at the academy. On February 16, the *Evening Bulletin* published a story headlined "Indignant Art Students: They Demand the Return of Mr. Eakins."

> Upwards of forty art students, members of the life class at the Academy of the Fine Arts, marched down Chestnut Street about 10 o'clock last night from Seventeenth street to the studio of Mr. Thomas Eakins.... Each man wore a large E on the front of his hat as a symbol that he was for Eakins first, last and all the time. On reaching this point they came to a halt and cheered lustily for their head instructor. After waiting a reasonable length of time for him to appear, and seeing no sign of his appearance, they dispersed to their homes. Prior to this demonstration they met at the rooms of one of their number and drew up a petition requesting the Board of Directors of the Academy to endeavor to persuade Mr. Eakins to withdraw his resignation, which was recently sent in, and return to his old place. The students allege that the disaffection in the class is confined to a comparative few who have exhibited a prudery that is, to say the least, unbecoming among those who pretend to make a study of art. The methods of Mr. Eakins are those followed in all the art schools abroad, and there has been, it is held, nothing ungentlemanly or indelicate in his actions, which is the gist of the charges that have been brought against him. The lady pupils of the Academy held a meeting this morning and drew up a petition similar to that signed by the gentlemen last evening, to which the names of all but a dozen were appended. It is said that should the directors refuse to comply with the request thus made, the students, with a few exceptions, will leave the Academy, and accept Mr. Eakins's offer to teach them outside the institution.[6]

Three days into the scandal, nudity clearly had emerged as the central issue in public coverage of the events. The directors, though irritated, refused to reinstate the artist.

Over the course of the next week, the threat of an alternative art academy provoked a great deal of notice in the press. Several papers quoted a board member who stated: "If all left, we could close the school and save money. Why, we have an annual deficiency of about $7,000, and are now trying to raise an endowment fund of $100,000, which it is hoped will keep the school running without a loss." The *Item* was quick to blame the academy's financial predicament on Eakins. "We imagine the reason why the school is *not* supporting itself is very clear.... Let the Directors arouse themselves. As for Mr. Eakins, does anyone imagine he will not sink into obscurity and leave the city?"[7] The hostile reporter at the *Item* certainly seems to have hoped so.

Instead, Eakins' supporters rose in dramatic support of their mentor, and on Friday, February 19, the papers reported that "nearly forty students" had met in one of the rooms "at the College of Physicians" to organize an Art Students' League. The *Philadelphia Press* offered a temperate account of the meeting: "H. C. [*sic*] Cresson, a fellow-student with Professor Eakins under Gerome [*sic*], called the meeting to order. He said that the charges against Eakins were that he was too much devoted to the nude and made unnecessary exposures of subjects in the anatomical class. As the students were studying art for art's sake he did not think it right that they should be hampered, in the pursuit by prudishness and false modesty, and therefore it would be wise to form a league."[8] By now, it was clear to all concerned, and to newspaper readers in the city, that exposure of bodies for the sake of art was the heart of the trouble at the academy. It probably is not an accident that the students met at the College of Physicians to assert their right to look at the nude. Only doctors enjoyed the privilege of looking at fully nude living bodies in nineteenth-century Philadelphia, and progressive young artists wanted that privilege as well.

On the same day, the 19th, the *Evening Bulletin* followed this relatively neutral account by chiding the rebellious students for their "failure to appreciate the fact that the Life School of the Academy is a benefaction established by the directors for the good of the students.... It is their School and nobody's else. It is for them to determine what shall and shall not be done in it." The echoes here of the conflict between Rembrandt Peale, fellow students, and the directors of the Pennsylvania Academy in 1810 are striking. The directors in both cases of course did in fact own the school and determine its fate. Art students in the 1880s, as in 1810, did not like taking direction about art matters from businessmen.

The reporter in the *Bulletin* was more explicit than previous authors in explaining the "general facts" that had led students to rebel. The story continued: "Mr. Eakins has for a long time entertained the most 'advanced' views, as they are often called, regarding the methods of study in life schools. Teaching large classes of women, as well as of men, he holds that, both to the living model in the drawing-room and the dead subject in the anatomical lecture and dissecting room, Art knows no sex. He has pressed this always-disputed doctrine with much zeal and with much success, until he has impressed it so strongly upon a majority of the young men that they have sided with him when he has pushed his views to their last logical illustration by compelling or seeking to compel the women entrusted to his direction to face the absolute nude both as to the living and the dead subject."[9] Although Eakins heartily would have agreed that "the absolute nude" was a logical manifestation of his principle that "Art knows no sex," the editor commenting on the situation was not impressed with the argument.

The essay went on to claim that the women of the academy had been the ones to "revolt at the tests forced upon them.... They appreciate the value of the privileges afforded by the Academy so much that there is probably not one among them who would have made open protest against any of its methods if there had been any legitimate room for two opinions on the subject. A woman is never entitled to any special praise for following her womanly instincts, as she is never entitled to much consideration when she ignores them." The women of the academy and the city here were forcefully instructed that they would never openly protest their (male) patrons, and that "womanly instincts" of course would rebel at the notion of equal education. The petition reportedly drafted in support of Eakins by female students never was mentioned again.

The women of the academy who had been involved in its most advanced study from the nude can have had little doubt that their reputations were in severe danger as they followed coverage of events in city newspapers. Rather than step forward and declare their right to equal education (as they had been reminded by the press they would never dare to do), they stayed out of the fray, or else perhaps were ignored. Reporters never revealed that female and male students and their professor were posing for and with each other nude, or that any nude photographs were made. Letters between Eakins and Coates, and some other players in the drama, suggest that the directors were effective at preventing the press from reporting details of the matter that would have compromised the reputations of female students. It also is possible that reporters themselves made the choice not to fully disclose the details of the matter due to their own sense of propriety. In either case, the result was that, publicly at least, women were reported to be proper, grateful to their (gentlemen) benefactors, and understanding that they should not be exposed to the male nude for their own sake.

The last gasps of the episode in city newspapers included hostile coverage of the rebellious students whom Eakins agreed to teach in the new Art Students' League. An inflamed academy board member speaking in the *Item* accused the students of staying with Eakins "to gratify their imagination." H. T. Cresson, the new president of the league, retorted in a front-page letter to the editor the next day that the students who stuck by their teacher were "as much to be respected for their virtues as any of the Pennsylvania Academy's directors. They desire to study THE ENTIRE NUDE FIGURE, not because it affords them pleasure to look at it, but because it is the only true way to obtain the necessary experience to represent a draped figure in its movement and proportion."

Cresson, who had studied with Gérôme, went on to mention the Parisian artist six times in defending Eakins and his method of study in his short essay. Toward the end of his defense, Cresson recounted that before leaving Paris, he "had the honor of asking our preceptor, I. L. Gerome [*sic*], whom he considered the best pupils among the Americans who studied in his atelier at the Ecole des Beaux Arts. His answer was, '[Frederick] Bridgman, George de Forrest Brush, of New York, and Thomas Eakins of Philadelphia.' ... [W]e have only our own voice to state that he said so, but if the public doubt it, probably Prof. Gerome would be willing to state his opinions of Mr. Eakins."[10] This appeal to French superiority of artistic understanding again reminds us of how little the core tensions in American art had shifted in seventy years. When Rembrandt Peale and John Vanderlyn came back from France with their "nudities," they also relied on American appreciation for the superiority of French culture and training to rationalize their productions. What had changed was that through the efforts of Eakins and many others, America did present a viable alternative for art students in the 1880s. The sense of jealousy and rivalry between Eakins, who often boasted of his French training, and others who never left home is redolent in the text of many letters exchanged.

Although the public phase of the academy scandal ended in February 1886, the retribution against Eakins next entered a very unpleasant private phase. Frank and Charley Stephens, and a few other former students of the artist, continued their agitation.[11] In a letter to Coates, Eakins wrote: "It was asked incredulously could refined ladies do such and such things, and the strong doubts reflected on my dear Susie and others of Maggy's friends who to me are sweet and refined above all others. The thing is a nightmare. My heart breaks for them, yet how can I defend them from the vicious attacks of those who never should have known what was [a] private professional matter. It seems to me that no one should work in a life class who thinks it wrong to undress if needful. About the hazard, that is another matter. Was ever so much smoke for so little fire? I never in my life seduced a girl, nor tried to, but what else can people think of all this rage and insanity? For years Miss Barber studied with me with enthusiasm and induced others, and with motives as pure as my own."[12] Eakins went on to stress that the women studying at the academy were not girls, but rather adults capable of making their own decisions.

The names of the women involved in the scandals were kept out of the newspapers, but Eakins complained bitterly to Coates and others that they were circulated widely among artists in New York and Philadelphia. Alice Barber and others who had taken part in the sessions—including Susan's sister Elizabeth "Lid" Macdowell—had few options as they struggled to salvage their reputations. The scandal served both in public and private realms to prove their powerlessness. The idea of equitable professional education must at the time have come to seem a bitter "advancement."

In the private sphere, Eakins' torment only deepened. In mid-March, the artist was informed that he had been expelled from the Philadelphia Sketch Club. Eakins' reply, which referred to the fact that he had never joined the club but rather been granted an honorary membership because he informally instructed students there free of charge, was understandably furious. "The action of the club in advising me as it has done, without stating what the charges are, or by whom they are preferred, is so inconsistent with the principles of plain and fair dealing that I can only regret that the club has permitted itself to be put in such an equivocal position."[13]

Ten days later, Eakins sent a statement to Emily Sartain expressing his hope that she might show it to "some persons" who it might "do a deal of good." It is likely that Eakins was referring to Emily's father, John Sartain, a prominent artist and engraver in the city who somehow was dragged into the mire. In the statement attached to his letter to Emily, Eakins reiterated that he used the naked model in his "business and professional studies," that "for economy" his students had "studied from each other's figures," and that he had used his male students as models frequently and his female students "very rarely ... and then with the knowledge and consent of their mothers." He went on to accuse Frank Stephens of being the one to bring shame on the female students. "One of the woman pupils, some years ago gave to her lover who communicated it to Mr. Frank Stephens a list of these pupils as far as she knew them, and since that time Mr. Frank Stephens has boasted to witnesses of the power which this knowledge gave him to turn me out of the Academy, the Philadelphia Sketch Club, & the Academy Art Club, and of his intention to drive me from the city."[14]

Frank Stephens bore a strong hatred for his famous and unconventional brother-in-law, and would have loved to see him leave Philadelphia. Ideological and temperamental differences combined with sheer jealously to doom the relationship from its start. Today it is impossible to determine all the causes Stephens might have had for his loathing, but we do know its outcome—he took every conceivable opportunity to humiliate Eakins, who in turn mounted a defense against his brother-in-law both professionally and at home. Stephens had appeared before the academy directors in February to encourage them to fire the artist, and then he had instigated the actions of the Sketch Club by accusing Eakins of incestuous relations with his sister Margaret, who had died of typhoid fever four years earlier.

Benjamin Eakins, along with his daughter and son-in-law Frances and Will Crowell, composed lengthy affidavits denying the charge, and asserting that Tom was never indecent or immoral. Their more personal letters to Tom demonstrate their sincere belief in his moral character, but they also complain that his habit of walking around the family home in his "shirttails" might have provided fodder for lewd magnification. These letters also imply that "one or more of the sisters," presumably Margaret, posed in the nude for the artist.[15]

There is no doubt that this situation was painful, depressing, and complicated for Benjamin and the entire family. Throughout the public phase of the scandal, Susan and Tom lived in his studio on Chestnut Street while Frank Stephens and his wife, Caroline, expecting her first child, were living in the family home on Mount Vernon Street. Tom insisted that their presence in the family home gave rise to the notion that Benjamin supported the actions and statements of his son-in-law. This does not appear to have been the case. After their baby was born, Frank and Caroline were asked to leave Mount Vernon Street, and they never were invited back. In their place, Tom moved back to his childhood home with his wife and stayed until his death thirty years later. Frank's ouster from his wife's home in favor of a man he considered immoral must have been especially galling.

Although Eakins experienced several more public scandals regarding exposure of the nude in anatomy classes in the decade that followed, in the public mind he always was associated with the "troubles" recounted in the press in 1886.[16] The dichotomy between this public knowledge and what really transpired in that year is a good reminder of just how restrictive the conventions governing middle-class female bodies were at the time. Even the most limited awareness of what had happened was enough to scandalize Philadelphia newspaper readers.

Although the most egregious charges against the artist can never be fully assessed, we do have copious evidence that at the very least Eakins willfully flouted the conventions of his age, and he put his female students in a terrible position while doing so. What seems most shocking today is Eakins' expectation that he could transgress such obvious boundaries and still maintain his elevated place in society. In an environment in which display of the nude male model before a female student was a problem, clearly display of the whole, naked, professorial body was unthinkable. And certainly, the idea that female students would pose for their male professor even today would be anathema even in the most liberal institutions. Eakins seemed to be taking his cultural cues from another world, and he caused enormous suffering on the part of those surrounding him in the process.

In concluding the defense of his conduct drafted to Coates on February 15, 1886, Eakins wrote:

> I am not in society nor skilled in the world's ways like you and Will MacDowell. My life has been spent with doctors and life students. If I am giving you trouble or have given you more than I ought, it is because I cannot keep everything to myself, and I hoped much from your power in appeasing wrath or making people see reason.
>
> Yours truly
>
> Thomas Eakins[17]

Eakins' grouping of doctors and life students in this letter is indicative both of his perception that they shared a similar body culture, and also of the source of his problems: he was wrong in assuming this to be the case. Doctors and life students were indeed not allowed the same license in nineteenth-century America; perhaps more to the point, women were not allowed to share the same privileges of freedom to see and study the human body in any arena.

Examination of Eakins' defense that he had "spent his life with doctors" reminds us that he meant that in a nearly literal sense; not only had Eakins spent much of his life in the halls of medical schools, painting and studying, but he also had modeled the Pennsylvania Academy of the Fine Arts on the paradigm of medical education. For Eakins, doctors were not only mentors but also role models. When it came time for Eakins to defend himself against the claims of his critics that his actions and conversations had crossed boundaries of propriety and convention, the artist had a plethora of examples from the medical and scientific communities to follow in gauging his response. We should not forget that in the same years that Eakins made his nude photographs and fought his public battles, Eadweard Muybridge was not far away, creating similarly unconventional images with the prospect only of celebratory acclamation. If Eakins ever expected to emerge from his conflict with the board as a champion of educational progress, he undoubtedly would have been influenced quite specifically by Muybridge, but perhaps even more so by the subject of his (later) portrait Dr. William Smith Forbes (fig. 65).

In 1905, near the end of his career, and with waning bravura in his style, Eakins painted a life-size portrait of the eminent William Smith Forbes in the year of his retirement as professor of anatomy. Today, the portrait hangs on a wall adjacent to *The Gross Clinic* and across Jefferson Medical College's Eakins gallery from the 1874 painting of Professor Benjamin Howard Rand. From Rand to Forbes, the gallery surveys thirty years of the artist's career, revealing the awkward characteristics of both the artist's youth and old age, and bracketing the undisputed glory of his mature career. At left, we look up at Rand at his desk, intent on chemistry apparatus and surrounded by distracting tools of his profession, like a supplicant student perhaps not worthy of attention, or not willing to interrupt.

Thirty years later, Eakins' relationship to Forbes represents a drastic shift in the artist's sense of his own standing. Whereas Eakins had studied with Rand as a teenager at Central High School, Forbes was a lecturer who informed Eakins during the course of his mature professional career. In contrast to the view looking up at Rand, the view looking down at Forbes in the later portrait is oddly disorienting—both because we do not see the picture from above in the gallery, but also because Eakins seems to have skewed the scale of Forbes' body in foreshortening the legs.

Despite its eccentricities, the heightened view in the 1905 portrait made some sense, as Eakins painted Forbes standing in the pit of a classroom amphitheater, lecturing as he had hundreds of times in the course of his long career. Forbes' white, receding hair, his deeply etched wrinkles, and the watch hanging around his neck all remind us of how much time Forbes had passed in this arena; it is hard to imagine, having recently turned sixty, that Eakins wasn't also thinking about how much time *he* had spent in this arena, listening to mentors including Gross, Agnew, and Forbes, as well as painting them.

But Eakins' portrait of Forbes was different from his dynamic images of Gross and Agnew; here, the acts of teaching and learning are alluded to in more subtle and symbolic ways. The clock and the skull place the painting in the category of a traditional memento mori, and perhaps we are meant to think on death as we look at it. If that is the association Eakins intended, then his choice was both brilliant and profound, for the life and career of Dr. Forbes raise provocative questions about nineteenth-century attitudes toward death that influenced both medical education and, by association, Eakins' career as well.

Forbes gestures not to a living patient, as in Eakins' previous medical amphitheater paintings, but rather rests his fingers gently on the Anatomy Act he famously drafted to ensure the availability of corpses for the use of medical education. Forbes, like Eakins, ignored societal conventions to further the study of anatomy, and left a path of hurt feelings, rebellious students, and public scandal in his wake. The human skull facing Forbes' hand is an eerie reminder of the macabre events leading to his arrest on conspiracy charges in the courts of Philadelphia in 1882, and his subsequent acquittal and laudation in 1883. Forbes' emergence from his trials as a heroic defender of medical education surely must have informed Eakins' response to

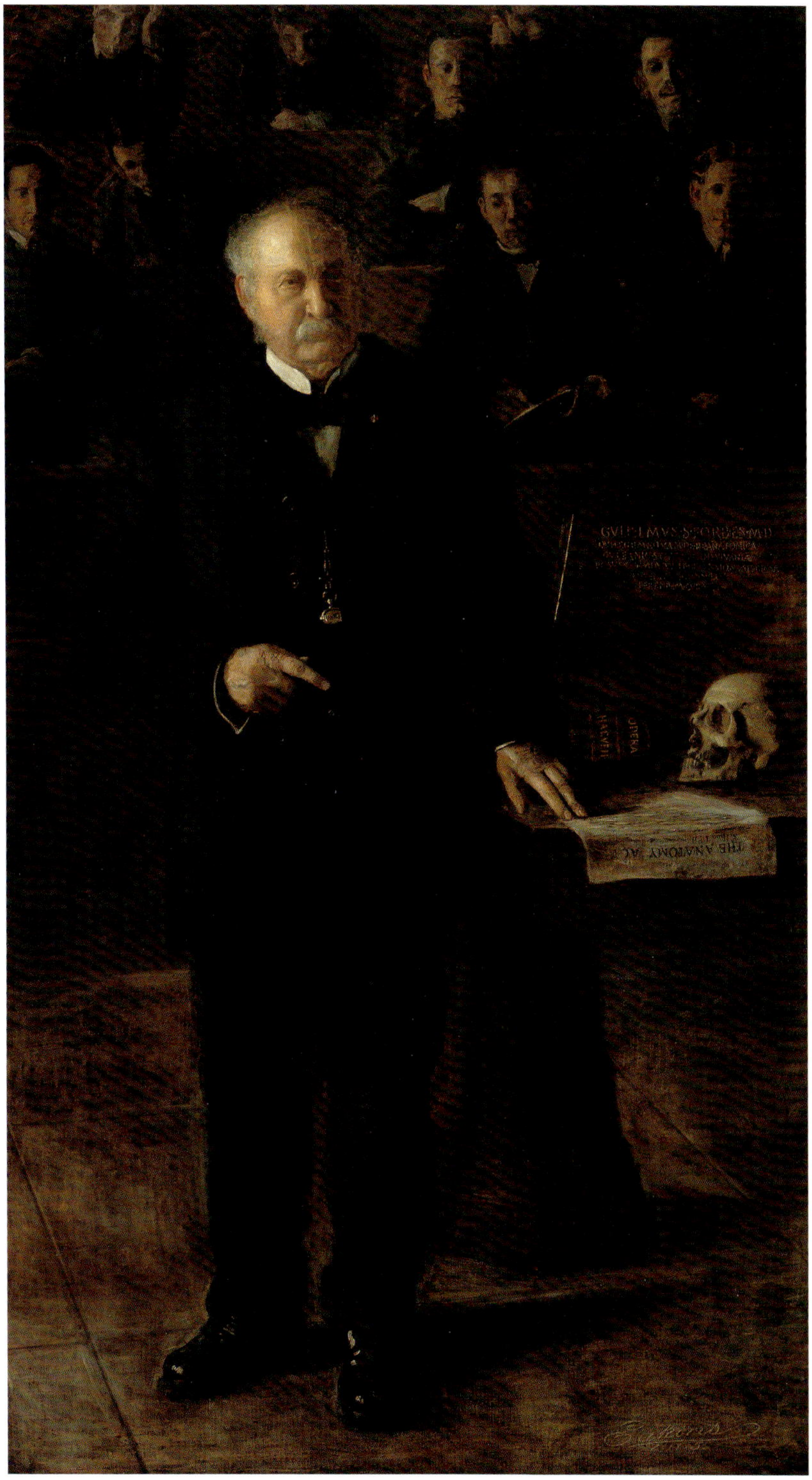

Fig. 65. Thomas Eakins, *William Smith Forbes, M.D.*, 1905. Oil on canvas, 84 × 48 in.

the scandals he faced just a few years later when he defended his actions by claiming that he had spent his life with doctors; certainly, the happy outcome of the earlier case may explain why Eakins seemed so shocked that his treatment was utterly the reverse of Forbes'.[18]

To understand the 1882 trial of Dr. William Smith Forbes requires that we delve a bit farther back in the history of anatomical education and its chief constraint over the course of centuries: in order to dissect a cadaver and study its intricate construction, one first had to obtain a cadaver, and many were required. The best nineteenth-century medical colleges required each student to fully dissect his own corpse.[19] Adding to the numbers required was the fact that bodies could not be reused; the process of dissection rendered the cadaver unusable by future students, as important parts had to be removed to get access to others. Burial practices and beliefs, far less diverse than today's, meant that few were willing to offer their own bodies, or those of relatives, to the anatomist's scalpel, and bodies mostly had to be purchased from unsavory vendors. Physicians of the nineteenth century, in both England and the United States, lamented their difficult legal status: they could face stiff fines for malpractice claims in civil lawsuits brought by disgruntled patients, yet the only way to acquire the requisite skills brought with it another possibility of prosecution. Dissecting an improperly obtained cadaver was "held to be a misdemeanor, punishable by fine and imprisonment."[20]

In response to the dearth of available corpses, physicians and professors were often drawn into the illegal world of body snatching. An example is provided in the following account of the son of Eakins' earlier portrait subject:

> In 1883, Samuel D. Gross, M.D., was a practicing surgeon in Easton, Pennsylvania. It came to his attention that a drunken soldier had committed suicide by hanging himself. Gross determined to have the body for anatomical study. Calling upon a student at the University of Pennsylvania named Green, he expressed his desire. Late in the evening of the day of burial, Gross and two students set out with digging equipment and a wheelbarrow to a resurrection party. The grave was located with no difficulty and the work of removing the soil was begun. The shovels made so much noise, however, that Gross elected to refill the grave and leave without disturbing the body. Several days later the brother of the deceased accosted Green and accused him of stealing the body. "Doctor," he said, "I believe you got my brother's body." Green neither admitted nor denied the charge and replied, "You can believe what you please."[21]

It was common knowledge that physicians not only knowingly purchased illegally dug bodies but also participated in their "resurrection" in the nineteenth century. Grave-robbing served in this era as the subject both of a great deal of outrage and of dark humor.

As the preeminent anatomist in the country, William Smith Forbes took action in 1867 to try to resolve cadaver distribution problems by authoring the seminal Pennsylvania Anatomy Act. Forbes' act directed mortuaries and prisons to release unclaimed bodies to medical colleges and chartered private anatomy schools for educational purposes. In his account of the passage of the bill, Forbes recalled his efforts to galvanize support for it after a first failure in the state senate. Hoping to present the bill with a more resounding voice, he offered a lengthy resolution at the meeting of the College of Physicians of Philadelphia on February 6, 1867:

> Resolved, that a Committee of three be appointed to present the views of this College to the Legislature of the State urging the passage of a law sanctioning the dissecting of dead human bodies....
>
> I trust it may not be thought impertinent in me to state, by way of preface, that after having been a teacher of anatomy and operative surgery in this city for ten years, to classes numbering in the aggregate near a thousand students, some of them now within the sound of my voice, I may be supposed to know something of the difficulties in the way of obtaining sufficient material for purposes of practically teaching so large a number of young gentlemen.
>
> In view of the fact that our city contains now three-quarters of a million inhabitants, I think it is idle to suppose there is not ample number of unclaimed dead bodies to satisfy the demands of all who may come for the purpose of cultivating a knowledge of anatomy, both healthy and morbid. In what then is the difficulty?
>
> I believe it consists entirely in the fact that as there is no law

> of the Commonwealth by which our physicians can claim these dead bodies, to be used for medical investigation, the authorities in whose hands they are lodged do not feel themselves at liberty to give them up for any purpose, however laudable....
>
> They are therefore buried, and are afterward obtained surreptitiously by a third party, the so-called "resurrectionists."[22]

Forbes went on to urge the organization of physicians to lobby the legislature for passage of his bill.

In assessing Forbes' actions and motivations, both in 1867 and at the time of his trial in the early 1880s, it is important to remember the economics and politics of nineteenth-century medical education, in addition to its pedagogic concerns. Forbes was vested in the cadaver trade not only as a physician and teacher but also as a businessman. The story of his professional successes and difficulties is by no means unique, and it reveals that the bleak business of the body trade threatened a great deal more than simply the ability of physicians to receive adequate training.

After early education at private academies, Forbes studied medicine at the University of Virginia from 1850 to 1851, and then attended Jefferson Medical College, where he received his medical degree in 1852. After working as an attending physician at Pennsylvania Hospital and serving abroad in the Crimean War, Forbes returned to Philadelphia, where he conducted the private College Avenue Anatomy School from 1857 until 1870, with the exception of the Civil War years during which the school was closed while Forbes performed surgery on the Union side. In 1879, he was appointed professor of anatomy and clinical surgery at Jefferson Medical College.

These different phases of Forbes' career demonstrate a variety of financial arrangements typical of the nineteenth-century surgeon and anatomy teacher. Although he began his training in his home state of Virginia, Forbes came to Philadelphia to receive a truly modern, and prestigious, medical education (thus tendering his tuition dollars in the larger city). Forbes' "anatomy school" was not exactly a competitor to the medical colleges in Philadelphia. Rather, it was a part-time program chiefly patronized by young men preparing for the rigors of medical school, supplementing, or continuing their medical education on a postgraduate basis.

Because Forbes was sole operator of an old-fashioned anatomy school in the ilk of that run by Caspar Wistar a century earlier, his financial success depended on his ability to attract paying students, and on his ability to procure bodies for them to dissect. When corpses were too expensive and paying students too few, such small anatomy shops closed. The growth of medical colleges as degree-granting institutions requisite for medical practice had a chilling effect on the prospects of such private schools, and they gradually died out by the turn of the twentieth century.

Although Forbes had much greater financial security at Jefferson Medical College a decade after his anatomy school closed, teaching as a professor at a mid-nineteenth-century medical college was not much less risky. Faculty members functioned largely as independent small business men within the college scheme, and they made their money by selling textbooks they had written, collecting fees for their classes, and sharing in the overall expenses and profits of the larger institution. Medical colleges like Jefferson and the University of Pennsylvania, and their vested faculty members, secured their position in part by drawing off students from smaller private anatomy schools and out-of-state institutions. Keen writes, for example, that he was forced to close the Philadelphia School of Anatomy when the University of Pennsylvania relocated to West Philadelphia, thus drawing away students who had been attending classes in both places. "The students from the Jefferson alone would not be sufficient to make the school a financial success."[23]

The body snatching problem changed the economics of medical education in a number of ways that would have prompted Forbes to begin his legislative work: first, the fines and mandatory jail term for body snatching were an important disincentive that threatened the physicians involved and raised the premium paid to "resurrectionists." But also, the relative availability of sufficient bodies in the hinterlands encouraged the flowering of smaller regional medical colleges, which threatened the flow of students into Philadelphia's premier (and relatively expensive-to-maintain) institutions. As long as there was no system for distributing cadavers, they would simply go to the highest—and nearest—

bidders. Forbes referred to "the injury of our city as a seat of medical learning" in his pitch to the College of Physicians.[24] Eakins held a similar vision of the Pennsylvania Academy of the Fine Arts and, by extension, Philadelphia, as the greatest center for American art education due to its availability of bodies for study.

The difficulties physicians faced in acquiring bodies for medical education made Forbes' resolution an easy sell, and the College of Physicians both approved it unanimously and appointed a committee of three members to push for passage of "An Act for the Promotion of Medical Science, and to Prevent the Traffic in Human Bodies." The committee included Dr. Forbes, Dr. S. D. Gross, and Dr. D. Hayes Agnew. It is noteworthy that Eakins applauded all these men by immortalizing them in paint during the course of his career, while enjoying precious few moments of acclaim for his own efforts on behalf of correct artistic anatomy education.

A few months after Forbes, Gross, and Agnew were commissioned to promote passage of the Anatomy Act, Forbes was able to report back to the College of Physicians on the success of their endeavor. Initial opposition to what was termed "the Ghastly Act" gradually gave way to "other arguments," including reminders that "the bodies of distinguished legislators themselves, after a life of good works, were no longer safe in their graves, but were liable to be rudely disturbed."[25] Forbes' aside here was not only vaguely threatening but also prescient. In 1878, the body of John Scott Harrison was "snatched." Harrison was a prominent congressman from Ohio, and also the son and father of the U.S. presidents William Henry Harrison and Benjamin Harrison.[26] Body snatching was no less gruesome and scandalous in 1878 than it had been a decade earlier.

The well-publicized Harrison scandal is a good reminder that the 1867 Anatomy Act in a small way improved, but by no means solved, the problem of body snatching. Forbes' persistence, if not an end to the business of "resurrection," at least regularized the collection and distribution of cadavers, but only within the bounds of Philadelphia; legislators had not been willing to extend the law to the entire state, and many other states had not attempted to address the problem at all. Even in Philadelphia, the fix was only partial: after 1867, a committee consisting of medical doctors and the coroner (who, interestingly, "owned and conducted" his own school of anatomy) made sure that bodies "required to be buried at public expense" first made their trip through the dissecting halls of the city, divided up equitably according to the number of students attending each institution.[27]

Forbes' prosecution in 1882 for conspiring to break the law he had written reveals that his legislation had by no means solved the problem. Even more disturbing and revealing is the issue of who was being snatched in the 1880s. As in the case of Muybridge, bodies were never equal in the nineteenth century, alive or dead, and the ways they were dealt with reveal the assumptions and fault lines in American culture in the late nineteenth century.

Years after Forbes' trial had ended, he recounted the circumstances leading up to his arrest: "In a few years it was discovered that in the Act of 1867 the words '*shall give permission* to take the bodies of deceased persons required to be buried at the public expense,' did not bind certain officials who had control of the bodies. Thus, when these bodies were asked for more than one of the officials said, 'Yes, go and take them, permission is given, that is the law,' it was found that these bodies now so civilly permitted to be taken, had already vanished. They could not be found."[28] Reading between the lines of Forbes' artful prose, one quickly gathers his assessment that the coroner himself had been sending bodies to his own anatomy school first, and then selling the rest.[29]

In 1882, the role of the coroner was hardly at issue, however. In the middle of the night on December 5, a group of *Philadelphia Press* reporters, working in conjunction with a private detective and city police, drove to the Lebanon cemetery on the outskirts of Philadelphia and caught three men in the act of transporting six bodies from the African-American burial ground to Jefferson Medical College. The bodies all had been exhumed that night from freshly laid graves, and they were quickly confiscated by police and taken to the city morgue to be identified by family members.

The scene in the streets outside the morgue was threatening after the story broke in the *Press* on the afternoon of

December 5. "An immense crowd of people surrounded the magistrates office" where the conspirators were being held on $5,000 bail, "and threatened to kill the resurrectionists. A squad of police was sent for, and by their aid the men were removed to a place of safety, although razors and revolvers were displayed."[30]

Thus began one of the most disturbing racial clashes of nineteenth-century Philadelphia. It was a scandal that forced city residents and readers across the country to think about the value they placed on medical education, the rights of African-Americans, and the sanctity of the human body. It was clear to most that some should be dissected for the sake of teaching doctors how to heal. The question was: whose dead should go under the knife?

In the days following the arrest of Frank McNamee, the hauler of the bodies, Robert Chew, superintendent of the cemetery and one of the gravediggers, and his brother Levi Chew, another "resurrectionist" (along with two more conspirators), the city of Philadelphia erupted in confrontations that often threatened violence. The connection to Jefferson Medical College was inarguable. McNamee had in his pocket the keys to the main door of the college and the room where corpses were embalmed; a drawing of the keys was published on the front page of the *Press* on December 6, with the headline: "Jefferson's Resurrection Keys: The Means by Which the Body Snatcher Gained Entrance to the College."[31] There was no doubt that these bodies were intended for Dr. Forbes' anatomy class.

The scene at the morgue was captured in dramatic detail in the columns of every city newspaper, as hundreds of African-Americans came to view the corpses, hoping not to find their loved ones. The bodies were rapidly identified, and the stories of the reactions to finding them recorded:

> A well dressed young colored man entered the morgue, and going up to the nearest coffin, drew back the covering, only to see the dead dull eyes of his brother gazing into his own. With one wild scream, he fell upon the coffin and cried to be left there alone, and begged that his friends would not attempt to take him away; calling on God to witness that he would avenge the wrong done him. His brother's name was Charlie Robinson, twenty-nine years of age, living at 1920 Kates street and known familiarly about town as the "hot corn man." "What is a man to do," exclaimed the living brother. "We live and work hard to earn an honest living, pay our debts and bury our dead and then they are not permitted to rest in peace, and even their grave clothes are stolen, oh! It is terrible! It is terrible![32]

Across town, the trustees of the college immediately denied any responsibility regarding the procurement of cadavers. Since faculty collected their own tuition, arranged for their own supplies, and hired and paid assistants as necessary, they felt no culpability whatsoever for any transgressions that might have taken place in Forbes' anatomy class.

It also was clear that there were few in the medical community who believed a sin had been committed. In a tense encounter, a reporter asked Jefferson trustee Henry C. Gibson about the incident and he replied that there was "no use to kick up such a fuss about nothing." "'Suppose the stolen bodies happened to be those of respectable white people?' the visitor suggested. Moving about uneasily in his chair, Mr. Gibson said something about imagining that the stolen bodies were those of paupers."[33] The threads between race and class in this case, never more than thinly veiled, were unraveling quickly. Whereas the Anatomy Act allowed any body "requiring burial at public expense" to be used for medical purposes, these bodies were in fact not remotely in that category.

An elderly "Aunty" interviewed at the morgue where she had discovered the body of her husband recounted how she had "paid twenty-two dollars to have him put in the ground. And how do you think I raised that money, sir? Why I went down along the wharves where my old man worked and begged a penny here and a penny there, and finally I got all the money and gave it to Mr. Foster, the undertaker, and he buried him for me, and now just to think these devilish fiends have been and robbed the grave and stole my old dead man away."[34]

With the body snatchers in prison, and the trustees and other faculty members of Jefferson Medical College pointing their fingers in Forbes' direction, investigators turned their full attention to the anatomy professor. Justice had to be done, if only to quell a potentially explosive outbreak of violence.

The students of Jefferson Medical College supported their professor avidly, but their violent threats against his detractors simply fueled the sensational accounts in the muckraking press. Two days after the initial arrests, hundreds of African-Americans gathered at Lebanon cemetery to open and inspect the graves of their loved ones, while at Liberty Hall another gathering of "Colored Citizens" was holding an "Exciting Indignation Meeting" during which the "ghouls" were "denounced." Violence was threatened, and the administrators at Jefferson were first on the list of scoundrels to be avenged.

Instead of expressing empathy for the families of the victims, Jefferson medical students unfortunately lived up to the reputation they previously had earned for their coarse manners. Waiting for Dr. Forbes' lecture to begin on December 7, the students yelled threats to the reporters who had shown up, physically expelled several, and sang racist songs threatening "niggers" with more body snatching.[35] When the story first broke at the college, one student was reported to have said, "I shouldn't mind if we were [mobbed]. There are 600 of us, and I guess we might have some fun. We might make a few fresh stiffs too."[36] Clearly, the Jefferson students Forbes addressed were no paragons of virtue. As Alan Braddock writes, some of them mockingly sang abolitionist songs and threatened black passers-by near the medical college with murder and dissection during the time of the trial.[37]

Dr. Forbes entered the amphitheater and made a short speech before lecturing on a skeleton: "Gentlemen," he said, "you are about to enter a noble career.... Your profession is one in which you welcome man into life, and when he is done with it, you are at his bedside, to make his departure easy. Therefore, taking into consideration the nobility of your future life, I hope you will pay strict attention to what I have to say—about anatomy."[38] The lecture then proceeded as usual, although Forbes was noticeably shaken. The following week, his situation grew increasingly dire. Frank McNamee confessed to the crimes of which he was accused, and implicated Dr. Forbes in a lengthy testimony, claiming that he had expressed concerns to the doctor directly and was told by him that digging and transporting bodies from the cemetery was perfectly legal. McNamee stated that another anatomist in the city had warned him to stop his trafficking and Forbes had countered: "He wants to get more students for his school and he does not like to see me get along."[39]

As several involved parties came forward over the course of the trial of McNamee, Chew, and the others, more damning revelations came out about Jefferson. Some students reported surprise at seeing any white bodies on the dissecting table, as the vast majority were dark-skinned. More stories of the robbery and dissection of black bodies around the country came to light, and more disturbances at Lebanon cemetery were discovered.[40] Descriptions by the grave robbers in the Forbes case of their methods were particularly inflammatory. The grave, never more than two weeks old, would be dug up, the lid removed, clothes torn off and thrown back in the coffin, and then a rope would be slipped around the neck of the naked victim and the body dragged up into the bed of McNamee's wagon.

The association of this practice with lynching must have been especially disturbing to African-Americans, and it can't have helped that medical students were so disrespectful and recalcitrant. For most newspaper readers, coverage of the shameless racist taunts of the students undoubtedly reinforced the idea that prejudice was publicly acceptable. For African-Americans, in contrast, the trial brought much-needed attention to the frequent robberies from their cemeteries, and provided an opportunity for the expression of solidarity. "A listener" wrote the following letter to the editor published in the *Philadelphia Inquirer* on December 12.

> SIR: In a sermon on Sunday night, delivered by Rev. T. Doughty Miller, of Cherry Street, one of the most cultured of the colored ministry of this city, occurs the following passage, which we commend to the attention of the Jefferson students, as an argument, hard to overcome:
>
> "Very many scientists and philosophers have written long and learned arguments to demonstrate the fact that, as a race, we were not really human beings, but only some remote connection therewith; were made and fit only for slaves—merchandise.

> Oh! bless God, through the dark cloud comes the sunshine. As high an authority as has ever spoken in denial of our manhood has spoken for it, proven it, by selecting the bodies of those declared by so many to be mere animals, as models upon which to base the study of human anatomy.... No, the same bones, ligaments, sinews run alike through the human frame, despite the outside hue. God's word is true; of one blood hath He made all nations.... The students of Jefferson, all unconscious, perhaps, of the source from which their subjects come, go forth to the world with a grander conception of the unity of the races, and the brotherhood of man.... Surely they cannot, they dare not join in the cry of race inferiority.... Thus our God overturns the acts and designs of men, and out of darkness brings light, out of sorrow brings joy."[41]

A "grander conception of the unity of the races" is still a work in progress, but the Forbes scandal contributed to a process through which racist assumptions were brought to light, articulated, and challenged.

Although tensions died down as the resurrectionists were forced to stand trial, for many African-Americans only the indictment of Dr. Forbes would guarantee that justice might be done. On the day after McNamee's confession, these desires were gratified as the "ghouls were committed" and Forbes was arrested and brought into court to stand trial on conspiracy charges. "By a singular coincidence, the first juror called was a colored man, and according to general usage, he took the first chair in the box and the position of foreman."[42]

In a packed courthouse, Forbes denied any knowledge of where the bodies had come from, admitting only to paying for them and arranging for their embalming by the staff once they were received. Forbes' father-in-law died that night, and his trial was put off for several months, a beneficially timed misfortune that allowed tensions to cool down in the city.

When the trial resumed on March 15, much more detail was recorded about the way Forbes organized his anatomy class. Cadavers were brought directly to his assistant for embalming, and discussion of their origins was avoided. They were brought in at night to avoid giving offense to passers-by. Once the bodies arrived in the building they generally, but not always, stayed there until reburial. "He had made a rule that no bodies should be taken out of the college, but the students were permitted to take the bones home after dissection." Students bought a ticket to the class for ten dollars from Forbes directly, and then paid roughly five dollars more for a "part of a body"—two students often shared a corpse, and Forbes typically taught three hundred students per year.[43] The almshouse and the prison simply did not produce enough bodies to satisfy the demands of city medical institutions.

In the end, the jury's decision amounted to a choice between the damning testimony of a convict and the sworn statements of an eminent physician. There was little surprise when, on March 18, Forbes was acquitted of all charges. "There was no proof produced worthy of a moment's consideration, or having a feather's weight, to show that Dr. Forbes knew whence the bodies delivered to the College came."[44] The story had already retreated to page two, and, with hindsight aplenty, the staff of the *Philadelphia Press* was criticized by many for having enflamed readers with their muckraking journalism. Attention in many quarters already had turned to revising the 1867 Anatomy Act, and in June 1883 the Pennsylvania legislature passed a greatly expanded version, directing that bodies "required to be buried at public expense" be collected from throughout the state and distributed on a pro rata basis throughout the commonwealth for medical education.[45]

The dramatic story of the trial of William Smith Forbes has been considered important mostly by medical historians, yet this public trial also helps to place Eakins' own troubles in context. Forbes was an educator whose practices put him on the front page, with students in the streets agitating in his favor—his trial and acquittal undoubtedly dominated discussion in the halls of Jefferson Medical College, the University of Pennsylvania (where Eakins was working on photographic experiments), and also at the Pennsylvania Academy, where dissections of cadavers regularly were taking place in basement classrooms. It is extremely unlikely that Eakins and his students did not follow every moment of the scandal and trial diligently and even avidly.

The outcome of Forbes' trial must have shaped Eakins' understanding of his problems at the academy three years later. Forbes not only was acquitted, but he was sanctified as well. In 1884, Agnew and his colleagues Richard J. Levis and J. William White circulated a letter on Forbes' behalf to raise money to pay his legal bills of several thousand dollars. The letter emphasized the doctor's "complete vindication" and that "he had acted not as a private teacher, but for the good of a public institution and medical science.... Honors and promotions" followed.[46] Eakins may well have similarly expected to be acquitted of the charges leveled against him, perhaps even to be celebrated as a pioneer in his field. Yet in the artist's case, as we have seen, the dynamic was far different. Like Forbes, Eakins believed that progress required free access to bodies, but artists lacked the privileged status of doctors; the concept of progress by any means necessary was certainly not acceptable in the artistic realm.

Further, because complaints about Eakins' program centered on the exploitation of female, white, and middle-class bodies as opposed to black bodies, the issue of *who* was involved—as both students and subjects—overwhelmed all other discussions about pedagogical purpose. The importance of race, class, and sex in all of this cannot be overstated; the affront to African-American bodies rather than female European-American bodies simply made all the difference between veneration and condemnation.

The dynamics of the scandal Thomas Eakins lived through in 1897 were far different, and not nearly as complex as his troubles of 1886, but they too were informed by a notorious and public scandal. In 1897, the cast of characters was more limited, the subtext of the drama not nearly so labyrinthine, but the plot just as tragic.

There is no way to convict or acquit a man who has been dead for ninety years, particularly without documented statements by the participants in an alleged crime. In a court of law at the time, the claim that Eakins abused his niece Ella Crowell when she lived in his home in the early 1890s would have been thrown out summarily for lack of evidence. What we do know is that the accusation of abuse arose at a moment of stress in dealings with family members when the alleged victim already was deceased—these were the same circumstances under which Frank Stephens accused Eakins of abusing his sister Margaret in 1886. There is no doubt that the accretion of claims against Eakins through all these years weighed like evidence against him. As Kathleen Foster writes, the artist "after 1886 moved through life with an aura of sexual disreputability."[47]

With both Margaret and Ella, it is impossible to determine whether any abuse in fact did occur, but it is certainly clear that the suspicion they had posed nude played a central role in the charges. As the scandals of 1886 demonstrated, nude posing by middle-class women was so controversial in the 1880s and 1890s that claims of sexual impropriety spun out quite naturally from that more benign practice, whatever their relation to the truth. One certainty is that Eakins does not seem to have learned anything from his experiences in 1886. And whatever the true facts of the case, there is little that is benign in what is known about this dark episode in the life of Eakins' family.

In 1897, Ella Crowell, Thomas Eakins' niece and the subject of his painting *Baby at Play*, shot herself at the farm owned by her parents, Will and Fanny (Frances Eakins) Crowell. Distraught exchanges between Eakins, Fanny, and Will following the suicide reveal that, as the family attempted to understand that tragedy, the artist increasingly was implicated in the events that led to her troubled end.

Ella, her sister Maggie, and her brother Ben all moved in with their Uncle Tom and Aunt Susie while studying to become painters during their early teen years. At the time, Eakins was still teaching at the Art Students' League. In those years in the early 1890s, the Mount Vernon Street house must have been quite crowded—Benjamin Eakins and his sister-in-law Eliza Cowperthwaite also still were in residence. Fanny and Will allowed their children to move to the city only hesitantly. Letters reveal their concern that the girls would be exposed to an inappropriate atmosphere at the league, and they adamantly insisted that the girls not pose in the nude themselves.

On the day the Crowell children moved into the house at Mount Vernon Street, Eakins wrote to his sister to allay her fears in a manner that demonstrates his misguided belief that rationalization of his practices made any difference:

The children arrived all right. Maggie is looking better than I should expect from her whooping. I hope the change of air will be beneficial.

That you should feel so anxious over … [illegible] having them go out from you, even as far as here, I will understand but you can be sure that they will have from me & Susie a watchful and loving care. Yet the dangers you have me guard against are not real ones until they pass from our control into the world, if they ever have to, and then I think the better educated and more refined they are the better they are armed can resist. I am sure the necessary art surroundings you mention are not coarsening & the society of the young men in the class room is better for them than that of a strictly girls school.

I am sorry for your comfort you wish so much that their studies lay in another direction & that you only accept the present opening as a last resort. It is not I think worse than the others [*sic*] openings type writing, music, nursing, & stove tending of which trained nursing would be my own choice next to art.

If it is not too early to wish, I should like Ella to be an animal painter, if not a great one at least a good honest one.

To do this she must learn well the naked figure, in some directions better than ordinary figure painters for much may be copied in a human model by the eyesight only, for human models must hold still to the light, but the animals must be constructed by understanding.

Now as soon as a certain dexterity is acquired in painting the children will need to supplement their school studies by closer examination of the joints & other machinery & they should model from one another occasionally. I should correct their work & they should see any time any part of my body or Susie's, or any professional or private model that I or Susie might have. In fact I should like them to have the free run of both of our studios.

Now every one who goes all into constructive art does just this thing & you will have to in time abate your prejudice far enough to see that the study of the naked body is either wholly right or wholly wrong.

If you should forbid your children to do what they see no harm in and see some others benefiting by but good they will come to be sour or rebellious.

With every facility many fail entirely, without facility no one succeeds. I shall see you soon and will tell you better than I write.[48]

Fanny Crowell must have wondered at how oblivious her brother was to send her this letter in response to her concerns. Did he really imagine she would appreciate that her daughters could see their aunt and uncle naked at any time as an aid to their education? Eakins' misreading of the situation was even more striking because this should have been a lesson the artist already had learned.

From his sister's perspective, Eakins' insistence on student posing already had cost the family dearly—Fanny and her sister Caroline never reconciled through 1889, when the younger sister died, and their reputations all had been marred by the 1886 scandals. After Caroline's death and throughout the early 1890s, Fanny and Will both wrote to denounce Eakins' insistence on nude posing, but they acceded to the wishes of their children to remain in the city and study with their uncle. After the Art Students' League disbanded in 1893, Ella and Maggie continued to study art and pose for each other and presumably their uncle in his Mount Vernon Street studio, even after such sessions had been forbidden expressly by Fanny.

Ella ultimately decided that art was not her guiding passion, and she followed her uncle's advice by enrolling at nursing school in the fall of 1895 while still living at Mount Vernon Street. This experience worked out even less well—in the first year of her course, Ella delivered a nearly fatal dose of laudanum to a patient and quit the program. After that time, she suffered from uncontrollable outbursts, attempted suicide with the same dose of laudanum, was institutionalized for a short time, and eventually shot herself in an unguarded moment in Avondale.

The details of the exchanges between Eakins, Fanny, Will, and other family members in letters written before and after Ella's suicide have been extensively reviewed by Kathleen Foster and other scholars, with no conclusive evidence about Eakins' involvement in contributing to Ella's mental illness. He might have touched her or asked her to touch him in a sexual manner, or simply misjudged her maturity and commitment as an art student. Dead people make poor defendants, and hearsay makes dubious history.

What can be gleaned from these exchanges is not guilt or innocence, but rather a sense of how the dialogue surrounding sexuality had shifted in the decade between 1886 and 1897. In his earlier trouble, Eakins demanded a full accounting of the claims against him, and then took some small satisfaction in refuting them over the course of the next year. In the later case, Eakins might have wished for such reserve. Now, the claims were much better articulated—and much more devastating. Fanny claimed that Ella was driven to a mental hospital to "escape Tom's approaches," and she accused him of touching her daughter in a "degrading manner." We know these accusations principally through a memorandum that Susan Eakins composed in 1897 in her husband's defense.[49] By that time, she already was practiced at defending her husband.

In October 1896, following Ella's institutionalization, Susan wrote to Fanny to complain that "Maggie is freely talking at the Academy against her Uncle Tom. The stories are that her sister Ella's insanity was brought on by the wearing effect of unnatural sexual excitements practiced upon her in the style of Oscar Wilde."[50] Jennifer Doyle comments on the assumptions implicit in Susan's letter to Fanny: "In this letter the phrase 'sexual excitements in the manner of Oscar Wilde' does not appear to give the author any pause. That she is not concerned that Fanny will not 'get' the drift of the rumors, and that the stories Maggie spread hinged on inference, demonstrates a shared understanding of sodomy as a thing not to be named, but as a thing everyone is presumed to understand."[51] In fact, it is entirely unclear what Philadelphians inferred when they talked about "sexual excitements in the manner of Oscar Wilde."[52]

Maggie's reference to Wilde is stubbornly ambiguous—Wilde never was accused of sodomy with women. It is also unclear from newspaper accounts in Philadelphia at the time that many specifically understood the trial to be about "sodomy"—itself a term with changeable definitions. Although it was precisely in this period that the terms of sexual definition were crystallizing, articulation of explicit terms happened much sooner in Europe than in America.

Eve Kosofsky Sedgwick argues that it was not until 1891 that a homosexual fully emerged in American literature—Melville's Billy Budd, who is "different in his essential nature than the men around him." Even in this novel, in which homosexuality is a major element in the narrative, that sexual orientation still was named only in coded phrases: "hidden nature," "peculiar," "natural depravity," and so on.[53] Four years later, coded language was still in use to describe the trial of Wilde for Philadelphia's newspaper readers. In London, newspapers were derided for printing the explicit testimony verbatim. In Philadelphia, not a single newspaper covering the trial ever even used the term "sodomy," which was in fact the accusation that caused the sordid and tragic affair. The story of Oscar Wilde's trial as told in Philadelphia illuminates the murky prelude to modern dialogues about sodomy and homosexuality.

The court proceedings that sent Oscar Wilde to prison in 1897 resulted from a lawsuit he himself had filed. Wilde was a married father of two, and an increasingly successful literary star in Europe and America, when the Marquess of Queensberry scrawled a fragment of a sentence on a visiting card and left it for Wilde with the hall porter at the Albemarle Club in London. Surprised by its message, the porter placed it inside an envelope addressed to the playwright and marked the date and time. The marquess had written: "For Oscar Wilde posing somdomite [*sic*]."

Wilde had been on "intimate" terms with Lord Alfred Douglas, son of the marquess, for several years, and this was only the most public of Queensberry's frequent, hostile invectives. The offense of the words scrawled on the card was in Wilde's mind so great that he sued the marquess for libel, thus initiating his own downfall. Interestingly, the marquess was so hated by his own family that his wife and son underwrote Wilde's legal expenses in order to encourage him to pursue the suit.

In Philadelphia, readers of local newspapers understood far less about the trial than their British counterparts did, although they were no less familiar with Wilde himself. In

1882, at the same time Philadelphia newspapers were filled with accounts of the trial of William Smith Forbes and the riots that surrounded it, they also were reading about a new "Apostle of Aestheticism." Only twenty-eight at the time, Wilde already was such a notable celebrity in America that he toured more than a hundred cities in the country, "paid to promote not only the aesthetic message but also the D'Oyly Carte American production of Gilbert and Sullivan's Patience, a light-hearted operetta based on the aesthetic movement in England."[54] Wilde's tour prompted a great deal of reaction in American cities. Newspapers reported at length on every element of Wilde's artful and outrageously dandyish dress, his "womanly" appearance and manners, and his prescriptions for decorative and elegant "aesthetic" living. In New York, writers also noted Wilde's following of boys and men, described with elusive references to a thriving underground homosexual subculture.[55] Thirteen years later, Wilde still was an important and celebrated player on the American cultural scene.[56]

A public fall is dramatic only if it occurs from the heights, and this one surely did. The first mention of the Queensberry incident in the Philadelphia press was unremittingly supportive: "Oscar Wilde Libelled—He Brings Suit Against the Marquis of Queensberry for an Offensive Remark." The story went on to say: "A lawyer who appeared on behalf of Mr. Wilde said the latter, who was on affectionate terms with his wife and child, had been the object ... of the most cruel persecution at the hands of the Marquis.... Oscar Wilde and his wife are both members of the Albemarle Club, and on February 28, it appears, one of the hall porters handed Mr. Wilde a card.... Written on this card were three most offensive and indecent words, implying that Mr. Wilde was *souteneur* and indicted to unnatural vices."[57]

The French term *souteneur* translates as "pimp" or "panderer." The phrase does not appear in any British reports of the trial, so we may assume the reporter in this case was choosing a less decipherable euphemism for "sodomite."

Philadelphians lacking a French-English dictionary may well not even have understood the term *souteneur*—using foreign languages, or dead ones in some cases, was a favorite way of limiting the conveyance of information to an educated elite. In following months, many more writers on this side of the Atlantic strained to find acceptable translations for the more explicit language used in the trial. As events unfolded, even the use of foreign terms subsided as the job of obfuscating facts of the trial grew increasingly difficult.

On April 4, the morning papers began their coverage of the libel suit in the Old Bailey. Wilde was witty and urbane and the marquess inflamed, satisfying expectations as the prosecution presented its case, but when the trial turned to the defense, the mood darkened. Queensberry's lawyer, Edward Carson, began efficiently and effectively demonstrating that the offending note had, in fact, been correct. In a "plea of justification," Queensberry accused Wilde not only of "immorality and sodomitical tendencies in his published work, especially *The Portrait of Dorian Gray*, but also of fourteen counts of gross indecency with young men."[58] Unbeknownst to Wilde and his attorney, private detectives working for the marquess already had supplied the defense with a large arsenal of statements and damning evidence from "rent boys," hotel personnel, "procurers," and others who could testify that young men had spent evenings with Wilde. The author's relationship with Queensberry's son, Alfred "Bosie" Douglas, was only sporadically at issue through the next two days of proceedings.

Philadelphia followers of the story never read about the "plea of justification," or understood as fully as court attendees just what was being discussed. On April 4, the *Evening Bulletin* led on page one with the headline: "WILDE SCORED ... The Testimony in the Case Not of a Choice Character." The specifics of the testimony were only hinted at: "Oscar Wilde ... admitted that he had attended tea parties in the rooms of a man named Taylor, which were artistically furnished, and in which perfumes were burning. He denied, however, that he had seen Taylor in a woman's costume." In the afternoon, the defense speech was termed "terribly denunciatory." Although the reporter would offer no proof of that other than the claim of perfumed rooms and an alleged cross-dressing host, the text included some discussion of why that was the case: "The nature of the evidence and the whole circumstances in the case prove to be of such a character that we cannot report it."[59] The *Philadelphia Press* and the *Inquirer* that day were slightly more willing to describe the testimony. The *Press* wrote:

> Mr. Carson began the presentation of the case for the Marquis by reading passages from "Dorian Gray," one of Oscar Wilde's novels of modern life, to show that he upheld an unnatural practice.
>
> The cross-examination brought out the great difference in ages of Oscar Wilde and Lord Alfred Douglas (the former was born in 1856, and the latter in 1870), how the two had visited various towns together, stopped at the Savoy Hotel together, and how Lord Alfred visited Wilde's chambers in St. James Place.[60]

On the same day, the *Inquirer* described the cross-examination as touching on "Wilde's relations with various boys and men." Wilde took one boy to a hotel at Brighton, was "intimate" with an eighteen-year-old newsboy, and gave the newsboy a cigarette case and a book that were presented in court as evidence.[61]

The recorded transcript of the trial reveals just how much was left out of these accounts. On that Wednesday afternoon, the second day of the trial, Carson cross-examined Wilde about his relations with a man named Wood:

> CARSON: Did you ever have any immoral practices with Wood?
> WILDE: Never in my life.
> CARSON: Did you ever open his trousers?
> WILDE: Oh, no!
> CARSON: Put your hand upon his person?
> WILDE: Never.
> CARSON: Did you ever put your own person between his legs?
> WILDE: Never.

In the course of the afternoon, Carson went on to pursue a further damning line of questioning about Wilde's relations with other young men, including eighteen-year-old Edward Shelley:

> CARSON: Did you kiss him?
> WILDE: Never.
> CARSON: Did you put your hand on his person?
> WILDE: Never.
> CARSON: And then bring him into your bedroom?
> WILDE: Never.
> CARSON: Sleep in the same bed with him all night?
> WILDE: Never.
> CARSON: Each of you having taken off all your clothes, did you take his person in your hand in bed?
> WILDE: My lord, is it not sufficient for me to give an entire denial without being exposed to the ignominy of detail after detail of an imaginary thing going on?[62]

Despite Wilde's consistent denial of "unnatural" acts with trousers and "persons," the defense was able to use its investigative files to bring forward numerous accounts of young men who had been alone with Wilde, and then been given money and gifts.[63] To those in attendance, it seemed impossible that there were any other explanations for what had taken place than the "sodomitical" acts alleged by Queensberry and Carson.

While the London papers printed the text of the trial in excruciating detail and followed up with excoriating editorials, newspapers in Philadelphia continued to find ways to allude to, rather than report, what was being said. The *Philadelphia Times* put the London press itself on trial with the headline: "Most of the London Newspapers Print Almost Verbatim Reports of the Evidence, Which is Glaringly Indecent."[64] American newsmen clearly did not want girls like Maggie Crowell to learn new words, foreign or otherwise.

On April 5, the newspapers reported the outcome of the trial: Wilde not only had withdrawn his case against the marquess, but he very quickly was arrested by police to stand trial under section 11 of the 1885 Criminal Law Amendment Act for committing acts of gross indecency with other male persons. Wilde spent that night in Scotland Yard, in a "cramped cell, neither bail nor servant's attendance being allowed him." Even worse perhaps, the same reporter noted, "His name has been expunged from all playbills of London theatres where his plays are currently running and his future is apparently blasted forever."[65]

The same reporters who had on April 4 condemned Queensberry for his "foul epithets," on April 6 sanctimoniously declared that of course the marquess had been right, and that Wilde's prosecution was important for public safety. Philadelphia editors leaped at the opportunity to scathingly rebuke Wilde, and suddenly the plays and witticisms that had been well loved were now harbingers of immorality.

> There was at one time a disposition to regard Wilde good-naturedly as a harmless charlatan. But his literary and dramatic career for several years past has furnished so many examples of abominable cynicism in social ethics that he had come to be looked upon as a moral nuisance.... If he shall be sent to prison for his odious offences, as now seems probable, his punishment will fittingly close the career of a fraud whose literary stock in trade has been to anger at morality and religion, and who in his private life has been such a creature as even the most hardened man of the world cannot now view but with loathing.[66]

In his second trial for "indecent acts" the following month (the first resulted in a hung jury), Wilde was convicted, and he then served two years of imprisonment "with hard labor."

The vagueness of Wilde's alleged "crimes" as reported in the Philadelphia press demanded that readers use their own imagination to fill in the blanks and determine whether the sentence was just. They knew that young men were involved, that things happened in hotel rooms that were "unnatural" and "indecent," but they were left to visualize on their own what those things might have been. For homosexuals reading the coverage, the condemnation had been as clear as it was for female art students reading news of Eakins' resignation, or African-Americans of the acquittal of Dr. Forbes. All of these scandals served as instruction on one's place in society, guided by its worst prejudices. In the case of Wilde, the cautionary tale was aimed not only, or even principally, at those who experienced homosexual desire.

Much more prominent in Philadelphia editorials than any condemnation of sexual acts was the conclusion that Wilde's trial vindicated critics of the aesthetic movement he had championed. Almost immediately, social critics used the outrage provoked by the trial to condemn every manner of unconventional social behavior. An editor at the *Philadelphia Times* wrote: "The hideous exposure of Oscar Wilde ... justifies those healthy-minded critics who have stood out against the whole fashionable and hysterical 'movement' as obscene, abnormal and diseased."[67] And an editorial in the *Bulletin*, titled "A Blow to Erotics," took the opportunity equally to condemn Wilde and all other threats to marriage, art, literature, theater, and dress:

> Within a comparatively few years a number of English writers, as well as a few Americans, have come forward in the field of literature and of the drama and posed as "cynics" or "reconstructors" of society. The chief object of their attack has been the marriage relation.... It may be noted that one of the most aggressive and dangerous of these pests is now posing as a prisoner in the dock, charged with crimes so infamous and so disgusting that the mind shrinks from contemplation of them and their author. Is not the conclusion obvious? ... It is too much to believe that so odious a creature as the downfallen aesthetic has numerous counterparts even among the writers of cynical books and plays. Yet, though the authors of certain novels which we have lately had presented to us and "boomed" openly on the score of their erotic nastiness may escape charges of personal turpitude of the Wilde stamp, it does seem as if the conditions which produced those books must have been similar, to more or less extent, with the conditions which produced some of the Wilde creations.... There is no way to convince many readers and theatre-goers of the wrong they are doing in giving ear to the specious arguments for free love and kindred creeds.... But it does seem as if the revelation of the vileness of the authors of some of these novels and plays, to which vileness the Wilde case has given clue, should make a proportion of our people hesitate before further being a party to the nourishment of a literature born in iniquity and of diseased minds.[68]

As this vitriolic text makes clear, the fallout from the trial of Oscar Wilde was not limited to condemnation of acts of "gross indecency committed with young boys." Instead, the trial came to stand for any acts, or advocacy, that threatened conventional roles regarding gender and sexuality. The reference here to "free love and kindred creeds" is a good reminder that Eakins was by no means the most committed opponent of Victorian prudery.

"Free love" advocates were vilified enough in late-nineteenth-century sources that it is likely that Thomas Eakins and many other Philadelphians were somewhat aware of their activities. From 1872 until 1907, these sexual revolutionaries published invectives against Victorian prudery in obscure journals named *Lucifer, the Light-Bearer* and *The Word.* In these journals, authors including Moses Harman, Ezra Hervey Heywood, and Angela Fiducia Tilton Heywood argued for public and explicit discussion of reproductive anatomy, normal sexual practices, "aberrant behavior," contraceptive options, and genital health. Harman wrote in his article "Heywood Again Under Arrest" in 1883: "Sexual health could be achieved … only after the prudishness, the false modesty that shrinks from open and fearless discussion of everything pertaining to the sexual nature of men and women had been overcome."[69] It is hard to imagine circumstances in which Eakins would have read this report, but it is striking that he and his students used the same phrase—"false modesty"—repeatedly to describe restrictions against the study of the nude.

If Eakins had come into contact with free love writings, he might well have agreed with many of their positions. The free love movement argued a relatively moderate platform by modern standards; they wanted greater availability of information about sexual matters, recognition that conjugal relations were natural and enjoyable for both men and women, and family planning. In the context of Victorian America, the language with which they expressed all of these ideas and hopes was starkly clear. In an essay titled "Penis Literature," Angela Heywood concluded: "Virtue, Chastity, Rectitude allwise suffer by *conventional falsehood;* so Gentlemen and Ladies, the sooner 'pure' hypocrisy ceases, the whole truth is out and afloat, the better for all Humankind."[70]

When the editors of Philadelphia's newspapers condemned Wilde for his aestheticism and indecency, they also were condemning the era's sexual revolutionaries, including not only the egalitarian free love adherents, but also a variety of other small but kindred creeds that threatened the Victorian social order. With conventional norms so narrowly defined, it is not surprising that subversives were plentiful in both America and Europe.

Parliament's impetus in 1885 for providing British courts with the power to punish "indecency between male persons in public or in private" (a law against homosexuality first fully enforced in Wilde's case) was public fear of the corruption of young people in the prostitution trade.[71] The desired effect was not achieved. As Kirby Farrell writes: "In mapping an underworld of criminal horrors, the law inevitably focused public attention on—and gave official weight to—the vices it sought to crush … the concern with 'private' crimes directed attention to what could not be measured or even seen. Moral panic, after all, is as shapeless as the 'unnamable horrors' it fears."[72] The accusations against both Eakins and Wilde are hard to understand if we fail to look at them within the dark and combative framework of Victorian sexual culture. We will never know the full story of Ella Crowell's troubled life, but we do know that her life—and death—occurred in a period of "moral panic" in which unseen private crimes increasingly caused anxiety.

It was not long before the aesthetic movement itself fell victim to the trial of Oscar Wilde. As Mary Warner Blanchard writes, after 1895 aestheticism in the arts was "cut off by Wilde's own fall from grace … and by the resurgence of a culture of virility and war in the nation at large (the rise of Teddy Roosevelt and the imperialist adventures of the late 1890s)."[73] Eakins benefited professionally from the demise of aestheticism, as his paintings stood out from the more decorative works he had always loathed. Personally though, both Wilde and Eakins endured devastating consequences from their scandals of the mid-1890s.

For Wilde, of course, the public and litigious nature of his scandal produced a far worse outcome. Wilde spent two years in a prison work camp in failing health. During that time, his plays were closed down in London, and his family went bankrupt. Constance Wilde, who had stood by her husband during the trial, oversaw the auction of her possessions, changed her last name and that of her sons to Holland, and moved the small family to Ireland. Wilde never saw them again. He was released from prison on May 19, 1897, and died in Paris on November 30, 1900, at the age of forty-six.[74]

In Pennsylvania, a lesser version of the same fate befell Eakins; he never again saw his sister, brother-in-law, nieces and nephews, nor ever again visited the Avondale farm that had been such an important part of his life. After 1897, Eakins continued to paint, and to exhibit his work around the country, but he gave up teaching entirely.

The trial of Oscar Wilde was, indeed, one of the great scandals of the nineteenth century, and it changed the lives of those who read about it in some cases as much as its celebrated victim. The unquestioned same-sex "companionships" of the nineteenth century thereafter would be called into question. Nude young men swimming together with their professor never would look quite the same. As James Saslow writes, "By exposing the mushrooming homosexual underworld, Oscar Wilde's trial galvanized society. It alarmed traditionalists, who mobilized against the new subculture; it energized gay people themselves, who realized how pernicious their oppression was and how potentially strong their voice; and it alerted entrepreneurs to an exploitable market for commercial art and entertainment."[75] Now, Baron von Gloeden and Fred Holland Day, among others, would redefine the male nude for a recognized audience.

Although Wilde and Eakins suffered greatly as a result of their trials in the 1890s, artists always have the last word—or picture, as the case may be. Even during his trial, Wilde spoke with an eloquence that stands the test of time, far beyond the forgettable pronouncements of his accusers. On the Thursday morning of his trial against Queensberry, Wilde came back to the courthouse with the best defense he and his attorney could offer—an extended reading from the novel that had been attacked as "sodomitic" and immoral the day before. In this portion of his defense, Wilde was brilliant, and his testimony stands as a moving and poignant statement of artistic integrity. Years after the trial, Eakins would respond to a request for biographical information and a philosophic statement: "My life is all in my work." Oscar Wilde took a similar approach at the moment when he was tied to the stake, the firewood piling up around him.

In answer to claims that Wilde's *Dorian Gray* was an "immoral" work, his lawyer Sir Edward Clarke asked the author to read aloud a letter he had written to the editor of the *Scots Observer* following its publication of a scathing review of the novel: "It was necessary, sir, for the dramatic development of this story to surround Dorian Gray with an atmosphere of moral corruption. Otherwise the story would have had no meaning and the plot no issue. To keep this atmosphere vague and indeterminate and wonderful was the aim of the artist who wrote the story. I claim, sir, that he has succeeded. Each man sees his own sin in Dorian Gray. What Dorian Gray's sins are no one knows. He who finds them has brought them."[76] If Eakins had been so articulate, he might have issued the same challenge to his own accusers—the naked body in Eakins' art and teaching provided the same "vague and indeterminate and wonderful" mirror for his audiences' "brought sins" that Wilde's ambiance in *Dorian Gray* presented to his readers.

Later in the trial, Clarke had Wilde read from the novel itself. In this passage, Dorian is defending himself against accusations of unhealthy relationships with boys and men: "I know how people chatter in England. The middle classes air their moral prejudices over their gross dinner-tables, and whisper about what they call the profligacies of their betters in order to try and pretend that they are in smart society, and on intimate terms with the people they slander. In this country, it is enough for a man to have distinction and brains for every common tongue to wag against him. And what sort of lives do these people, who pose as being moral, lead themselves? My dear fellow, you forget that we are in the native land of the hypocrite."[77] Eakins' repeated condemnation of "false modesty" was not as eloquent as Wilde's, but it was every bit as venomous against the prejudices of Victorian society. And both men spurned the idea that the untrained should be permitted the liberty of criticizing artistic accomplishment, as the following prosecutorial exchange reveals.

CARSON: May I take it that no matter how immoral a book was, if it was well written it would be a good book?

WILDE: If it were well written it would produce a sense of beauty, which is the highest feeling that man is capable of. If it was badly written, it would produce a sense of disgust.

CARSON: A well written, immoral book would—

WILDE: I beg your pardon—I say if a book is well written, that

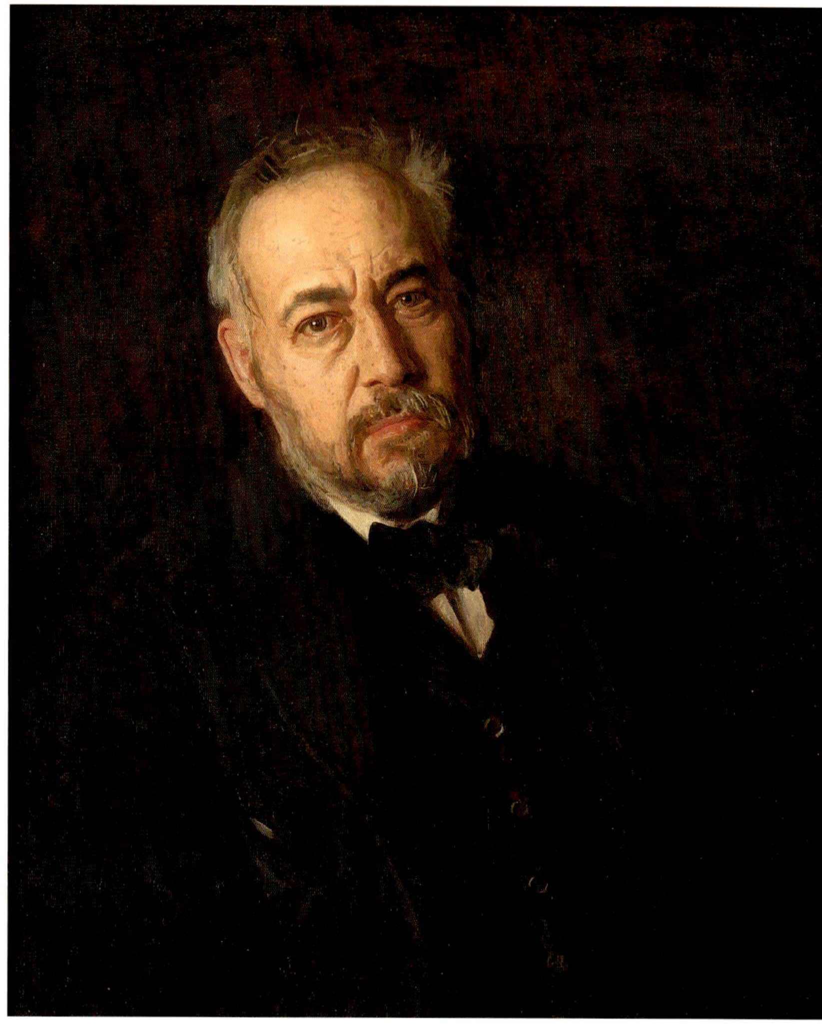

Fig. 66. Thomas Eakins, *Self-Portrait*, 1902. Oil on canvas, 30 × 25 in. National Academy Museum, New York.

is if a work of art is beautiful, the impression that it produces is a sense of beauty, which is the very highest sense that I think human beings are capable of. If it is a badly made work of art, whether it be a statue or whether it be a book, it produces a sense of disgust; that is all....

CARSON: We will say a sodomitical novel might be a good book according to you.

WILDE: I don't know what you mean by a sodomitical novel.

CARSON: Don't you?

WILDE: No.

CARSON: I will suggest to you *Dorian Gray*. Is that open to the interpretation of being a sodomitical book?

WILDE: Only to brutes—only to the illiterate; perhaps I should say brutes and the illiterate.

CARSON: An illiterate person reading *Dorian Gray* might consider it a sodomitical book?

WILDE: The views of the Philistine on art could not be counted: they are incalculably stupid. You cannot ask me what misinterpretation of my work the ignorant, the illiterate, the foolish may put on it. It doesn't concern me. What concerns me in my art is my view and my feeling and why I made it; I don't care twopence what other people think about it.[78]

Eakins was similarly severe in his proclamations about how little he thought of his critics. In 1893, he wrote to Dr. Jacob Mendez DaCosta, who presumably had criticized his portrait and suggested some revisions.

It is I believe to your interest and to mine that the painting does remain in its present condition....

As to your friends, I have known some of them whom I esteem greatly to give most injudicious art advice and to admire what was ignorant, ill constructed, vulgar and bad; and as to the concurrent testimony of the newspapers, which I have not seen, I wonder at your mentioning them after our many conversations regarding them.

I presume my position in art is not second to your own in medicine, and I can hardly imagine myself writing to you a letter like this: Dear Doctor, The concurrent testimony of the newspapers and of friends is that your treatment of my case has not been one of your successes. I therefore suggest that you treat me a while with Mrs. Brown's Metaphysical Discovery.

Yours truly,

Thomas Eakins[79]

During a life often spent defending himself, by the 1890s Eakins clearly had grown weary of even the slightest pretension to politeness. His acerbic witticisms may not have risen to the erudition of Wilde's, but they shared a spirit of indignation that the untrained would presume to criticize the work of a master. In the end, each man's best comfort was the art he already had committed to future generations.

Looking once more, and finally, at the portrait of William Smith Forbes, I am struck again by the differences between this portrait and the Rand and Gross portraits hung with it in the Jefferson Medical College gallery. Rand, absorbed in his experiments, and Gross, mid-sentence as he teaches the students around him, are depicted as active agents, in the process of creating their contributions to society. We may hypothesize on the sum of what those will be, but Eakins can't exactly make that clear. These are portraits about the thrill of making history and of forging progress.

The Forbes portrait, in contrast, is a eulogy. The doctor was ill at the time, and in fact he died six months later; he already had stopped teaching. His hand rests on the Anatomy Act and behind him are a copy of his favorite anatomical text (the historic *Opera Harveii* by William Harvey), a pointer used in lecturing, and of course the oddly smiling skull, which looks in some ways more vigorous than Forbes. The doctor is adorned with mementos of his success: a gold chain and watch he received from students following his acquittal in 1883, and the "lapel pin of the Military Order of the Loyal Legion of the United States."[80] In the seats behind him, students visibly record Forbes' words. This is a portrait about history already "in the bag."

Eakins was ready in 1905 to meditate on what it meant to summarize a lifetime of achievement. Scandals long behind him, he was beginning to accrue a fine collection of his own badges of success: for the past several years, he had been invited to serve as juror for several art competitions (including the Pennsylvania Academy in 1901), he was elected as both associate and academician of the National Academy of Design in 1902 (a rare double honor), and he won gold medals and other distinguished prizes in exhibitions across the country. And although Eakins never received the laudation Forbes did for his efforts to further the cause of modern education, the passage of time at least had served to rehabilitate him as a painter.

The self-portrait Eakins painted for the National Academy of Design to mark his election as an academician in 1902 bears no visible symbols of accomplishment such as medals or certificates—Eakins never would have been so self-congratulatory (fig. 66). Instead, he painted himself with simply gorgeous gravitas, presumably staring out at his own visage in a mirror, but also meant to stare down at the Americans who would assess his life's work for generations to come. Eakins' slightly disheveled, grayed hair, bow tie somewhat askew, and heavy eyes and brow serve to demand respect for an individual so determined to paint what his trained eye saw. And for Eakins, this was always the goal, without compromise. Those who condemned Oscar Wilde and Thomas Eakins during their lives have long since died, leaving behind a trail of documents for historians to recover and debate. The reputations of these men may never quite be recoverable for some, but the plays, novels, and paintings they obstinately created survive untarnished for new generations to scrutinize. The last word, the last impression, always has rested with the artist rather than the critic.

Conclusion
Thomas Eakins' Family Values

What made him a bit of a rebel, and later much more of one, was his inbred resistance to establishment authority. Not awed by rank … he continued in his writings and letters to extol the diligence of the middling class of tradesmen, shopkeepers and leather-aprons.

—WALTER ISAACSON, on Benjamin Franklin

For Benjamin Franklin, resisting authority and extolling the middle class were the basis for a strident patriotism that shaped a young democracy. For Thomas Eakins, the same ideology informed his sensibilities, but resisting the establishment and its pretensions was better business for a revolutionary than it was for a high-end portrait painter.

Given the obvious fault lines that existed in the society in which he lived and studied the nude, one has to ask why Eakins insisted on carrying on as he did. Why was compromise with Victorian norms so difficult to accept? Eakins might well have conducted his classes as he did but limited them to male students, or merely segregated his audiences more diligently. He might have sought out and hired more models from impoverished circumstances instead of asking students to pose. Eakins might even have slightly improved the features of his portrait subjects on occasion. He steadfastly refused to compromise on any of these points. Instead, he spent much of his life pointedly provoking the hostility of those who disagreed with his own version of strident patriotism.

The staying power of a maverick is greatly enhanced when room and board and social support are in place. Eakins never lacked any of these, and the story of his life would be unthinkable without the contributions of his family—most noticeably his father Benjamin and his wife Susan. Caroline Cowperthwaite died early in her son's career, but Thomas Eakins was a natural descendant of her "leather-apron" Quaker ancestors (including a mapmaker and printer for whom the artist was named), and the influence of that inheritance is omnipresent in his life. The artist's strong convictions and sense of self were nourished by his understanding of both his father's and mother's place in the social fabric of nineteenth-century Philadelphia. Continuity in habits and values through three generations provided the strong background for Eakins' self-possession.

Although little is known about Caroline Cowperthwaite, who died in 1872, Benjamin Eakins lived a long and relatively well documented life.[1] He was raised on a farm in Valley Forge, Pennsylvania, in the home of his father, Alexander, a weaver who had emigrated from Ireland shortly before the War of 1812. Like most early-nineteenth-century weavers, Alexander Eakins produced cloth from his working farm. As midcentury neared, however, industrialization in textiles had made farms like his increasingly unprofitable. Benjamin hoped to increase his fortunes by choosing a new, more

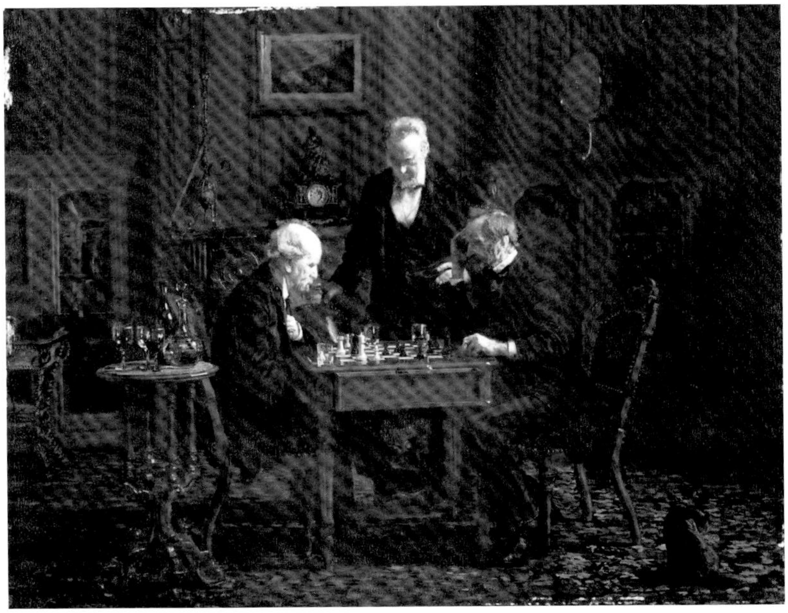

Fig. 67. Thomas Eakins, *The Chess Players*, 1876. Oil on wood, 11¾ × 16¾ in. The Metropolitan Museum of Art, New York. Gift of the Artist, 1881.

lucrative career in the city, and indeed he enjoyed far greater economic benefits as a result of his manual labors than his father. Benjamin's career as a writing master included more than fifty years as calligraphy instructor at the Friends' Central School, in addition to abundant commissions for marriage certificates and graduation diplomas.[2]

Benjamin's fortunes also were improved by his own shrewd skills in managing money. Investments in railroads and real estate provided financial security for the family during his life and support for them after his death.[3] Although Thomas Eakins did not often earn a steady income as an artist and teacher, he lived his entire life in the "modestly affluent" middle-class surroundings he grew up in and celebrated in such paintings as *The Chess Players* (fig. 67). In this painting, we see Benjamin Eakins observing his friends playing chess, surrounded by the fashionable comforts of the family's large home on Mount Vernon Street. As Kathleen Foster writes, "from such an interior, with its new piano, globe, and framed engraving over the mantel, would come an artist to express the values of this culture, so comfortable with its materialism, so confident about its own progress and artful civilization."[4] Alexander, Benjamin, and Thomas Eakins all were the type of "middling" men Benjamin Franklin viewed as the greatest strength of American society.

Thomas paid tribute to his father by emulating his life in many ways. He directed equal effort to teaching and practicing art as his father did, spent most of his life in the family home, and enjoyed similar recreational activities. Benjamin in turn encouraged his son to pursue art, and then sustained him financially.[5] The strength of this support is especially evident in the document Benjamin Eakins penned in 1883:

> This paper made double witnesses an agreement between Thomas Eakins (painter and sculptor, Director of the Schools of the Pennsylvania Academy of the Fine Arts) and Benjamin Eakins his father, owner of the premises 1729 Mount Vernon St. In consideration of the sum of Twenty dollars per month (this until changed or broken by sufficient notice) paid by Thomas Eakins to Benjamin Eakins, Thomas Eakins received his board, lodging, and the exclusive use of the 4th story studio.
>
> Thomas Eakins will have the right to bring to his studio his models, his pupils, his sitters, and whomsoever he will, and both Benjamin Eakins and Thomas Eakins recognizing the necessity and usage of professional secrecy [*sic*], it is understood that the coming of persons to the studio is not to be the subject of comment or question by the family.
>
> B. Eakins
>
> Thomas Eakins
>
> This agreement without date was entered into in the presence of the family in 1871 shortly after my sons [*sic*] return from his studies in Europe but was put into writing in 1883. B. E.[6]

With this lease agreement, Benjamin in effect told his son that he respected and trusted him, and that he needn't worry about supporting himself in another home. It is impossible to know whether Benjamin Eakins agreed with the nude posing that took place in the fourth-floor studio, and we will never know what was said between them in private in 1886, but what happened on record is strong testimony of shared respect. In following years, Benjamin stood by his son through every scandal, even at the expense of relationships with his other children.

Thomas' paintings of his father provide evidence that Benjamin's reverence for his son was amply returned. In *The Writing Master*, Benjamin's head and hands, and the document he is constructing, emerge radiantly from an impenetrable black background—he is center stage, the only player in the drama (fig. 68).[7] We are equally drawn to respect the craft of writing, as all lines in the painting point toward the document, including the axis of the calligrapher's gaze. Overall, the painting is a tribute to the mind, hand, and craft of the aging writing master.

The strong bond between father and son entailed more than just familial loyalty. Thomas Eakins not only resisted aspirations to higher class status than his father enjoyed, he also conducted his personal and professional life in a manner that affirmed the superiority of the middle class. When he wrote to Benjamin in 1866 to complain about Howard Roberts, the artist referred to his fellow école student as a "rich disagreeable young man."[8] The adjectives resonate as synonymous in the construction of the sentence.

In a letter to his Aunt Eliza in the following year, Eakins demonstrated that observation of class relations in Paris only hardened his stance against the rich: "The washwoman goes home in an omnibus and my lady in a state carriage mounted by flunkeys. These footmen and coachmen dress up like monkeys always with long white stockings and high hats with pom poms in them and they often powder their hair. They are low dogs and very insolent to honest people.... They are the only men I can never respect."[9]

Thirty years later, Eakins was no less disgruntled on the subject of class. In February 1897, he wrote to decline an invitation extended by a ladies club to lecture on the academy exhibition for "working people."

> Dear Mrs. Benson,
> With regard to the matter of your letter of the 2d., I do not see my way very clear to comply. The artist's appeal is a most direct one to the public through his art, and there is probably too much talk already.
>
> The working people from their close contact with physical things are apt to be more acute critics of the structural qualities of pictures than the dilettanti themselves and might justly resent patronage.
>
> In my own case, I have not yet found time to examine the Academy exhibit, and would be puzzled indeed to tell anybody why most of the pictures were painted.[10]

Such dismissive comments about the "dilettanti" hardly can have been helpful to Eakins' standing in the eyes of potential patrons. His class prejudices were evidently a problem in other aspects of his career as well.

In some cases, art critics identified leather-apron sensibilities in Eakins' works and rejected them on that ground. When a tony reviewer in the *Art Interchange* of 1879 complained that *The Gross Clinic* was "revolting to the last degree, with the repulsiveness of its almost Hogarthian detail," it was a signal to readers that the painting was not appropriate for "refined" upper-class viewers.[11] Just as Hogarth's world of undisciplined working-class children and uncouth adults was not the proper addition to a drawing room, so Eakins' portrait of Gross also was the province of lower sorts.

The physician who was the painting's portrait subject might have found the association apt, and not unwelcome. Throughout the nineteenth century, medicine strove to treat bodies without regard to class. Gross himself wrote in 1868: "It is the glory of our profession that the ragged pauper, feeding upon the husks of the rich man's table, receives as much care and sympathy, when the subject of disease or injury, as the millionaire, the merchant prince, or the chief magistrate of a nation."[12] This was an appropriate goal for a profession populated mostly by middle-class men.

Eakins never painted ragged paupers, and he didn't like to hire them as models, instead focusing on Philadelphia's social segment between the realms of pauper and merchant

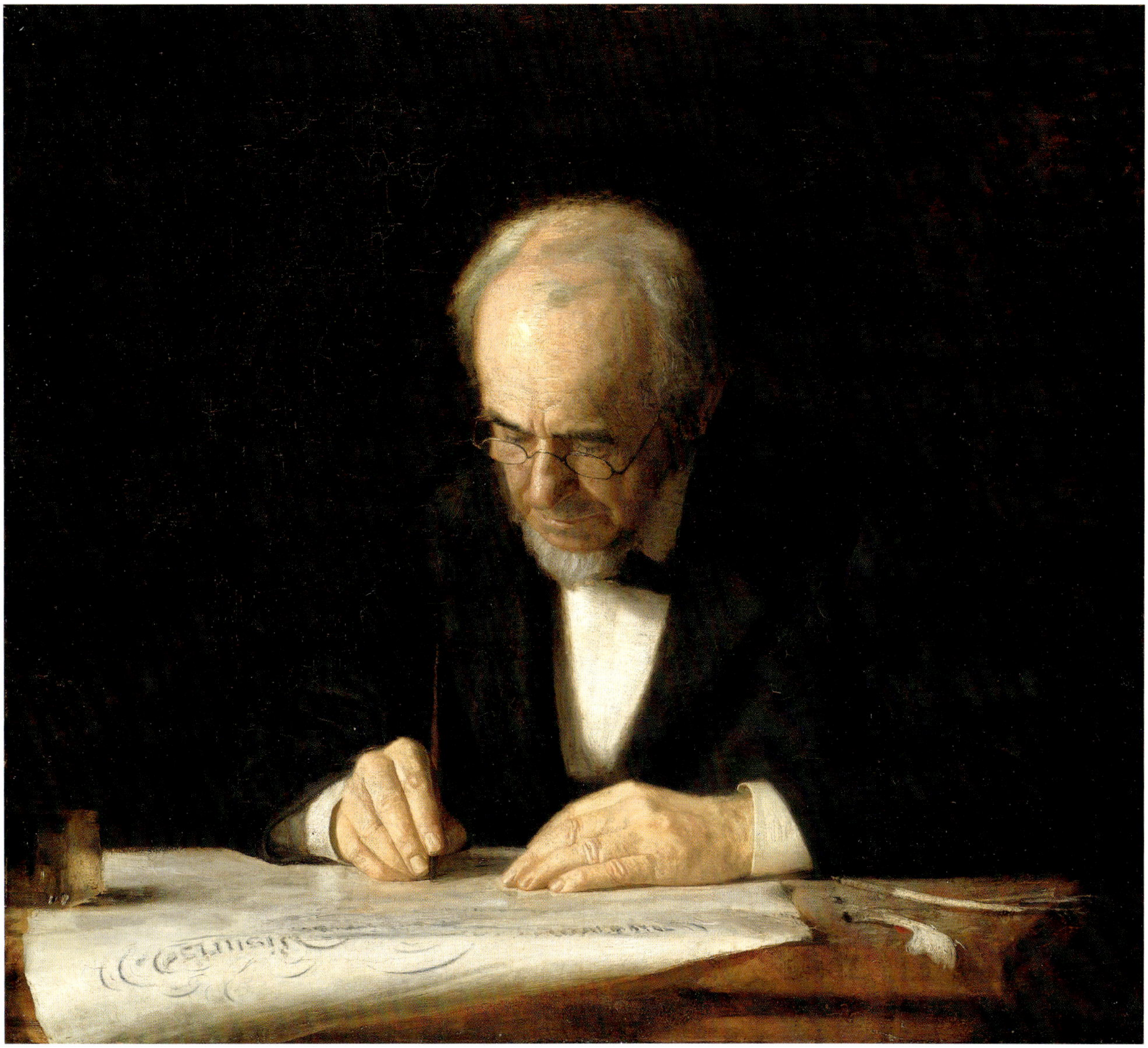

Fig. 68. Thomas Eakins, *The Writing Master (Portrait of Benjamin Eakins)*, 1882. Oil on canvas, 30 × 34¼ in. The Metropolitan Museum of Art, New York.

prince. His canvases are peopled with fishermen, athletes, doctors, scientists, and performers, most of whom fell into the increasingly stratified middle class of the city. Following in the footsteps of his father, Eakins throughout his career also maintained a leather-apron style in which hourly labor always could be comprehended and respected. James McNeill Whistler, in contrast, commented in the introduction to his exhibition "Notes—Harmonies—Nocturnes" in London in 1884: "To say of a picture, as is often said in its praise, that it shows great and earnest labour, is to say that it is incomplete and unfit for view.... Industry in Art is a necessity—not a virtue—and any evidence of the same, in the production, is a blemish, not a quality—a proof, not of achievement, but of absolutely insufficient work."[13] Unlike Whistler, Eakins maintained an old-fashioned embrace of labor in art, and his efforts never were hidden (except in the rare shortcut of using projected images). As a teacher, Eakins expected his students to do the same.

When Fairman Rogers described the curriculum of the Pennsylvania Academy in 1881 following the language supplied by his director of schools, he stressed that the program was designed to produce artists who would work for pay in the trade: "In an examination of the system of the schools of the Pennsylvania Academy of the Fine Arts, it is necessary to bear in mind distinctly that they are supported in the interest of those who intend ... to devote themselves to the production of pictures and statuary as a business or means of livelihood.... [T]he system pursued is not that best adapted to the teaching of drawing as an accomplishment, or to cultivating artistic taste among amateurs."[14] The assumption here was that anyone who did not need to earn a living from art would forever be condemned to the rank of "amateur"—the dilettanti were not welcome because they sought "cultivation" rather than "accomplishment." Eakins' academy instead was going to be the Central High School or the Jefferson Medical College of the art world—scientific, professional, labor intensive, and designed to provide the distinctive hallmarks of specialized and advanced education for employment-seeking graduates.

When students left the academy to form the Art Students' League five years after Rogers' article, class was an obvious fault line dividing Eakins' supporters and detractors. This dimension was blatant in the justifications put forth by H. T. Cresson, the president of the league, as Alan Braddock notes: "Defending his teacher and announcing the new independent organization, Cresson praised what he called the 'young men' who had formed the League, proudly identifying them as 'bohemian' in contrast to the men of 'wealth' in charge of the Academy. Cresson further distanced their clique from notions of aristocracy or bourgeois privilege by calling Eakins a 'conscientious and hard working artist.'"[15] Cresson also stated: "The Art League cordially invites the press to see its methods of study, which will be carried on in the same manner as the French ateliers are conducted. Its members—more especially in the night classes—are composed of that element from whence spring the back-bone and sinews of America. We refer to the laboring classes."[16] This was an art class Benjamin Franklin would have approved. It must have been enormously gratifying for Eakins to have such strident support and advocacy of his views among his students.

It is impossible to know whether Caroline Cowperthwaite Eakins contributed to the class prejudices her son maintained through his life, but we do know that her family fell squarely into the "middling" category of Pennsylvanians shared by her husband and immortalized by her son.[17] Caroline's father was a shoemaker, and among her uncles were an upholsterer named Emmor and her uncle Thomas, a publisher and mapmaker. All of these men undoubtedly bore strong arms and well-stained fingers.[18]

Another familial influence on the Cowperthwaite side is pertinent to study of Thomas Eakins as well. Among the slight documentation of the Cowperthwaites is an interesting comment by Thomas Eakins' early biographer Margaret McHenry, who wrote: "Margaret Jones [Cowperthwaite, Eakins' maternal grandmother], herself an Episcopalian, had married a stern Quaker, and her Cowperthwaite daughters, Eakins' mother and Aunt Eliza, had had a difficult time being fashionable. Eliza would have to take her scarlet crepe dress and jewelry out of the house in her reticule and put them on at a friend's. Another sister was permitted a few tucks in her bonnet and used to wear a pink bow on the side of it that would be away from her father as they sat in meeting house."[19] Caroline's Quaker ancestry raises the question of religious philosophy and influence, for Eakins was descended from practicing Quakers and spent his life in the City of Brotherly Love.

Although it may seem an obvious historical connection, in fact Eakins' religious views have not been extensively discussed. This lacuna undoubtedly is a result of the artist's lack of obvious spiritual practice. In this sense, Eakins again shared a similarity with his predecessors Benjamin Franklin and Charles Willson Peale. As Walter Isaacson writes, "[Franklin] fit squarely into the tradition—indeed, was the first great American exemplar—of the Enlightenment and its Age of Reason. That movement, which rose in Europe in the late seventeenth century, was defined by an emphasis on reason and observable experience, a mistrust of religious orthodoxy and traditional authority, and an optimism about education and progress."[20]

Charles Coleman Sellers situates Peale within the same French, deistic Enlightenment tradition in which God played a rather small role in daily thought. "Young Peale, rather quaintly regarding his Huguenot grandmother as of one heart with the *philosophes*, felt he had his own kinship with France, with Rousseau and Montesquieu.... God was the 'Great First Cause,' but not an ever-active presence."[21] Although surrounded by religious sects, Franklin, Peale, and Eakins all operated on rather secular assumptions following on the ideology of the philosophes.

The brief accounts of Christian influence on Eakins in earlier scholarship are appropriate given the absence of religious study or practice in his immediate family.[22] Benjamin, Caroline, and their children are not known to have attended religious services, and the same is true of many other relatives as well. The only evidence of practice is quite attenuated: the artist's maternal grandfather, Mark Cowperthwaite, came from a family of Friends, but he married a non-Quaker, thus ending his ability to take part in religious worship within his "guarded" community. The only member of Mark's family who seems to have attended a Monthly Meeting is his brother Samuel Cowperthwaite, who received a certificate to worship in the Northern District (Philadelphia) Monthly Meeting in 1793. Eakins' Quaker great-uncle, born in 1765, probably did not live long into the artist's life.[23]

Even more powerful proof of the small place of religion in Eakins' life is his own recorded sentiment on the subject. Late in his life, Eakins painted a series of portraits of Catholic clerics he admired. One of his sitters, however, Cardinal Dennis Dougherty, recalled that "[Eakins] told me he was a man who didn't believe in the divinity of Christ."[24] Earlier in his life, the artist revealed more heated feelings on the subject. He wrote to his sister in 1868: "Think of the comtemtible [*sic*] catholic religion the three in one & one in '3' 3=1 1=3 3x1=1 which they call a mystery & if you don't believe it be damned to you & the virgin mother that afterwards married a man look at it isnt it rediculous [*sic*] ... It is beyond all belief."[25] Despite such powerful irreligious feeling, many aspects of Eakins' ideology—even, surprisingly, statements such as this—reflect the influence of Quaker culture. The historians Hugh Barbour and William Frost write: "What [liberal Quakers] sought was a clear, reasonable, and benevolent deity who would appeal to human intellect.... Early Quakers had opposed the term Trinity as unscriptural; liberal Quakers thought the whole concept was absurd ... just to attempt to conceive of an eternal being dividing into three persons and then deciding to sacrifice one part to another made no sense."[26] Such rationalist thinking is clearly present in Eakins' condemnation of Catholic math.

Despite his weak family history of Quaker relations, and his outspoken irreligious sentiments, parallels like this one reveal that Thomas Eakins grew up so steeped in Quaker culture that a lack of documentary evidence seems beside the point. Whether or not Eakins' own family included practicing Quakers, he lived his life surrounded by Friends. His neighborhood was home to many Quakers.[27] More important, Benjamin Eakins, his most revered mentor, spent most of his professional life deeply involved in the Quaker community.

Benjamin Eakins' fifty-one years of teaching at Friends' Central School was quite uncommon—non-Quakers rarely were employed there in the nineteenth century. Joseph Haines writes in *A History of Friends' Central School:* "In length of service on the faculty, he stands first.... It is a tradition that in [*The Writing Master*] Benjamin Eakins is engraving a Friends' Central School diploma, although it may have been a

Quaker wedding certificate, since Benjamin Eakins' craftsmanship was much sought after by many Quaker brides and grooms."[28] In addition to Benjamin's significant Quaker employment, his "close friends and hunting partners, George Morris and William Hallowell, were from Quaker families."[29]

Long after his death, Benjamin Eakins still was remembered in the context of his Quaker connections. David Wilson Jordan, a pupil and a portrait subject of the artist, recalled in a 1930 interview that Benjamin "was known to everyone in Philadelphia as 'Master Benjamin'—a Quaker phrase, not because he was a Quaker, but because he taught at Quaker schools." Jordan also recalled, as has everyone else who ever wrote about Benjamin Eakins, that he was "very much beloved."[30] Benjamin's admired status may have been a response to the Quaker manner in which he seems to have parented and run his home. As Walter Homan writes, "Quaker parents held authority, but they were to command in love and justice.... The single word which seemed to define the parental authority and express its methods was LOVE."[31] Certainly, no one familiar with the story of Thomas Eakins' life could describe his father with any greater precision. Thomas Eakins' own life followed a very different course, but it was informed by values that can be seen as similarly influenced by the Society of Friends—his scientific bent can be explained as a Quaker habit, as can his carefully observed humanist realism.

As historians note, the empirical basis for Quaker spirituality led many Friends to become scientists or to engage in scientific experimentation as a hobby. In Philadelphia, the prominence of Quaker scientists and physicians among Eakins' colleagues and portrait subjects is especially striking. Edward Coates and Harrison Allen were Quakers, as were Horatio C. Wood, the physician and arachnologist, and Edward Drinker Cope, who attended Friends' School in Westtown, Pennsylvania, and went on to make contributions to the fields of geology, paleontology, herpetology, ichthyology, mammalogy, and comparative anatomy. John Hill Brinton was a Quaker surgeon, and Dr. Benjamin Sharp was a zoologist specializing in marine biology.[32] Eakins' original contribution to the study of motion in humans and animals using photographic equipment, and his publication on equine anatomy, are projects truly Quaker in their objectivity and attention to the details of the natural world.

Eakins also paid close attention to details of nature in the human subjects he portrayed. Scholars, critics, and artists for decades have praised the sense of individualism and humanity in Eakins' portraits. At a deep level, the artist appears to have absorbed the Quaker concept of "Inner Light." In Quaker philosophy, each person is equally and highly valued because of his (or, notably, her) ability to speak directly with God. Direct experience of God is the basis for emphasizing empirical experience in the classroom, as well as in the meetinghouse. "To them it was clear that everyone is endowed at birth with an Inner Light. We can deny this divinity within us as well as outside of us. We can ignore it. We can minimize it. But it is always there ready to be released. And that light, seed or aspect of the Divine is present in everyone, regardless of age, sex, race, nationality, or economic or social status."[33] In the public realm, Quakers put this ideology into practice through their deep involvement in the causes of abolition and suffrage, and through their establishment and support of progressive educational institutions.

A typical example of this activism in Philadelphia was the establishment of the Woman's Medical College of Pennsylvania. The idea for the college originated with Dr. Bartholomew Fussell, a member of the Society; the first two generations of male faculty at the college consisted primarily of Friends; and Joseph Longshore, a "radical Quaker physician," gave the valedictory address at the first commencement of the college. Significantly, Steven J. Peitzman also notes that the founders of the college were not members of "old Philadelphia families," but rather "belonged to a new medical meritocracy of middle-class origins," including several graduates of Central High School.[34]

Eakins' efforts on behalf of equal education for women, despite their uneven results, fit into the same model of radical, egalitarian, middle-class, Quaker, and Central High School alumni ventures. He also demonstrated these influences in teaching his one African-American student—Henry Ossawa Tanner. As in the case of his female students, Eakins welcomed Tanner into his class at the Pennsylvania Academy despite controversy, and then held him to the same high standards as his other students. Tanner recalled in his autobiography: "Mr. Thomas Eakins, under whom I was studying at the Pennsylvania Academy of Fine Arts, gave me a criticism which aided me then, and ever since; and, as it may apply to all walks of life, I will 'pass it along.' I had made a start on a study, which was not altogether bad, but very probably the best thing I had ever done. He encouraged me; but, instead of working to make it better, I became afraid I should destroy what I had done, and really did nothing the rest of the week. Well, he was disgusted. 'What have you been doing? Get it, get it better, or get it worse. No middle ground of compromise.' With this advice in mind, I did all sorts of things."[35] For Eakins, Tanner's race did not diminish his capacity to push himself to the highest level of achievement as an artist. As with his female students, Eakins gave Tanner the gift of attention and high expectations.

The artist also may be credited with portraying the individuality in each of his portrait subjects with a rigorous gaze, whether his sitter was African-American, as in his portrait of Tanner, young, as in *Baby at Play*, or old. Mrs. Mary Hallock Greenewalt recalled that when she sat for Eakins he exclaimed, "How beautiful an old woman's skin is—all those wrinkles!"[36] In 1881, Eakins explained to William Brownell his policy at the academy to "change the model as often as possible … because it is only by constant change that pupils learn that one model does not look at all like another. There is as much difference in bodies as in faces, and the character should be sought in its complete unity."[37] Eakins' ability to portray the subjects before him with individuality, humanity, anatomical rigor, dignity, and meticulous craftsmanship mark his art as reflective of Quaker and middle-class ideology. In a sense, Eakins was Gross' ideal physician—treating every patient equitably without regard to financial circumstances.

In spite of his profound abilities, Thomas Eakins' Quaker and leather-apron disdain for pretension often was expressed to an off-putting extreme. Eakins preferred, for example, to paint his subjects in their "plain" dress, a preference that recalls Quaker resistance to clothing that was decorative and boastful, rather than simply utilitarian. In Eakins' version, however, the requirement for plainness often was translated into slovenliness—hardly a Quaker tenet. Portrait subject Leslie Miller recalled: "When he painted my portrait he not only wanted me to wear some old clothes but insisted that I go and don a little old sack coat,—hardly more than a blouse,—that he remembered seeing me in, in my bicycle days, and which I certainly never would have worn facing an audience which the portrait presents me doing. He did much the same thing with Dean Holland,—see the picture 'The Dean's Roll-call.' … He made the poor Dean go, too, and put on a pair of old shoes that he kept to go fishing in, and painted him, as you know, shod in this way when he faced a distinguished audience on a very impressive occasion."[38]

Miller also writes about a botched commission Eakins had obtained from the Union League Club to paint U.S. president Rutherford B. Hayes: "He painted the President as he found him, working with the stub of a lead-pencil in the White House, in his shirt-sleeves, with sweat running down his face. I have no doubt he enjoyed doing it, but the League refused to receive it."[39] The Union League Club eventually did take the portrait, but never hung it—the painting has since been lost. Stories of other rejected commissions are numerous. Even more common are stories of sitters who accepted their portraits but never really liked them.

The negative reaction to Eakins' unflinching portrayals of his subjects in their plain dress and manners was matched by the reception of his own clothing and habits. As he grew older, Eakins increasingly took delight in protesting conventions, including the polite niceties and dress codes of bourgeois culture. As Leslie Miller told Lloyd Goodrich: "He really seemed to prefer things that are outside the range of what are usually reckoned as constituting not only the charms but even the amenities of existence.… [I]f you could have seen how he kept his studio and even his house, and on what terms he lived with his monkey and other pets, you would know what I mean. This was one of the things that alienated the inclinations of some of the sitters to whose want of sympathy you allude in your monograph. Mrs. Gillespie, for instance, refused to go near him again after he received her one blistering hot day in his studio up three or four flights of stairs … dressed only in an old pair of trousers and an *undershirt*!"[40] Another portrait subject, Beatrice Fenton, "thought Tom Eakins looked very unconventional. He wore carpet slippers when he came down to her house.... Dr. Fenton, Beatrice's father, ignored the carpet slippers, but not everybody did."[41] Another sympathetic sitter was David Wilson Jordan, who similarly remembered Eakins' "exaggerated sloppiness," with his "shirt coming out of his trousers, pantaloons unpressed, and shoes down at the heel."[42]

Thomas Eakins' shocking dress (or undress) should not be blamed on anyone save himself, and yet there is something oddly, perhaps not-so-vaguely, Quaker about his unconventional choices. Howard H. Brinton writes: "At home and at school the Quaker child came to have a sense of belonging to a 'peculiar people.' His plain dress and special code of behavior reiterated that lesson. He learned to be loyal to his group. He learned not to fear the mockery of the world for his peculiarities. An unmentioned reason for Quaker co-education was the facilitation of this requirement of like-mindedness by making possible acquaintances resulting in marriage within the society. Such apparent tribalism may seem undesirable today."[43]

Once again, Eakins' connections to this religion he undoubtedly never practiced are striking. Eakins never minded his "peculiarity" enough to actually change his behavior, despite the repeated loss of teaching jobs and portrait commissions. His father never seems to have admonished him for behaviors or perceptions that must certainly have been known to him. And Susan Eakins appears to have been a stalwart and like-minded companion. Peculiarity, loyalty, and even tribalism all were values Thomas Eakins and his closest family members and friends maintained with strength and reserve. While certainly Eakins' subversive behavior is in no way a reflection of Quaker cultural values, the artist's willingness to play the part of "scientific" outsider throughout his career certainly found some sanction in the example of the "peculiar" families that surrounded him.[44]

Eakins' tribe included more than just his immediate circle. Because he consistently submitted his work for public exhibition, Eakins attracted the attention of admirers as well as critics. Even *The Gross Clinic* received some good reviews in the 1870s: "The entire picture is a serious, thoughtful work, and we can readily understand what a fascination a subject like this must have for an artist who is himself a profound student of reality. There is thought and feeling of a high order in this painting, and in this respect it is in marked contrast with many of the paintings that surround it."[45] This reviewer was not the only source of moral support the landmark surgical portrait generated for Eakins. As a young woman, Susan Macdowell saw it in 1875 at the Haseltine Gallery, where the painting was exhibited briefly before its forlorn installation at the Centennial Exhibition with the latest bedpans and mosquito netting. She later told Lloyd Goodrich that it was in front of that painting that she first fell in love with Thomas Eakins.[46] Their relationship, including a marriage of thirty years, is by far the happiest storyline of the artist's biography.

Susan Eakins was an ideal partner for Thomas Eakins. Her father, William Macdowell, "was a distinguished reproductive engraver, a well-travelled free-thinking atheist who permitted his daughters to develop their own way."[47] Susan attended Friends' Central School, where Benjamin Eakins taught her the beautiful penmanship she used throughout her life. After graduation, she enrolled at the Pennsylvania Academy, where she joined the inner circle of female artists who dissected and depicted the nude, and frequently posed nude themselves. In the early 1880s, Susan is known to have earned substantial sums selling copies of paintings and her own work as well.[48] She thus fit squarely into the category of working artists who were Thomas Eakins' ideal students, and in fact she was the first recipient of the school's Mary Smith Prize. In 1884, Susan Macdowell and Thomas Eakins were wed in a Quaker ceremony.

The story of the marriage is not entirely positive to modern readers. Susan, one of Eakins' most talented students at the academy, largely gave up painting between the time she married and the time of her husband's death.[49] She did paint during the years of her marriage—Thomas Eakins refers to "both" their studios in a letter of 1890, and we also know that

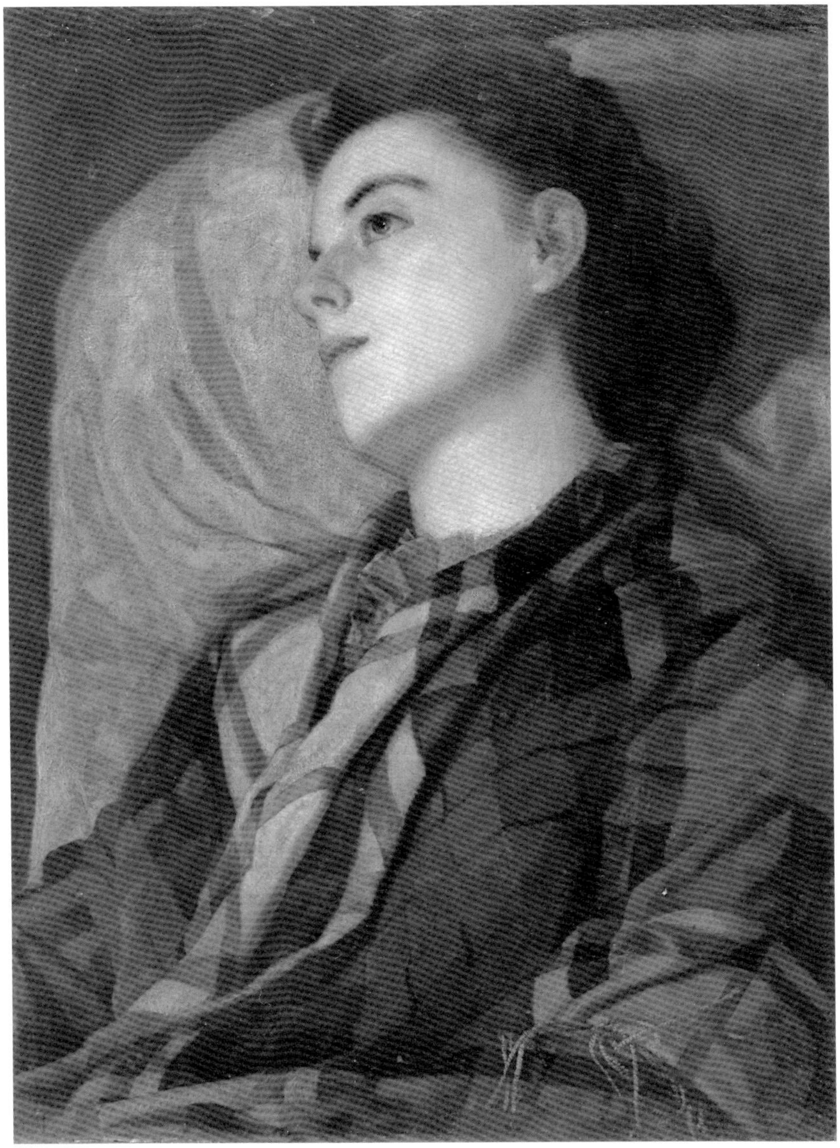

Fig. 69. Susan Macdowell, *Woman in a Plaid Shawl*, c. 1872. Oil on canvas mounted to panel, 28 1/16 × 21 in. Courtesy of the Pennsylvania Academy of the Fine Arts, Philadelphia, Charles Bregler's Thomas Eakins Collection. Purchased with the partial support of the Pew Memorial Trust and the John S. Phillips Fund and the Henry C. Gibson Fund.

she contributed to works including *The Agnew Clinic*.[50] But there are few paintings by Susan that date to her married years. She rather spent a great deal of that time managing the household for not just Thomas but for other members of the Eakins family as well, and writing in her husband's defense when necessary. A painting she made in the early 1870s or 1880s, *Woman in a Plaid Shawl*, demonstrates the promising talent she never fully developed (fig. 69).[51]

Susan Eakins' contributions to her husband's career were not limited to nurturing him while alive. After his death, Susan spent much of the last years of her life promoting the legacy of her husband, with the help of Charles Bregler, who briefly had been his student. Bregler wrote of the marriage: "It may not be amiss to say a few words about Mrs. Eakins, as it is to her untiring devotion for the preservation of his paintings, sculpture, drawings, and other works, that the students of art owe a debt of gratitude, she being an artist and understanding the intrinsic value of his work more fully than would otherwise have been the case, and being the life-long, loving wife and companion of Tom, as Mr. Eakins was affectionately known to her. They first met in the classroom of the Pennsylvania Academy of the Fine Arts, she being a student and he a Professor. Their loves were intertwined with a tenderness, affection and understanding broken only by his death."[52] One especially telling incident reflective of the nature of Susan Eakins' affections is her decision, after her husband's death, to box letters related to his many public and private scandals—many of them quoted here—and to write a note on the box, "Burn These."

Several points are interesting about this moment, when so much of the historical record so easily could have been destroyed. After all, the scandals themselves were long gone, their participants mostly dead. Why had Susan saved these letters? And then, what impulse led her not to burn them herself, but to leave that job for a family friend, who then left it to Eakins' most devoted student Charles Bregler, who also declined to destroy them? Bregler's widow kept the documents under a bed for thirty years along with the refuse of the artist's studio—drawings, manuscripts, oil sketches, and many of the photographs considered so shocking in his time. Susan Eakins would not have left the burning of those documents to fate had she not believed in their exculpatory capacity. She clearly was a true believer, as were the others who also declined to destroy the written records of the artist's darkest hours. Another true believer was Lloyd Goodrich.

In 1982, Goodrich published a revised version of his original 1933 biography of Thomas Eakins. In the later study, Goodrich spent much more time than in the earlier edition politely, though not explicitly, describing the scandals that plagued the artist's life. He disregarded the claims of homosexuality in his broader treatment, writing "there is no reason to get involved in moral issues about this"—even in 1982 he didn't have much interest in discussing the idea.[53] After briefly addressing other claims about the artist, Goodrich summarized his reaction: "Personally, I find it difficult to picture Eakins as a participant in extramarital affairs, in view of his seriousness, dedication to work, scorn of 'silliness,' and incapacity for the customary idealization and illusion—even his abstention from spirituous liquor and his habit of going to bed early and getting up early. He had married relatively late in life, and perhaps his earlier relations with Emily Sartain and Kathrin Crowell had held more youthful ardor; but in his marriage to Susan Macdowell there was complete mutuality of interests, ideas, and beliefs, and, judging by his letters to her from Dakota, deep emotional attachment."[54] Goodrich's heartfelt belief in the depth of Thomas and Susan Eakins' feelings for each other was informed by his own interviews with Susan in the 1930s, and with a variety of people who knew them. Of course, Susan's documented (and lengthy) defense of her husband through his many troubles is a testimony to the strength of their bond as well. Susan without a doubt always believed that his art was worth her sacrifice.

Ultimately, what people believe about Eakins depends on how they feel about his art, and then on what they need to believe about the artist to justify their reactions to the art. For Susan, the seduction of Eakins' paintings was enough to trigger her love, and then to sustain and nourish it through terrible ordeals. For those who respond passionately to art in any era, the process of being seduced is not altogether different, even though the object of our admiration may be long dead. Some of us prefer to fall for transgressive rebels, and others for virtuous innocents. Our fundamental priorities and values may be altered by our attraction to compelling images. For every artist, the ability to seduce viewers and sway critical assessment extends far beyond death. Inevitably, an artist's appeal varies from era to era as each generation applies its own definitions of greatness and depravity.

In the nineteenth century, those who promoted the veneration of our nation's greatest heroes could not imagine that Americans could still admire the author of the following letter:

> June 25, 1745
>
> My dear Friend,
>
> I know of no Medicine fit to diminish the violent natural Inclinations you mention; and if I did, I think I should not communicate it to you. Marriage is the proper Remedy. It is the most natural State of Man, and therefore the State in which you are most likely to find solid Happiness.... But if you will not take this Counsel, and persist in thinking a Commerce with the Sex inevitable, then I repeat my former Advice, that in all your Amours you should prefer old Women to young ones. You call this a Paradox, and demand my Reasons. They are these:
>
> 1. Because as they have more Knowledge of the World and

their Minds are better stor'd with Observations, their Conversation is more improving and more lastingly agreable.

2. Because when Women cease to be handsome, they study to be good. To maintain their Influence over Men, they supply the Dimunition of Beauty by the Augmentation of Utility. They learn to do 1000 Services small and great, and are the most tender and useful of all Friends when you are sick. Thus they continue amiable. And hence there is hardly such thing to be found as an old Woman who is not a good Woman.

3. Because there is no hazard of Children, which irregularly produc'd may be attended with much Inconvenience.

4. Because thro' more Experience, they are more prudent and discreet in conducting an Intrigue to prevent Suspicion. The Commerce with them is therefore safer with regard to your Reputation. And with regard to theirs, if the Affair should happen to be known, considerate People might be rather inclin'd to excuse an old Woman who would kindly take care of a young Man, form his Manners by her good Counsels, and prevent his ruining his Health and Fortune among mercenary Prostitutes.

5. Because in every animal that walks upright, the Deficiency of the Fluids that fill the Muscles appears first in the highest Part: the Face first grows lank and wrinkled; then the Neck; then the Breast and Arms; the lower Parts continuing to the last as plump as ever: So that covering all above with a Basket, and regarding only what is below the Girdle, it is impossible of two Women to know an old from a young one. And as in the dark all Cats are grey, the Pleasure of corporal Enjoyment with an Old Woman is at least equal, and frequently superior, every Knack being by Practice capable of Improvement.

6. Because the Sin is less. The debauching of a Virgin may be her Ruin, and make her for Life unhappy.

7. Because the Compunction is less. The having made a young Girl miserable may give you frequent bitter Reflections; none of which can attend the making an old Woman happy.

8. They are so grateful!!

Thus much for my Paradox. But still I advise you to marry directly; being sincerely

Your affectionate Friend,

Benjamin Franklin.[55]

At a time when America was a scant one hundred years old, Benjamin Franklin was an important part of its founding mythology. Some Americans felt it their patriotic duty to hide the fact that the conqueror of electricity and continental congressman also was a raunchy (and probably unfaithful) lout. His "Advice on Choosing a Mistress" was actively blocked from publication until the twentieth century.

Today, we are less inclined to censor our heroes to boost their stature. More often now, we seek to debunk the inflated images we may have of them. Eakins lived his life and created art in a way that has made him an easy target for modern debunking. But our historical subjects deserve the same common courtesies we hope for the living—the privilege of self-definition to the extent feasible, an effort to understand context and point of view, a presumption of innocence, and finally, not to be neutered, outed, demonized, or similarly categorized to suit the intellectual fashions of our own times. Whatever we may believe, say, or write, no historian or critic can have the last word on a consummate artist whose life was "all in his work." That privilege will reside with Thomas Eakins for as long as his art compels viewers to look deeply.

CHAPTER ONE

From Benjamin Franklin to Thomas Eakins

1. Walter Isaacson, *Benjamin Franklin: An American Life* (New York: Simon and Schuster, 2003), 243.
2. CWP to George Washington, Philadelphia, February 27, 1787, in *The Selected Papers of Charles Willson Peale and His Family*, ed. Lillian Miller, Sidney Hart, and Toby Appel (New Haven: published for the National Portrait Gallery, Smithsonian Institution, by Yale University Press, 1983), 1:473.
3. Eakins' use of photography "for gathering and studying subject matter" was shared by many other artists of the era; Mark Tucker and Nica Gutman, "Photographs and the Making of Paintings," in *Thomas Eakins*, ed. Darrel Sewell (Philadelphia: Philadelphia Museum of Art, 2001), 225.
4. Henry Adams, *The Education of Henry Adams: An Autobiography* (Boston: Houghton Mifflin, 1918), 385.
5. Isaacson, *Benjamin Franklin*, 124. Franklin used the phrase "we, the middling people" in declaring the intentions of shopkeepers to save the colony from expected Native American attacks by gathering a militia. Abandonment of reliance on British military troops was an important step toward revolutionary organization.
6. Jules David Prown, *Art as Evidence: Writings on Art and Material Culture* (New Haven: Yale University Press, 2001), 134.
7. Charles Peale (the elder) taught at the Kent Country School at Chestertown, Maryland. Benjamin Eakins taught at Friends' Central School in Philadelphia.
8. Charles Coleman Sellers, *Mr. Peale's Museum: Charles Willson Peale and the First Popular Museum of Natural Science and Art* (New York: W. W. Norton, 1980), 8.
9. David C. Ward, *Charles Willson Peale: Art and Selfhood in the Early Republic* (Berkeley: University of California Press, 2004), xxiii.
10. The most recent contribution to this scholarship is Henry Adams, *Eakins Revealed: The Secret Life of an American Artist* (New York: Oxford University Press, 2005).
11. For a full recounting of Eakins' correspondence with Sartain, see Patricia Likos Ricci, "*Bella, Cara Emilia:* The Italianate Romance of Emily Sartain and Thomas Eakins," in *Philadelphia's Cultural Landscape: The Sartain Family Legacy*, ed. Katharine Martinez and Page Talbott (Philadelphia: Temple University Press, 2000), 120–37.
12. The story of Lillian Hammitt is recounted by Kathleen A. Foster in Kathleen A. Foster and Cheryl Leibold, *Writing About Eakins: The Manuscripts in Charles Bregler's Thomas Eakins Collection* (Philadelphia: University of Pennsylvania Press, 1989), 95–104.
13. Sellers, *Mr. Peale's Museum*, 8.
14. Elizabeth Johns' excellent biography elucidates this point; *Thomas Eakins: The Heroism of Modern Life* (Princeton: Princeton University Press, 1983).
15. "For these people, science provided access to networks of intellectual and social exchange that crossed boundaries of rank and class, as well as national or colonial borders." Brandon Brame Fortune with Deborah J. Warner, *Franklin and His Friends: Portraying the Man of Science in Eighteenth-Century America* (exh. cat., National Portrait Gallery, Smithsonian Institution, 1999), 4.
16. The prestige Franklin obtained through his many experiments and discoveries (particularly his work with electricity) undoubtedly influenced the happy outcome of French alliance with the Americans during his tenure as delegate from the colonial Congress to France.
17. For a wonderful summary of these portrait conventions, see Fortune and Warner, *Franklin and His Friends.*
18. Benjamin Rush, *Two Essays on the Mind* (New York: Brunner/Mazel, 1972), 96, quoted in Fortune and Warner, *Franklin and His Friends*, 62.
19. Kathleen A. Foster reviews Eakins' "Portraits of Teachers and Thinkers," in *Thomas Eakins*, ed. Sewell, 307–15.
20. Isaacson, *Benjamin Franklin*, 127.
21. Isaacson, *Benjamin Franklin*, 130.
22. Margaret McHenry, *Thomas Eakins Who Painted* (privately printed for the author, 1946), 103.
23. Brooke Hindle, "Charles Willson Peale's Science and Technology," in *Charles Willson Peale and His World*, by Brooke Hindle, Edgar Richardson, and Lillian Miller (New York: Harry N. Abrams, 1983), 110, 148–49, 155. For an excellent overview of Peale's science and engineering, see also Sidney Hart, "To encrease the comforts of Life: Charles Willson Peale and the Mechanical Arts," in *New Perspectives on Charles Willson Peale*, ed. Lillian B. Miller and David C. Ward (Pittsburgh: University of Pittsburgh Press, 1991), 237–65.
24. Hindle, "Charles Willson Peale's Science and Technology," 185.
25. "Advertisement of Moving Pictures, *Pennsylvania Packet*," Philadelphia, May 19, 1785, in *Selected Papers of Charles Willson Peale and His Family*, 1:431.
26. Sidney Hart and David C. Ward, "The Waning of an Enlightenment Ideal: Charles Willson Peale's Philadelphia Museum, 1790–1820," *Journal of the Early Republic* 8, no. 4 (Winter 1988), 401.

27. Hart and Ward, "The Waning of an Enlightenment Ideal," 412.

28. Lillian B. Miller, "Charles Willson Peale as History Painter: The Exhumation of the Mastodon," in *New Perspectives on Charles Willson Peale*, ed. Miller and Ward, 150–51.

29. Edgar Richardson, "Charles Willson Peale and His World," in *Charles Willson Peale and His World*, by Hindle, Richardson, and Miller, 86.

30. Miller, "Charles Willson Peale as History Painter," 160.

31. "Address Delivered by Charles W. Peale to the Corporation and Citizens of Philadelphia, of the 18th day of July, in Academy Hall, Fourth Street" (Philadelphia, 1816), 9–10, quoted in Sellers, *Mr. Peale's Museum*, 18. Peale's egalitarian *intentions* never have been questioned, but David Brigham suggests that the museum ultimately encoded and reified existing patterns of class and gender division in early republican culture. David R. Brigham, *Public Culture in the Early Republic: Peale's Museum and Its Audience* (Washington, D.C.: Smithsonian Institution Press, 1995).

32. Quoted in Sellers, *Mr. Peale's Museum*, 19.

33. Hart and Ward, "The Waning of an Enlightenment Ideal," 394.

34. Lee L. Schreiber reviews the history of early squabbles in the academy in "The Academy: School for Artists or Private Art Club?" *Pennsylvania History* 46, no. 4 (October 1980), 331–50.

35. Lillian B. Miller, *In Pursuit of Fame: Rembrandt Peale, 1778–1860* (exh. cat., National Portrait Gallery, Smithsonian Institution, 1992), 103.

36. Edward J. Nygren, "The First Art Schools at the Pennsylvania Academy of the Fine Arts," *Pennsylvania Magazine of History and Biography* 95, no. 2 (April 1971), 222.

37. William T. Oedel, "After Paris: Rembrandt Peale's Apollodorian Gallery," *Winterthur Portfolio* 27, no. 1 (Spring 1992), 12.

38. E. McSherry Fowble, "Without a Blush: The Movement Toward Acceptance of the Nude as an Art Form in America, 1800–1827," *Winterthur Portfolio* 9 (1974), 113.

39. Fowble, "Without a Blush," 105.

40. Philadelphia Museum of Art, *Philadelphia: Three Centuries of American Art* (exh. cat., Philadelphia Museum of Art, 1976), 165.

41. Quoted in Oedel, "After Paris," 9–10.

42. Fowble, "Without a Blush," 116–17. Rembrandt Peale bid on *Danaë* when it was put up for auction in 1812, but the painting sold for $1,550 (an outrageous sum at the time) to William Hamilton, who leased the painting to a "Mr. Dorsey"—clearly another entrepreneur engaged in the flesh-on-canvas trade. Peale, ever the cup-half-full entrepreneur, described the outcome as beneficial: "Dorsey prepared to exhibit his picture to great advantage, and I hastened to display my *Dream of Love* in my own gallery. Our advertisements were together. Visitors came from his room to mine, and went from my room to his—and I was satisfied with the result." Quoted in David Sellin, *The First Pose: 1876, Turning Point in American Art—Howard Roberts, Thomas Eakins, and a Century of Philadelphia Nudes* (New York: W. W. Norton, 1975), 26.

43. Oedel, "After Paris," 9.

44. Sellers, *Mr. Peale's Museum*, 8.

45. Oedel, "After Paris," 14. For a recent psychoanalytic and poetic reading of this painting, see Alexander Nemerov, *The Body of Raphaelle Peale: Still Life and Selfhood, 1812–1824* (Berkeley: University of California Press, 2001), 163.

46. Oedel surveys critical response to the painting in "After Paris," 9–10.

47. Quoted in Oedel, "After Paris," 23.

48. Hart and Ward, "The Waning of an Enlightenment Ideal," 229.

49. CWP to Thomas Jefferson, Germantown, Pa., October 3, 14, 1811, in *Selected Papers of Charles Willson Peale and His Family*, 1:117.

50. CWP to Rembrandt Peale, Germantown, Pennsylvania, June 4, 8, 1815, in *Selected Papers of Charles Willson Peale and His Family*, 1:330–31.

51. John Vanderlyn was simultaneously trying the same approach in New York, with his own gallery and racy history painting, *Ariadne Asleep on the Island of Naxos*. For a great review of Peale and Vanderlyn, see Oedel, "After Paris."

52. Fowble, "Without a Blush," 118.

53. Quoted in Helen Lefkowitz Horowitz, *Rereading Sex: Battles over Sexual Knowledge and Suppression in Nineteenth-Century America* (New York: Random House, 2003), 214.

54. Oedel, "After Paris," 26.

55. Quoted in Horowitz, *Rereading Sex*, 218. Even in 1842, the New York producers and vendors of obscene materials such as these, indicted in a series of well-publicized arrests, served no more than a month in jail. Most states at midcentury still had few statutes to assist in the prosecution of obscene materials. After 1842, new federal tariff laws were enacted to stop the importation of pornography from Europe. Soon, American writers produced their own "home-grown" works. It is doubtful that Philadelphians were any less able to buy this type of materials than their better-researched New York cousins.

56. Horowitz, *Rereading Sex*, 226–27.

57. Horowitz, *Rereading Sex*, 241, 369, 373.

58. "At this time the term gay referred to those who did not adhere to strict moral standards,

and the gay life meant prostitution or dissipation, not homosexuality." John D'Emilio and Estelle B. Freedman, *Intimate Matters: A History of Sexuality in America* (New York: Harper and Row, 1988), 133, 381 n. 48.

59. Lloyd Goodrich's transcription of TE to Benjamin Eakins, January 16, 1867, The Lloyd Goodrich and Edith Havens Goodrich Archive, Philadelphia Museum of Art.

60. TE to Fanny Eakins, April 1, 1869, Archives of American Art, Smithsonian Institution, Washington, D.C.

61. For a thorough review of Rembrandt Peale's life and work, see Miller, *In Pursuit of Fame.*

62. G. Q. Colton, *A History and Description of Peale's Great National Painting of the Court of Death* (New York: G. Q. Colton, 1859).

63. Quoted in Miller, *In Pursuit of Fame,* 132.

64. These assignments of character are based on the diagram included in *A History and Description of Peale's Great National Painting.*

65. Miller, *In Pursuit of Fame,* 137.

66. See Colton, *A History and Description of Peale's Great National Painting.*

67. C. Edwards Lester, *Artists of America: Rembrandt Peale, Thomas Crawford* (New York: Baker and Scribner, 1846), 226–27.

68. Sylvester Graham, *A Lecture to Young Men* (Providence: Weeden and Cory, 1834), title page.

69. Graham, *A Lecture,* 20.

70. Graham, *A Lecture,* 75–76.

71. Graham, *A Lecture,* 33.

72. Graham, *A Lecture,* 43.

73. Graham, *A Lecture,* 72. Graham was followed as high priest of the sexual reform domain, oddly enough, by another food inventor. John Harvey Kellogg, M.D., of later breakfast cereal fame, published another best-selling cold-shower promoting tome in 1877, *Plain Facts About Sexual Life.* Kellogg's view of sexuality was even darker than Graham's, amplified by a crude conception of genetics. Licentiousness, Kellogg believed, could be passed down to future generations and lead to "the downfall of the nations." One can only hope that Kellogg's cures for masturbation—including circumcision without anesthesia for boys, and carbolic acid applied to the clitoris for girls—never were applied. M. E. Melody and Linda M. Peterson, *Teaching America About Sex: Marriage Guides and Sex Manuals from the Late Victorians to Dr. Ruth* (New York: New York University Press, 1999), 27–32.

74. Melody and Peterson, *Teaching America About Sex,* 46.

75. Graham, *A Lecture,* 73.

76. Anonymous student notebook (1859), unpaginated. Collection, Archives of Central High School.

77. Peale's canvas was not the only evidence of moral reform sentiment still alive and well in the city in 1860. The following October, Beale recorded attending a rousing event: "This morning the United Order of Cadets of Temperance paraded & had a tremendous turnout. Their procession formed in Broad street, & was composed of boys, all sizes." Quoted in Nicholas B. Wainwright, "Education of an Artist: The Diary of Joseph Boggs Beale, 1856–1862," *Pennsylvania Magazine of History and Biography* 97, no. 4 (October 1973), 493.

78. Wainwright, "Education of an Artist," 495.

79. Harry Jacob, personal ms., October 1877, Archives of Jefferson Medical College.

80. William A. Alcott, M.D., *The Physiology of Marriage* (Boston: Dinsmore, 1866; reprinted with an introduction by Charles E. Rosenberg, New York: Arno Press and the New York Times, 1972), 221.

81. See Franklin Spencer Edmonds, *History of the Central High School of Philadelphia* (Philadelphia: J. B. Lippincott, 1902), 27, and Amy Werbel, "Perspective in the Life and Art of Thomas Eakins" (Ph.D. dissertation, Yale University, 1996).

82. Edmonds, *History of the Central High School,* 4.

83. Edmonds, *History of the Central High School,* 27.

84. Edmonds, *History of the Central High School,* 169.

85. Bache served as Central High School's first principal, from 1839 until 1842. See Alexander Dallas Bache, "Report to the controllers of the public schools on the reorganization of the Central High School of Philadelphia" (Philadelphia: Board of Controllers, 1839).

86. Merle M. Odgers, *Alexander Dallas Bache, Scientist and Educator* (Philadelphia: University of Pennsylvania Press, 1947), 99.

87. Rush in particular saw a link between utility and science in education. As an early proponent of public schools, Rush "urged a genuinely useful education, pointedly addressed to the improvement of the human condition. At its heart would be the new sciences, through which citizens might come to know the immutable laws governing nature and humankind and on the basis of which they might build a society founded on reason and conformity to moral truth." Lawrence A. Cremin, *American Education: The National Experience, 1783–1876* (New York: Harper and Row, 1980), 3–4.

88. "Thirty-Ninth Annual Report of the Controllers of the Public Schools of the First District of Pennsylvania" (Philadelphia: Board of Controllers, 1858), 128.

89. "Thirty-Ninth through Forty-Third Annual Reports of the Controllers of the

Public Schools of the First District of Pennsylvania" (Philadelphia: Board of Controllers, 1858–61).

90. Peter Marzio, "The Art Crusade: An Analysis of American Drawing Manuals, 1820–1860," *Smithsonian Studies in History and Technology* 34 (1976), 12.

91. Amy B. Werbel, "Thomas Eakins: Last of the Art Crusaders," in *A Drawing Manual by Thomas Eakins*, ed. Kathleen A. Foster (New Haven: Philadelphia Museum of Art in association with Yale University Press, 2005), 34, 38.

92. In all these ways, Eakins' drawing manual clearly reflected Peale's sensibilities. His own text, however, was far less influential—Eakins' drawing manual never was completed, and it was published only ninety years after his death, while tens of thousands of copies of *Graphics* flooded American schools and homes in the mid-nineteenth century.

93. Edmonds, *History of the Central High School*, 108.

94. Isaacson, *Benjamin Franklin*, 120.

CHAPTER TWO

The Agnew Clinic, *The Gross Clinic*, *The Crucifixion*, and *Swimming*

1. The names of the portrait subjects, most of them members of the class of 1889, are recorded in "The Unidentified Student in the Agnew Painting," *Old Penn Weekly Review*, October 30, 1915, University of Pennsylvania Archives.

2. J. William White, M.D., "Memoir of D. Hayes Agnew, LL.D.," *University of Pennsylvania Medical Magazine* (February 1893), 10.

3. Margaret McHenry writes: "Mrs. Eakins told Dr. Nitzsche of the University of Pennsylvania that she herself had done the actual painting of that small portrait of her husband." Margaret McHenry, *Thomas Eakins Who Painted* (privately printed for the author, 1946), 143.

4. TE to Caroline Eakins, February 28, 1867, Archives of the Pennsylvania Academy of the Fine Arts.

5. Elizabeth Johns, *Thomas Eakins: The Heroism of Modern Life* (Princeton: Princeton University Press, 1983), 53.

6. Julie S. Berkowitz, *Adorn the Halls: History of the Art Collection at Thomas Jefferson University* (Philadelphia: Thomas Jefferson University, 1999), 124–25.

7. See John Harley Warner, *Against the Spirit of System: The French Impulse in Nineteenth-Century American Medicine* (Princeton: Princeton University Press, 1988).

8. Berkowitz, *Adorn the Halls*, 126–27.

9. Thomas Eakins, "The Differential Action of Certain Muscles Passing More than One Joint," *Proceedings of the Academy of Natural Sciences of Philadelphia* (1894), 172–80.

10. D. Hayes Agnew, "An Introductory Lecture delivered in the Philadelphia School of Anatomy" (Philadelphia: Joseph M. Wilson, 1859), 4.

11. This photograph is catalogued in Berkowitz, *Adorn the Halls*, 97.

12. "Fifty-Seventh Annual Announcement of the Jefferson Medical College of Philadelphia" (1881–82), 9.

13. Kenneth M. Ludmerer, *Learning to Heal: The Development of American Medical Education* (New York: Basic, 1985), 55.

14. Although Jefferson prided itself in its literature on offering "practical," "clinical" demonstration in the many hospitals with which it was affiliated, in fact the pedagogical model in both didactic and clinical classes required listening, watching, and memorizing enormous texts, written chiefly by the school's professors. The "Laboratory of Practical and Manipulative Obstetrics," for example, relied principally on the use of cadavers, "and, in addition, models, diagrams and the manikin." "Fifty-Seventh Annual Announcement," 11.

15. David Y. Cooper III and Marshall A. Ledger, *Innovation and Tradition at the University of Pennsylvania School of Medicine: An Anecdotal Journey* (Philadelphia: University of Pennsylvania Press, 1990), 116.

16. William Williams Keen, "Personal Recollections," typed manuscript, undated, Archives of the College of Physicians of Philadelphia, 2–3.

17. John Ruskin, *The Art Criticism of John Ruskin*, ed. Robert L. Herbert (Gloucester, Mass.: Peter Smith, 1969), 34.

18. Ruskin, *The Art Criticism*, 28.

19. TE to Benjamin Eakins, October 29, 1868, Archives of the Pennsylvania Academy of the Fine Arts.

20. See various pages in *Prospects* 11 (1987).

21. Margaret Supplee Smith, "*The Agnew Clinic*: 'Not Cheerful for Ladies to Look At,'" *Prospects* 11 (1987), 161.

22. TE to Society of American Artists, May 7, 1892, The Lloyd Goodrich and Edith Havens Goodrich Archive, Philadelphia Museum of Art.

23. Quoted in Marc Simpson, "The 1880s," in *Thomas Eakins*, ed. Darrel Sewell (Philadelphia: Philadelphia Museum of Art, 2001), 120.

24. See Amy B. Werbel, "Art and Science in the Work of Thomas Eakins: The Case of *Spinning* and *Knitting*," *American Art* 12, no. 3 (Fall 1998).

25. Werbel, "Art and Science."

26. William C. Brownell, "The Younger Painters of America: First Paper," *Scribner's Monthly* 20, no. 1 (May 1880), 4, and "The Society of American Artists," *Art Interchange* 2, no. 6 (March 19, 1879), 42.
27. W. Clark, "The Fine Arts: Eakins' 'Portrait of Dr. Gross,'" *Philadelphia Daily Evening Telegraph* (April 28, 1876), 4.
28. Clark was irate when the painting was relegated to the exhibition's United States Hospital Building, writing, "It is rumored that the blood on Dr. Gross's fingers made some of the members of the Committee sick but judging from the quality of the works exhibited by them we fear that it was not the blood alone that made them sick." W. Clark, "The Centennial. The Art Department: American Section—Eakins," *Daily Evening Telegraph* (June 16, 1876), 2. For a thorough account of these events, see Gordon Hendricks, "Thomas Eakins's *Gross Clinic*," *Art Bulletin* 51 (March 1969), 57–64.
29. See Werbel, "Art and Science."
30. See Charles Frankenberger, "The Collection of Portraits Belonging to the College," *Jeffersonian* 17, no. 132 (November 1915), 1, and "The Unidentified Student in the Agnew Painting," *Old Penn Weekly Review* (October 30, 1915), 171. Elizabeth Johns writes, "Gross supported [his] picture so completely that when Eakins submitted the painting to the jury of the art section of the Centennial exhibition and the jury rejected it as unsuitable for public display, he arranged to have it exhibited at the medical building under his sponsorship." She also writes of *Agnew:* "With the participation of the surgical community at Penn in bringing the picture into being, another powerful group agreed with the artist that the essence of surgery was not 'decorum' but detailed knowledge, precise skill, and commitment to the alleviation of human suffering." Elizabeth Johns, "'These Men Ought to Be Painted': The Social Context of Eakins' *Portrait of Professor Gross (The Gross Clinic)* and *The Agnew Clinic*," in *Thomas Eakins: Image of a Surgeon* (exh. cat., Walters Art Gallery, 1989), 10–11.
31. Frankenberger, "The Collection of Portraits Belonging to the College," 1.
32. TE to Benjamin Eakins, September 8, 1868, transcript by Lloyd Goodrich, The Lloyd Goodrich and Edith Havens Goodrich Archive, Philadelphia Museum of Art.
33. TE to Earl Shinn, January 30, 1875, Cadbury Papers, Swarthmore College.
34. "Art at the Academy," *Philadelphia Press* (November 25, 1880), 5, and Edward Strahan, "The Pennsylvania Academy Exhibition," *Art Amateur* 4, no. 6 (May 1881), 114–15.
35. "Pennsylvania Art Exhibit," *Public Ledger* (January 16, 1893).
36. Carolyn Kinder Carr, "Prejudice and Pride: Presenting American Art at the 1893 World's Columbian Exhibition," in *Revisiting the White City: American Art at the 1893 World's Fair* (exh. cat., Smithsonian Institution Press, 1993), 104.
37. "The Anorexe Exhibition—Suggestive Pictures—Christ Crucified by Eakins," *New York Times* (May 4, 1882), 5.
38. "The Fine Arts," *Philadelphia Evening Bulletin* (November 13, 1882), 8.
39. "Fine Arts. Exhibition Notes," *Independent* (May 11, 1882), 99.
40. "The Modern Athenian," *Boston Daily Advertiser* (October 7, 1887), 4.
41. "Remarkable Paintings," *Boston Evening Transcript* (October 27, 1887), 4.
42. M. G. Van Rensselaer, "The Society of American Artists, New York, II," *American Architect and Building News* (May 20, 1882), 231; M. G. Van Rensselaer, "Art Matters, New York," *Lippincott's Magazine* n.s. 4 (July 1882), 106. For an excellent discussion of Van Rensselaer's critique, see Lois Dinnerstein, "Thomas Eakins' *Crucifixion* as Perceived by Mariana Griswold Van Rensselaer," *Arts Magazine* 53, no. 9 (May 1979), 140–45.
43. Elizabeth Milroy, "Consummatum Est . . . : A Reassessment of Thomas Eakins' *Crucifixion* of 1880," *Art Bulletin* 71, no. 2 (June 1989), 271.
44. TE to Benjamin Eakins, May 9, 1868, transcribed manuscript, Thomas Eakins Research Collection, Philadelphia Museum of Art, Collection of Daniel W. Dietrich II.
45. Milroy, "Consummatum Est."
46. Quoted in Milroy, "Consummatum Est," 273.
47. McHenry, *Thomas Eakins Who Painted*, 53–54. Marc Simpson also discusses the creation and reception of *The Crucifixion* in "The 1880s," in *Thomas Eakins*, ed. Sewell, 108–9.
48. Goodrich, *Thomas Eakins* 1:190.
49. "With this destination in view, *Swimming* became a catalogue of Eakins's academic techniques, including photographic sessions, wax modeling of the figures, and landscape sketches." Kathleen A. Foster, "Eakins and the Academy," in *Thomas Eakins*, ed. Sewell, 100.
50. Quoted in Simpson, "The 1880s," 114.
51. For a full review of the painting's exhibition history, see Kathleen A. Foster, "The Making and Meaning of *Swimming*," in *Thomas Eakins and the Swimming Picture*, ed. Doreen Bolger and Sarah Cash (exh. cat., Amon Carter Museum, Fort Worth, 1996), 25–27.

52. Kathleen A. Foster, *Thomas Eakins Rediscovered* (New Haven: Yale University Press, 1997), 179.

53. Foster, *Thomas Eakins Rediscovered,* 188.

54. Elizabeth Johns, "*Swimming:* Thomas Eakins, the Twenty-ninth Bather," in *Thomas Eakins and the Swimming Picture,* ed. Bolger and Cash, 68. Martin Berger's interpretation of the painting as a portrait of the professional and personal bond between teacher and students is somewhat similar. Martin A. Berger, *Man Made: Thomas Eakins and the Construction of Gilded Age Manhood* (Berkeley: University of California Press, 2000), 96–97.

55. Johns, "*Swimming:* Thomas Eakins, the Twenty-ninth Bather," 69.

56. Johns, "*Swimming:* Thomas Eakins, the Twenty-ninth Bather," 77–78.

57. Whitney Davis, "Erotic Revision in Thomas Eakins's Narratives of Male Nudity," *Art History* 17, no. 3 (September 1994), 311.

58. Davis, "Erotic Revision," 332.

59. Michael Fried, *Realism, Writing, Disfiguration: On Thomas Eakins and Stephen Crane* (Chicago: University of Chicago Press, 1987), 68. For those who would enjoy reading Fried psychoanalyzed in turn, see Marcia Pointon, "Psychoanalysis and Art History: Freud, Fried, and Eakins," in *Naked Authority* (Cambridge: Cambridge University Press, 1990). She writes: "Fried deploys psychoanalytic theory in a dense analysis that serves to reaffirm a third institution, that of art history, and the role of the male writer within that institution" (p. 58).

60. Jennifer Doyle offers a fine critique of gender and sexuality in Eakins' art and life in "Sex, Scandal, and Thomas Eakins's *The Gross Clinic,*" *Representations* 68 (Fall 1999), 1–33. She summarizes the difficulty of analyzing sexual traits of nineteenth-century individuals along a "diacritical axis homo/hetero": "The terms of his ostracization speak directly to the particular character of late-nineteenth-century sexual politics, as they were *not* defined by a gay/straight distinction but rather as they wove together terms like art, virtue, sexual interest, and sodomy" (p. 8).

61. Carroll Smith-Rosenberg, *Disorderly Conduct: Visions of Gender in Victorian America* (New York: Alfred A. Knopf, 1985), 53–54.

62. Allen Ellenzweig writes that in the 1880s, "close physical intimacy, even between unclothed participants, was available as an expression of the abiding loyalties of colleagues, comrades, and companions." Allen Ellenzweig, *The Homoerotic Photograph: Male Images from Durieu/Delacroix to Mapplethorpe* (New York: Columbia University Press, 1992), 17.

63. TE to unknown recipient, November 26, 1866, transcribed in Lloyd Goodrich papers.

64. Fairman Rogers, "The Schools of the Pennsylvania Academy of the Fine Arts," *Penn Monthly* 22 (June 1881), 456.

65. Warner, *Against the Spirit of System,* 314.

66. Joseph LoPiccolo, "Introduction to the Arcade Edition," in Richard von Krafft-Ebing, *Psychopathia Sexualis: A Medico-Forensic Study,* trans. from the 12th German ed. and with an introduction by Franklin S. Klaf (New York: Arcade, 1998), ix.

67. Krafft-Ebing, *Psychopathia Sexualis,* xxi.

68. Krafft-Ebing, *Psychopathia Sexualis,* xxii.

69. Franklin S. Klaf, "Introduction," in Krafft-Ebing, *Psychopathia Sexualis,* xiv.

70. Klaf, "Introduction," xv; LoPiccolo, "Introduction to the Arcade Edition," x.

71. After chronicling these practices in his case studies, Krafft-Ebing summarized his study of this "pathological" condition with a somewhat sympathetic appraisal, writing that "the majority of homosexuals are happy in their perverse sexual feeling and impulse, and unhappy only in so far as social and legal barriers stand in the way of the satisfaction of their instinct towards their own sex," and that "the sexual life of these homosexuals, with due alteration of details, is entirely like that in normal hetero-sexual love." After chronicling truly violent, often criminal behavior, mutually gratifying sexual experiences would have stood out as a thoroughly different "pathology." Krafft-Ebing, *Psychopathia Sexualis,* 224, 240. While not going so far as to remove the stigma of pathology from homosexuality, the author, on the other hand, emphasized in his text that homosexuality only very rarely led to violent or pederastic behavior. Further, his research proved the relative frequency of such proclivities. In determining percentages of homosexuals (which he sometimes referred to as "urnings"), Krafft-Ebing noted "the subject of one of my cases knows personally, at his home (13,000 inhabitants), fourteen homosexuals. He further declares that he is acquainted with at least eighty in a city of 60,000 inhabitants." Krafft-Ebing, *Psychopathia Sexualis,* 231.

72. J. William White, "Memoir of D. Hayes Agnew, M.D., LL.D.," reprinted from *University Medical Magazine* (February 1893), Archives of the College of Physicians of Philadelphia.

73. Clara Marshall, *The Woman's Medical College of Pennsylvania: An Historical Outline* (Philadelphia: P. Blakiston, 1897), 29.

74. Marshall, *The Woman's Medical College,* 30.

75. Marshall, *The Woman's Medical College,* 31.

76. Bridget L. Goodbody, "The Present

Opprobrium of Surgery: *The Agnew Clinic* and Nineteenth-Century Representations of Cancerous Female Breasts," *American Art* 8, no. 1 (Winter 1994), 39. Here, Goodbody clearly was drawing on the writing of David Lubin a decade earlier, in which he wrote that "the painting depicts an almost exclusively masculine universe whose Cartesian center is male desire, focused and pinpointed. *The Agnew Clinic* permits—in fact, encourages—the spectator to take a 'penis-eye' view of the world." David Lubin, *Act of Portrayal: Eakins, Sargent, James* (New Haven: Yale University Press, 1985), 74. Another source for Goodbody is Pointon, "Psychoanalysis and Art History." For a less strident reading of the meaning of the patient's body and the presence of Nurse Clymer, see Judith Fryer, *The Female Body: Figures, Styles, Speculations* (Ann Arbor: University of Michigan Press, 1991), 235–54.

77. Goodbody, "The Present Opprobrium of Surgery," 43.

78. Goodbody, "The Present Opprobrium of Surgery," 44–45.

79. White, "Memoir of D. Hayes Agnew," 19.

80. Diana E. Long, "The Medical World of *The Agnew Clinic*," *Prospects* 11 (1987), 190–93, 197.

81. White, "Memoir of D. Hayes Agnew," 14, 16.

82. Patricia Hills, "Eakins's *Agnew Clinic* and Sargent's *Four Doctors*," *Prospects* 11 (1987), 226–27.

83. Lubin, *Act of Portrayal*, 34.

84. Michael Fried writes extensively on the "anomalous, baffling, discomfiting" composition of the *Gross Clinic* in *Realism, Writing, Disfiguration*, 61.

85. "The figure embodying reception within the picture, the woman, suggests disease in her very response to the 'actual' medical problem being corrected. Attenuated emotional response, behavior that could be characterized as other to order, maturity, and reason, and the extent to which these signs coalesce as something like epileptic constriction, the physical manifestation of the woman's psychological duress in *The Gross Clinic*, were all associated with hysteria at this time." Eric M. Rosenberg, "'One of the Most Powerful, Horrible, and Yet Fascinating Pictures': Thomas Eakins's *The Gross Clinic* as History Painting," in *Redefining American History Painting*, ed. Patricia M. Burnham and Lucretia Hoover Giese (Cambridge: Cambridge University Press, 1995), 183.

86. Eventually the Pennsylvania Hospital accepted the trainees, who later, in 1884, established the Pennsylvania Hospital Training School for nurses. Thetis M. Group and Joan I. Roberts, *Nursing, Physician Control, and the Medical Monopoly* (Bloomington: Indiana University Press, 2001), 81–82.

87. Mary Virginia Stephenson, R.N., *The First Fifty Years of the Training School for Nurses of the Hospital of the University of Pennsylvania* (Philadelphia: J. B. Lippincott, 1940), 49.

88. Unpublished ms., Mary V. Clymer Papers, Center for the Study of Nursing, University of Pennsylvania, 1888–89.

89. Mary V. Clymer Papers, various pages.

90. Henry Gray, *Anatomy, Descriptive and Surgical* (Philadelphia: Henry C. Lea, 1878), 876–77.

91. Berkowitz, *Adorn the Halls*, 211.

92. Eve Kosofsky Sedgwick, *Epistemology of the Closet* (Berkeley: University of California Press, 1990), 26.

93. Warner, *Against the Spirit of System*, 264.

94. Kenneth Klein, M.D., *Getting Better: A Medical Student's Story* (Boston: Little, Brown, 1981), 30.

95. Klein, *Getting Better*, 47, 53.

96. Perri Klass, *A Not Entirely Benign Procedure: Four Years as a Medical Student* (New York: G. P. Putnam's Sons, 1987), 37.

97. Klein, *Getting Better*, 56.

98. Klein, *Getting Better*, 56–57.

99. Klass, *A Not Entirely Benign Procedure*, 39.

100. Charles LeBaron, *Gentle Vengeance: An Account of the First Year at Harvard Medical School* (New York: Richard Marek, 1981), 171–75.

101. Klass, *A Not Entirely Benign Procedure*, 39.

102. Klein, *Getting Better*, 48. There has recently been a great deal of discussion about the waning of education in gross anatomy—several medical schools have begun to replace cadavers with computerized models. Abigail Zuger, "Anatomy Lessons, A Vanishing Rite for Young Doctors," *New York Times* (March 23, 2004), http://www.nytimes.com/2004/03/23/health/23CADA.html.

103. Cecil Helman, *The Body of Frankenstein's Monster: Essays in Myth and Medicine* (New York: W. W. Norton, 1991), 116.

104. Michel Foucault, *The Birth of the Clinic: An Archaeology of Modern Perception*, trans. A. M. Sheridan Smith (New York: Pantheon, 1973), xiii.

105. Michael Sappol, *A Traffic of Dead Bodies: Anatomy and Embodied Social Identity in Nineteenth-Century America* (Princeton: Princeton University Press, 2002), 3.

CHAPTER THREE
Body Casts and "Anatomical Eyes"

1. *Keen of Philadelphia: The Collected Memoirs of William Williams Keen, Jr.*, ed. W. W. Keen James (Dublin, N.H.: William L. Bauhan), 176–83. The College of Physicians of Phila-

delphia, Mütter Museum, "History and Overview," http://www.collphyphil.org/mutter_hist.htm, n.d. (retrieved June 28, 2006).

2. Object File "Anatomical Casts," many entries dated 1976, Department of American Art, Philadelphia Museum of Art.

3. Catherine Kimock, "Anatomical Drawings," in Kathleen A. Foster, *Thomas Eakins Rediscovered* (New Haven: Yale University Press, 1997), 308–9.

4. It was not until the 1930s that Samuel Murray, a close friend and colleague of the artist, "persuaded Mrs. Eakins to carry out the long deferred wishes of Mr. Eakins" and "have them cast in bronze." Samuel Murray to R. Sturgis Ingersoll, "November 28th," Object File "Anatomical Casts," Department of American Art, Philadelphia Museum of Art.

5. Fairman Rogers, "The Schools of the Pennsylvania Academy of the Fine Arts," *Penn Monthly* 22 (June 1881), 461.

6. Murray to Ingersoll, "November 28th."

7. Maria Jo Chamberlin-Hellman, "Thomas Eakins as a Teacher" (Ph.D. dissertation, Columbia University, 1981), various pages.

8. Chamberlin-Hellman, "Thomas Eakins as a Teacher," 136.

9. Board Minutes, Pennsylvania Academy of the Fine Arts, January 30, 1879, quoted in Chamberlin-Hellman, "Thomas Eakins as a Teacher," 145.

10. Jules David Prown, *Art as Evidence: Writings on Art and Material Culture* (New Haven: Yale University Press, 2001), 12–25.

11. Prown, *Art as Evidence*, 12–25.

12. For a comprehensive survey of the parallels between Rimmer and Eakins, see Chamberlin-Hellman, "Thomas Eakins as a Teacher," 240–43.

13. Anonymous, "American Art Schools: The Pennsylvania Academy Schools," *Art Union* 1, nos. 6–7 (July 1884), 133.

14. For a recent review of art anatomy training since the Renaissance, see Martin Kemp and Marina Wallace, *Spectacular Bodies: The Art and Science of the Human Body from Leonardo to Now* (Berkeley: University of California Press, 2000).

15. In 1879, it was reported that "on the average, a student would spend about six months in the second antique class, a period longer than that usually spent in the first class." Chamberlin-Hellman, "Thomas Eakins as a Teacher," 173.

16. Quoted in Chamberlin-Hellman, "Thomas Eakins as a Teacher," 201.

17. Louise Lippincott, "Thomas Eakins and the Academy," in *In This Academy: The Pennsylvania Academy of the Fine Arts, 1805–1976* (exh. cat., Pennsylvania Academy of the Fine Arts, 1976), 170.

18. See Jennifer Hardin, "The Nude in the Era of the New Movement in American Art: Thomas Eakins, Kenyon Cox, and Augustus Saint Gaudens" (Ph.D. dissertation, Princeton University, 2000), for an excellent review of classical influences in the PAFA curriculum.

19. William C. Brownell, "The Art Schools of Philadelphia," *Scribner's Monthly* 18, no. 5 (September 1879), 742.

20. Kathleen A. Foster, "Eakins and the Academy," in *Thomas Eakins*, ed. Sewell, 96.

21. "An Object-Lesson in Artistic Anatomy," *Art Amateur* 14, no. 2 (January 1886), 32.

22. "55th Pennsylvania Academy of the Fine Arts Annual Catalogue of Classes, Season of 1884–1885" (Philadelphia: Pennsylvania Academy of the Fine Arts).

23. Rogers, "The Schools of the Pennsylvania Academy," 454.

24. Marchal E. Landgren, *Years of Art* (New York: Robert M. McBride, 1940), 27–29.

25. Doreen Bolger, "The Education of the American Artist," in *In This Academy: The Pennsylvania Academy of the Fine Arts, 1805–1976* (exh. cat., Pennsylvania Academy of the Fine Arts, 1976), 59–60.

26. Brownell, "The Art Schools of Philadelphia," 743.

27. John Gadsby Chapman, *The American Drawing-Book* (New York: J. S. Redfield, 1858), 205–7. Eakins did adopt Chapman's perspective system fairly closely in contrast. See Amy Werbel, "Perspective in the Life and Art of Thomas Eakins" (Ph.D. dissertation, Yale University, 1996).

28. John Rubens Smith, *A Compendium of Picturesque Anatomy, Adapted to the Arts of Design, Painting, Sculpture, and Engraving* (Boston: published by the author, 1827), unpaginated.

29. William Rimmer, *Art Anatomy* (Boston: Little, Brown, 1877), unpaginated.

30. Anonymous, "Dr. William Rimmer," pencil notation above: "Transcript," Friday, August 22, 1879.

31. William Williams Keen, "For a Book on Artistic Anatomy or Better Anatomy for Artists," unpublished manuscript (undated), College of Physicians of Philadelphia, 4.

32. Keen, "For a Book on Artistic Anatomy," 17.

33. Henry Gray, *Anatomy, Descriptive and Surgical* (Philadelphia: Henry C. Lea, 1878).

34. Keen, "For a Book on Artistic Anatomy," 42.

35. Brownell, "The Art Schools of Philadelphia," 742.

36. William Wrenshall McCullough, Jr., "Thomas Eakins and American Art Instruction in the Later Nineteenth Century" (M.A. thesis, University of North Carolina at Chapel Hill, 1968), 30. McCullough cites

"Dr. Keen's reports, Archives of the Pennsylvania Academy of the Fine Arts." "While particularly fine specimens were not always available, cadavers were obtained regularly for study at the art school. Academy disbursement records indicate that they were brought to the school through the 1880s." Chamberlin-Hellman, "Thomas Eakins as a Teacher," 220.

37. Quoted in Chamberlin-Hellman, "Thomas Eakins as a Teacher," 217.

38. Brownell, "The Art Schools of Philadelphia," 742–43.

39. Keen, "For a Book on Artistic Anatomy," 12, 29–30.

40. Wm. W. Keen, "On the Systematic Use of the Living Model as a Means of Illustration in Teaching Anatomy," *Transactions of the International Medical Congress* (London: J. W. Kolckmann, 1881), 3–4.

41. Luther Holden, "Landmarks: Medical and Surgical," in Gray, *Anatomy, Descriptive and Surgical*, 913–14.

42. William Sartain, unpublished manuscript, transcribed copy in Thomas Eakins Research Collection, Philadelphia Museum of Art, 20, 35.

43. For a thorough review of Eakins' early demands for better models, see Chamberlin-Hellman, "Thomas Eakins as a Teacher," 134–35, 137.

44. Letter, TE to Committee on Instruction, dated January 8, 1876, but the minutes of the board of the academy for January 8, 1877, prove the date to actually be 1877 and not 1876. Pennsylvania Academy of the Fine Arts.

45. Linda Bantel, *William Rush: American Sculptor* (exh. cat., Pennsylvania Academy of the Fine Arts, 1982), 111. See also Alexander Nemerov, *Mammoth Scale: The Anatomical Sculptures of William Rush* (exh. cat., The Wistar Institute, University of Pennsylvania, 2002).

46. "Fifty-Seventh Annual Announcement of the Jefferson Medical College of Philadelphia: The Session of 1881–1882" (Philadelphia: Jefferson Medical College), 7, 13.

47. "Body Snatching," *Taggart's Philadelphia Sunday Times* (December 10, 1882), unpaginated.

48. See H. Barbara Weinberg, *The Lure of Paris: Nineteenth-Century American Painters and Their French Teachers* (New York: Abbeville, 1991).

49. John Harley Warner, *Against the Spirit of System: The French Impulse in Nineteenth-Century American Medicine* (Princeton: Princeton University Press, 1988), 314.

50. John B. Blake, "Anatomy," in *The Education of American Physicians: Historical Essays*, ed. Ronald L. Numbers (Berkeley: University of California Press, 1980), 36.

51. Quoted in Landgren, *Years of Art*, 29–30.

52. For a good review of these developments in medical education, see William G. Rothstein, *American Physicians in the Nineteenth Century: From Sects to Science* (Baltimore: Johns Hopkins University Press, 1972).

53. Ruth J. Abram, "Soon the Baby Died: Medical Training in Nineteenth-Century America," in *"Send Us a Lady Physician": Women Doctors in America, 1835–1920*, ed. Ruth J. Abram (New York: W. W. Norton, 1985), 20.

54. Harvard introduced faculty salaries subsidized by the university in 1870, and the Jefferson Medical College followed in the early 1880s. See Martin Kaufman, "American Medical Education," in *The Education of American Physicians: Historical Essays*, ed. Ronald L. Numbers (Berkeley: University of California Press, 1980), 16.

55. Kenneth M. Ludmerer, *Learning to Heal: The Development of American Medical Education* (New York: Basic, 1985), 54.

56. TE to the "Board of Directors," April 8, 1885, Archives of the Pennsylvania Academy of the Fine Arts.

57. William Williams Keen, "The Contrast Between the Surgery of the Civil War and That of the Present War," reprint from the *New York Medical Journal*, April 24, 1915. Collection of the College of Physicians of Philadelphia.

58. Brownell, "The Art Schools of Philadelphia," 744–47.

59. Foster, "Eakins and the Academy," in *Thomas Eakins*, ed. Sewell, 103.

60. Even William Rimmer had opened some art education to women in Boston in the 1850s, declaring that "Art is as independent of sex as thought itself." Quoted in Chamberlin-Hellman, "Thomas Eakins as a Teacher," 242.

61. The only co-educational "medical" school in Philadelphia in the 1880s was the sectarian Penn Medical University, which provided education by "eclectic" physicians who were widely viewed as cranks. Penn Medical did not award regular medical degrees and in fact closed due to financial pressures in 1881, after graduating 100 women from its "Female" Department. Regina Markell Morantz-Sanchez, *Sympathy and Science: Women Physicians in American Medicine* (New York: Oxford University Press, 1985), 69.

62. Ludmerer, *Learning to Heal*, 14. Although by 1930 there were only six remaining same-sex programs in the country, "the numbers of women in medical schools fluctuated between 4 and 5% until the beginning of the 1960s." Morantz-Sanchez, *Sympathy and Science*, 65, 314.

63. Michael Sappol, *A Traffic of Dead Bodies: Anatomy and Embodied Social Identity in Nineteenth-Century America* (Princeton: Princeton University Press, 2002), 62.
64. John S. Haller and Robin M. Haller, *The Physician and Sexuality in Victorian America* (New York: W. W. Norton, 1974), 59.
65. Administrators of women's medical colleges and hospitals often sent faculty members to Paris "as an investment in a school's future." Warner, *Against the Spirit of System*, 319.
66. Pioneering female medical professors created their own hospitals for women in New York in 1857, Boston and Philadelphia in 1862, and San Francisco in 1875. Ludmerer, *Learning to Heal*, 14.
67. Clara Marshall, *The Woman's Medical College of Pennsylvania: An Historical Outline* (Philadelphia: P. Blakiston, 1897), 17–20.
68. Marshall, *The Woman's Medical College*, 22–23.
69. Marshall, *The Woman's Medical College*, 25.
70. Marshall, *The Woman's Medical College*, 25.
71. Marshall, *The Woman's Medical College*, 30.
72. Steven J. Peitzman, *A New and Untried Course: Woman's Medical College and Medical College of Pennsylvania, 1850–1998* (New Brunswick, N.J.: Rutgers University Press, 2000), 99.
73. Peitzman, *A New and Untried Course*, 85.
74. "55th Pennsylvania Academy of the Fine Arts Annual Catalogue of Classes, Season of 1884–1885."
75. Quoted in Chamberlin-Hellman, "Thomas Eakins as a Teacher," 141.
76. Keen, "For a Book on Artistic Anatomy," 27.
77. Rogers, "The Schools of the Pennsylvania Academy," 455.
78. McCullough, Jr., "Thomas Eakins and American Art Instruction," 27.
79. TE to Edward Hornor Coates, February 15, 1886, quoted in Kathleen A. Foster and Cheryl Leibold, *Writing About Eakins: The Manuscripts in Charles Bregler's Thomas Eakins Collection* (Philadelphia: University of Pennsylvania Press, 1989), 215.
80. Elizabeth Macdowell to TE, January 31, 1882, Archives of the Pennsylvania Academy of the Fine Arts.
81. Carroll Smith-Rosenberg, *Disorderly Conduct: Visions of Gender in Victorian America* (New York: Oxford University Press, 1986), 247.
82. Anna Sellers to George Corliss, November 24, 1877, Archives of the Pennsylvania Academy of the Fine Arts.
83. Quoted in Peter Marzio, "The Art Crusade: An Analysis of American Drawing Manuals, 1820–1860," *Smithsonian Studies in History and Technology* 34 (1976), 9. Marzio here quotes John Rubens Smith, in *A Key to the Art of Drawing the Human Figure* (Philadelphia: Samuel M. Stewart, 1831).
84. Joseph Pennell, *The Adventures of an Illustrator, Mostly in Following His Authors in America and Europe* (Boston: Little, Brown, 1925), 50.
85. Letter from Diana Franklin, quoted in the minutes of the Committee on Instruction, March 24, 1884, quoted in Chamberlin-Hellman, "Thomas Eakins as a Teacher," 215.
86. Quoted in Landgren, *Years of Art*, 50–51.
87. Helen Lefkowitz Horowitz, *Rereading Sex: Battles over Sexual Knowledge and Suppression in Nineteenth-Century America* (New York: Random House, 2003), 384.
88. Horowitz, *Rereading Sex*, 409–10, 439.
89. Smith-Rosenberg, *Disorderly Conduct*, 250.
90. Smith-Rosenberg, *Disorderly Conduct*, 252.
91. Gray, *Anatomy*, 856–57.
92. Chamberlin-Hellman, "Thomas Eakins as a Teacher," 380, and Foster and Leibold, *Writing About Eakins*, 69, 132.
93. TE to Edward Hornor Coates, February, 1886, Archives of the Pennsylvania Academy of the Fine Arts.
94. Rogers, "The Schools of the Pennsylvania Academy," 455.
95. Quoted in Margaret McHenry, *Thomas Eakins Who Painted* (privately printed for the author, 1946), 30.
96. Keen, in Gray, *Anatomy*, 12.
97. Quoted in Chamberlin-Hellman, "Thomas Eakins as a Teacher," 213.
98. Sappol, *A Traffic of Dead Bodies*, 84.
99. McHenry, *Thomas Eakins Who Painted*, 67.
100. Foster and Leibold, *Writing About Eakins*, 88, 134.
101. Keen, "For a Book on Artistic Anatomy," 16.
102. Sappol, *A Traffic of Dead Bodies*, 81.
103. Quoted in Chamberlin-Hellman, "Thomas Eakins as a Teacher," 247.
104. Holly Pyle Connor, "Not at Home: The Nineteenth-Century New Woman," in *Off the Pedestal: New Women in the Art of Homer, Chase, and Sargent* (exh. cat., The Newark Museum, 2006), 25.
105. TE to E. Mitchell, October 27, 1888, transcript in Lloyd Goodrich and Edith Havens Goodrich Archive, Philadelphia Museum of Art.
106. Edwin H. Blashfield to TE, December 19, 1894, transcript in Lloyd Goodrich and Edith Havens Goodrich Archive, Philadelphia Museum of Art.
107. TE to Edwin H. Blashfield, December 22, 1894, transcript in Lloyd Goodrich and Edith Havens Goodrich Archive, Philadelphia Museum of Art.
108. "A Revolt at Drexel Institute," *Philadelphia Times* (March 14, 1895), 1.
109. "An Object Lesson in Artistic Anatomy,"

Art Amateur 14, no. 2 (January 1886), 32, 34.

110. Sappol, *A Traffic of Dead Bodies*, 313.

111. Brownell, "The Art Schools of Philadelphia," 749.

112. Quoted in Marc Simpson, "The 1880s," in *Thomas Eakins*, ed. Darrel Sewell (Philadelphia: Philadelphia Museum of Art, 2001), 108.

113. Kathleen Foster makes a compelling argument for Eakins' position during this change in tastes, in Kathleen A. Foster, "Realism or Impressionism? The Landscapes of Thomas Eakins," *Studies in the History of Art* 37 (1990), 69–91.

114. E., "Mr. Inness on Art-Matters," *Art Journal* n.s. vol. 5 (1879), 374.

115. "Mr. Inness on Art-Matters," 374–75.

116. Cecilia Beaux, *Background with Figures: Autobiography of Cecilia Beaux* (Boston: Houghton Mifflin, 1930), 96.

117. Lloyd Goodrich, transcripts of interviews with Mrs. Elizabeth M. Corliss, May 21 [no year given], Ms. Montgomery [undated], and Mrs. James Mapes Dodge, May 20 [no year given]. Lloyd Goodrich and Edith Havens Goodrich Archive, Philadelphia Museum of Art.

118. Keen, "For a Book on Artistic Anatomy," 59–60.

119. Michel Foucault, *The Birth of the Clinic: An Archaeology of Modern Perception*, trans. A. M. Sheridan Smith (New York: Pantheon, 1973), 196.

120. S. D. Gross, "The Glory and the Hardships of the Medical Life. Valedictory Address at the 49th Jefferson Medical College Commencement" (Philadelphia, 1875), Collection of the College of Physicians of Philadelphia, 9, 17.

121. Louise Lippincott, "Thomas Eakins and the Academy," in *In This Academy: The Pennsylvania Academy of the Fine Arts, 1805–1976* (exh. cat., Pennsylvania Academy of the Fine Arts, 1976), 170.

122. TE to Edward Hornor Coates, September 11, 1886, Archives of the Pennsylvania Academy of the Fine Arts, quoted in Foster and Leibold, *Writing About Eakins*, 235–38.

123. Jennifer Doyle summarizes this position: "Women, Eakins suggested, could handle looking at and studying naked men, even dissecting cadavers without any jeopardy to either their virtue or their mental stability. This was not an acceptable hypothesis at the time: It was incomprehensible that a woman would exhibit that kind of control over her emotions—to ask her to conquer her feelings, furthermore, amounted to the demand that she overcome femininity itself." In "Sex, Scandal, and Thomas Eakins's *The Gross Clinic*," *Representations* 68 (Fall 1999), 11.

124. TE to Amelia Van Buren, July 9, 1887, Archives of the Pennsylvania Academy of the Fine Arts.

125. W. W. Keen James to Amy B. Werbel, July 23, 2002, collection of the author.

126. Eakins in fact worked with four out of six of the society's founders—he painted Spitzka, and collaborated with William Pepper, Harrison Allen, and Francis X. Dercum on the committee that oversaw Eadweard Muybridge's work at the University of Pennsylvania. The other two founding members of the American Anthropometric Society were Spitzka's father, Edward Charles Spitzka, and Joseph Leidy. Brian Burrell, "The Strange Fate of Whitman's Brain," in *Walt Whitman Quarterly Review* 20, nos. 3–4 (Winter–Spring 2003), 109.

127. Edward Anthony Spitzka, M.D., "A Study of the Brains of Six Eminent Scientists and Scholars Belonging to the American Anthropometric Society" (Philadelphia: The American Philosophical Society, 1907), 176, 177, 211. "Dr. White" was J. William White, the surgeon depicted as assistant in *The Agnew Clinic*. The society also possessed the brains of Napoleon III and Hermann Helmholtz.

CHAPTER FOUR

Art, Pornography, Freak Shows, Medical Pictures, and the Guilty Pleasures of Photography in Nineteenth-Century Philadelphia

1. Letter in response to "questions about the method of study pursued by Thomas Eakins," Susan Eakins to Alfred R. Mitchell, October 26, 1930, Archives of American Art.

2. For a full discussion of Eakins' projections, see Mark Tucker and Nica Gutman, "Photographs and the Making of Paintings," in *Thomas Eakins*, ed. Darrel Sewell (Philadelphia: Philadelphia Museum of Art, 2001), 225–38.

3. "New Discovery in the Fine Arts," *New Yorker* (April 13, 1839), quoted in Mary Warner Marien, *Photography: A Cultural History* (New York: Harry N. Abrams, 2002), 25.

4. François Arago, quoted in Alan Trachtenberg, *Reading American Photographs: Images as History, Mathew Brady to Walker Evans* (New York: Hill and Wang, 1989), 5. For a lovely overview of the invention of photography, see Maria Morris Hambourg, et al., *The Waking Dream: Photography's First Century* (exh. cat., Metropolitan Museum of Art, 1993).

5. Arthur C. Danto, "Men Bathing, 1883: Eakins and Seurat," *ARTNews* 94, no. 3 (March 1995), 96.

6. *A Drawing Manual by Thomas Eakins*, ed. Kathleen A. Foster (New Haven: Philadelphia Museum of Art in association with Yale University Press, 2005), 103.
7. For an excellent discussion of Eakins' process, see W. Douglass Paschall, "The Camera Artist," in *Thomas Eakins*, ed. Sewell, 242–44.
8. Paschall, "The Camera Artist," 248; see also Marien, *Photography: A Cultural History*, 168.
9. Kenneth Finkel, in organizing a publication of nineteenth-century photographs in the collection of the Library Company of Philadelphia, used the categories people, places, objects, events, and views. Loved ones and the famous, mundane views and prestigious buildings, unique objects and important events, all were recorded in photographs of the era. Kenneth Finkel, *Nineteenth-Century Photography in Philadelphia: 250 Historic Prints from the Library Company of Philadelphia* (New York: Dover, 1980).
10. Susan Danly and Cheryl Leibold, eds., *Eakins and the Photograph* (Washington, D.C.: published for the Pennsylvania Academy of the Fine Arts by the Smithsonian Institution Press, 1994), 2.
11. Paschall, "The Camera Artist," 240.
12. Numerous examples of these transactions are discussed in Eakins' letters home, including a letter to Emily Sartain: "Your photograph is far the best I have ever seen of you and I am very thankful for it. I will soon have mine taken and will send it to you." TE to Emily Sartain, November 16, 1866, Archives of the Pennsylvania Academy of the Fine Arts. Eakins' accounts also list several photographic purchases, for example, two entries for "Photographs for Stereoscope" and a "Photograph of Couture" in a letter from TE to Benjamin Eakins, March 17, 1868, Charles Bregler's Thomas Eakins Collection, Pennsylvania Academy of the Fine Arts.
13. Jorge Lewinski, *The Naked and the Nude: A History of Nude Photography* (London: Weidenfeld and Nicolson, 1987), 30.
14. Thomas Waugh, *Hard to Imagine: Gay Male Eroticism in Photography and Film from Their Beginnings to Stonewall* (New York: Columbia University Press, 1996), 61.
15. TE to Caroline Cowperthwaite Eakins, August 30, 1869, Charles Bregler's Thomas Eakins Collection, Pennsylvania Academy of the Fine Arts.
16. Waugh, *Hard to Imagine*, 62. Registered and unregistered life studies in France in the second half of the nineteenth century were produced in several formats, the most popular of which were daguerreotypes, and stereoscopic cards on salted paper in pocket size and larger format. Serge Nazarieff, *Early Erotic Photography* (Cologne: Benedikt Taschen, 1993), 8–11.
17. Anne McCauley points out that by the time Eakins arrived in Paris, few photographers of the nude even were bothering with this small formality. Anne McCauley, "'The Most Beautiful of Nature's Works': Thomas Eakins's Photographic Nudes in Their French and American Contexts," in *Eakins and the Photograph*, ed. Danly and Leibold, 29.
18. Waugh, *Hard to Imagine*, 63.
19. Fragment of letter from TE to Benjamin Eakins, c. October 1867, Charles Bregler's Thomas Eakins Collection, Pennsylvania Academy of the Fine Arts; see also McCauley, "The Most Beautiful of Nature's Works," 34–35, for a full discussion of this letter.
20. TE to Frances Eakins, November 12, 1868, Archives of American Art.
21. Francis Wayland, D.D., *The Elements of Moral Science* (Boston: Gould and Lincoln, 1856), 295.
22. Capt. M. G. Tousley to Abraham Lincoln, March 23, 1864, copy of typescript in Vertical File, Institute for the Study of Sex, Gender, and Reproduction, Indiana University, Bloomington, Indiana; quoted in John D'Emilio and Estelle B. Freedman, *Intimate Matters: A History of Sexuality in America* (New York: Harper and Row, 1988), 132–33.
23. The large number of prostitutes that toured with Civil War soldiers, along with high rates of venereal diseases, indicate that pornography was not the only means by which soldiers satisfied sexual urges. Thomas P. Lowry, M.D., *The Story the Soldiers Wouldn't Tell: Sex in the Civil War* (Mechanicsburg, Pa.: Stackpole, 1994), 55.
24. D'Emilio and Freedman, *Intimate Matters*, 133. See also William H. Gerdts, *The Great American Nude: A History in Art* (New York: Praeger, 1974), 103, and Susan Sontag, who writes: "Photographs can abet desire in the most direct, utilitarian way—as when someone collects photographs of anonymous examples of the desirable as an aid to masturbation." Susan Sontag, *On Photography* (New York: Anchor, 1990), 16–17.
25. Danly and Leibold, eds., *Eakins and the Photograph*, 2.
26. "While nudes had formed a part of the French repertoire of academic studies, or *academies*, they were unknown in the United States until Eakins." Danly and Leibold also note that the "willingness to display photographs of himself and his wife at the Art Students' League was unprecedented in the Victorian period." Danly and Leibold, eds., *Eakins and the Photograph*, 14.
27. Marc Simpson comprehensively traces Eakins' classical references in "Thomas

Eakins and His Arcadian Works," *Smithsonian Studies in American Art* 1, no. 2 (Fall 1987), 71–95. Simpson notes that the painting *Arcadia* from 1883 marks the only time Eakins paired male and female nudes in a canvas. "The painting becomes an affirmation of art's asexual innocence seen through the double remove of childhood and mythical time."

28. Danly and Leibold, eds., *Eakins and the Photograph*, 48–49.

29. The Free Lovers were so outspoken in their attacks on Victorian reticence that Whitman, in a letter to William D. O'Connor (November 12, 1882), expressed his desire to distance himself from the "Free religious and lover folk" who challenged Comstock's attempts to imprison the publishers of his poetry. Rejecting their offers of assistance as well as their flagrant violations of the Comstock Act, Whitman refused to "do any thing to identify myself specially with free love." See Edwin H. Miller, ed., *Walt Whitman: The Correspondence* (New York, 1964), 3:314–15, 335. See also Jesse F. Battan, "The Word Made Flesh: Language, Authority, and Sexual Desire in Late Nineteenth-Century America," in *American Sexual Politics: Sex, Gender, and Race Since the Civil War*, ed. John C. Fout and Maura Shaw Tantillo (Chicago: University of Chicago Press, 1993), 111 n. 55.

30. Elizabeth Johns, "An Avowal of Artistic Community: Nudity and Fantasy in Thomas Eakins's Photographs," in *Eakins and the Photograph*, ed. Danly and Leibold, 82.

31. Jonathan Weinberg, *Male Desire: The Homoerotic in American Art* (New York: Harry N. Abrams, 2004), 18. Johns, "An Avowal," 86, discusses *Swimming* photos as a recreation of Plato's Academy.

32. Allen Ellenzweig, *The Homoerotic Photograph: Male Images from Durieu/Delacroix to Mapplethorpe* (New York: Columbia University Press, 1992), 35.

33. Waugh, *Hard to Imagine*, 42.

34. Another obvious exclusion from Eakins' nudes is the sight of penises in an aroused state, female genitals (at all), or sexual acts. Overt sexual scenes and narratives indelibly marked photographs as destined only for private use or underworld trade.

35. Quoted in Chamberlin-Hellman, "Thomas Eakins as a Teacher," 211.

36. Gérôme "freely advocated that students surround themselves with photographs." Paschall, "The Camera Artist," 240.

37. McCauley, "The Most Beautiful of Nature's Works," 47.

38. Daniel M. Fox and Christopher Lawrence, *Photographing Medicine: Images and Power in Britain and America Since 1840* (New York: Greenwood, 1988), 23.

39. Jacob Mendez DaCosta, "Modern Medicine. A Lecture Delivered October 7, 1882, Introductory to the Course at Jefferson Medical College" (Philadelphia: Lippincott, 1882), 18–19.

40. Fox and Lawrence, *Photographing Medicine*, 51, 142.

41. Robert Bogdan, *Freak Show: Presenting Human Oddities for Amusement and Profit* (Chicago: University of Chicago Press, 1988), 6.

42. Bogdan, *Freak Show*, 12.

43. Bogdan, *Freak Show*, 157.

44. The interesting story of Tom Thumb and his wife is reviewed by Robert Bogdan in *Freak Show*, 148–61.

45. Bogdan, *Freak Show*, 13.

46. Medical photography evolved rapidly in the second half of the nineteenth century, and turned toward interior as well as exterior imaging techniques. Charles Lester Leonard, one of Eakins' portrait subjects, worked with J. William White (Agnew's assistant in *The Agnew Clinic)* to develop X-rays beginning in 1896. Leonard "was the first person to demonstrate the presence of stones in the kidney and other parts of the urinary tract." Unfortunately, Leonard was unaware of the dangers of X-rays and radiation. "By the time he left Penn, his hands were so severely burned that his finger had to be amputated, later his hand, and finally his arm." He died in 1923 from squamous cell cancer. David Y. Cooper III and Marshall A. Ledger, *Innovation and Tradition at the University of Pennsylvania School of Medicine: An Anecdotal Journey* (Philadelphia: University of Pennsylvania Press, 1990), 100.

47. Fox and Lawrence, *Photographing Medicine*, 26.

48. Fox and Lawrence, *Photographing Medicine*, 25–26.

49. Martin Kemp, "'A Perfect and Faithful Record': Mind and Body in Medical Photography Before 1900," in *Beauty of Another Order: Photography in Science*, ed. Thomas Ann (exh. cat., National Gallery of Canada, Ottawa, 1997), 124.

50. Kemp, "A Perfect and Faithful Record," 148.

51. Paschall, "The Camera Artist," 243.

52. Danly and Leibold, eds., *Eakins and the Photograph*, 200.

53. This series is carefully chronicled in Ellwood C. Parry III, "Thomas Eakins's 'Naked Series' Reconsidered: Another Look at the Standing Nude Photographs Made for the Use of Eakins's Students," *American Art Journal* 20, no. 2 (1988), 53–77.

54. Mary Warner Marien discusses Duchenne's

work in *Photography: A Cultural History* (New York: Harry N. Abrams, 2002), 138–39.

55. W. W. Keen, "Report to the Board of Directors of the Penna. Academy of the Fine Arts," unpublished manuscript (April 2, 1878), Archives of the Pennsylvania Academy of the Fine Arts.

56. Chamberlin-Hellman, "Thomas Eakins as a Teacher," 228–29.

57. Keen, "For a Book on Artistic Anatomy," 24.

58. Bogdan, *Freak Show*, 29.

59. Bogdan, *Freak Show*, 29.

60. Trachtenberg, *Reading American Photographs*, 54–57.

61. Trachtenberg, *Reading American Photographs*, 59.

62. As Martin Kemp writes, "it is easy to be dismissive of such pseudo-science, and to exclude it from even the fringes of medical science, but the quantifiable criteria for the definition of race and character possessed an obvious appeal in an age obsessed with the promotion of all branches of the study of humanity into domains of measured certainty." Kemp, "A Perfect and Faithful Record," 128, 130. Alan C. Braddock also discusses the use of gridded backdrops by the British ethnologist John Lamprey, Eadweard Muybridge, and, in another format, Eakins. Alan C. Braddock, "Eakins, Race, and Ethnographic Ambivalence," *Winterthur Portfolio* 33, nos. 2–3 (Summer–Autumn, 1998), 156. Eakins' fanatical devotion to linear perspective demonstrates his comparably intense desire for "measured certainty." For an extensive review of Eakins' perspectival practices see *A Drawing Manual by Thomas Eakins*, ed. Foster; and Werbel, "Perspective in the Life and Art of Thomas Eakins" (Ph.D. dissertation, Yale University, 1996).

63. Parry compares Eakins' photographs with anthropological versions in Parry III, "Thomas Eakins's 'Naked Series' Reconsidered," 68.

64. Alan C. Braddock offers a fascinating discussion of Eakins' relationships with famed anthropologists and portrait subjects Stewart Culin (1899) and Frank Hamilton Cushing (1895). Braddock writes that "the object" of Eakins' portrait of Cushing was "not simply to portray an eminent scientist but to mimic Native American culture, thereby demonstrating ethnographic knowledge and colonial control of that culture." Braddock also writes: "Eakins's emblematic title for the *Culin* portrait emphasized the curator's status as an exemplary type of the modern anthropologist specifically engaged in the scientific excavation, collection, and cataloguing of antiquities." Alan C. Braddock, "Displacing Orientalism: Thomas Eakins and Ethnographic Modernity" (Ph.D. dissertation, University of Delaware, 2002), 308, 329.

65. David M. Lubin, *Picturing a Nation: Art and Social Change in Nineteenth-Century America* (New Haven: Yale University Press, 1994), 220.

66. Douglas R. Nickel, *Dreaming in Pictures: The Photography of Lewis Carroll* (exh. cat., San Francisco Museum of Art, 2002), 11.

67. Morton N. Cohen, *Lewis Carroll: A Biography* (New York: Alfred A. Knopf, 1995), 165–74.

68. Cohen, *Lewis Carroll*, 171.

69. Nickel, *Dreaming in Pictures*, 11.

70. Cohen, *Lewis Carroll*, xxiii. An elegant statement of the Freudian take on Eakins' photographs is provided by Sarah Burns in her book on the subject of the gothic imagination in nineteenth-century America. Viewing the Naked Series as a kind of "visual dissection," Burns reads the subjects of the series "as if they were specimens in some anatomy laboratory ... stripped and exposed from all angles." Burns notes that Eakins includes himself in the experiment, but fails to explain how this fundamentally changes the "eye of power" into "anatomist's eyes." Through the Freudian lens, it makes sense that Eakins treated the body as "a puzzle, to be taken apart and put back together, time and again.... In so doing, he was able to assuage his own repressed fears. Like the bodies he so single-mindedly dismantled and then reassembled in perfect working order, Eakins was haunted by deep-seated anxieties about disintegration, both physical and mental. His fetishism, indeed, may have had something to do with the need for reassurance and defense against unease about sexual potency and function." Sarah Burns, *Painting the Dark Side: Art and the Gothic Imagination in Nineteenth-Century America* (Berkeley: University of California Press, 2004), 214–15.

71. Carol Mavor, *Pleasures Taken: Performances of Sexuality and Loss in Victorian Photographs* (Durham: Duke University Press, 1995), 9.

72. David Lubin makes the case that we are not as good at understanding the therapeutic preventative of visual eroticism as our Victorian ancestors. "What we in our superior wisdom have come to regard as the Victorians' pure sexual desire masquerading as something else may at yet another level symptomize a nonsexual need that those Victorians understood extremely well: the need for irrepressibility in a time of deadening physical and emotional repression." Lubin, *Picturing a Nation*, 262.

73. Nickel, *Dreaming in Pictures*, 13.

74. TE to Benjamin Eakins, March 1866, transcribed copy, Lloyd Goodrich and Edith Havens Goodrich Archive, Philadelphia Museum of Art.
75. Lubin, *Picturing a Nation*, 211–15.
76. Jules David Prown, *Art as Evidence: Writings on Art and Material Culture* (New Haven: Yale University Press, 2001), 209, 213.
77. Martin Berger, *Man Made: Thomas Eakins and the Construction of Gilded Age Manhood* (Berkeley: University of California Press, 2000), 97–98.
78. Keen, "For a Book on Artistic Anatomy," 43.
79. Linda Nochlin, "Issues of Gender in Cassatt and Eakins," in *Nineteenth Century Art: A Critical History*, ed. Stephen F. Eisenman (London: Thames and Hudson, 1994), 267.
80. [Edward Strahan], "Collection of D. O. Mills," *Art Amateur* 3, no. 4 (September 1880), 73.
81. McCauley, "The Most Beautiful of Nature's Works," 37.
82. Rebecca Solnit, *River of Shadows: Eadweard Muybridge and the Technological Wild West* (New York: Penguin, 2003), 78.
83. TE to Eadweard Muybridge, 1879 transcribed draft, Lloyd Goodrich and Edith Havens Goodrich Archive, Philadelphia Museum of Art.
84. Fairman Rogers, "The Zootrope: Action of Animals in Motion—The Muybridge Photographs of Horses—The Instrument as a Factor in Art Studies," *Art Interchange* (July 9, 1879); reprinted in *Eadweard Muybridge: The Stanford Years, 1872–1882* (exh. cat., Stanford University Museum of Art, 1972), 117–19. Janine A. Mileaf provides a thorough assessment of the relation of Eakins' photographs to Muybridge's in "Poses for the Camera: The Muybridge Motion Studies, 1884–1885," *American Art* 16, no. 3 (Fall 2002), 30–53.
85. Charles Bregler to Henri Marceau, April 20, 1943, Philadelphia Museum of Art Archives.
86. "Wonders of the Camera," *New York Times* (March 5, 1888).
87. T. Anshutz to J. L. Wallace, June 18, 1884, typed transcript, Collection of David Sellin.
88. William Pepper, in *Animal Locomotion: The Muybridge Work at the University of Pennsylvania—The Method and Its Result* (Philadelphia: J. B. Lippincott, 1888), 5.
89. Pepper, in *Animal Locomotion*, 6.
90. Paschall, "The Camera Artist," 252.
91. Gordon Hendricks, *Eadweard Muybridge: The Father of the Motion Picture* (New York: Grossman, 1975), 161.
92. William Inness Homer, with John Talbot, "Eakins, Muybridge, and the Motion Picture Process," *Art Quarterly* 26, no. 2 (Summer 1963), 197.
93. Francis X. Dercum, M.D., Ph.D., "A Study of the Normal and Abnormal Movements Photographed by Muybridge," in *Animal Locomotion*, 130–32.
94. Dr. Francis X. Dercum to George E. Nitzsche, May 10, 1929, University of Pennsylvania Archives.
95. Harrison Allen, M.D., "Materials for a Memoir on Animal Locomotion," in *Animal Locomotion*, 35.
96. Allen, "Materials for a Memoir," 36.
97. Dercum, "A Study," 114.
98. T. Anshutz to J. L. Wallace, August 1884, typed transcript, Collection of David Sellin.
99. Edward H. Coates to William Pepper, September 27, 1886, copy of letter, Van Pelt Library, University of Pennsylvania.
100. Untitled, *University Magazine* 10, no. 16 (May 5, 1885), 214–15. University of Pennsylvania Archives.
101. Hendricks, *Eadweard Muybridge*, 168.
102. "Wonders of the Camera," *New York Times* (March 5, 1888).
103. Marta Braun, *Picturing Time: The Work of Etienne-Jules Marey, 1830–1904* (Chicago: University of Chicago Press, 1992), 247.
104. Muybridge changed his name several times before arriving at the final version—Eadweard Muybridge—in 1882. Solnit, *River of Shadows*, 7.
105. Braun, *Picturing Time*, 247.
106. Jennifer Hardin recounts Comstock's raids on a bookstore selling prints in 1883 and on Knoedler's in 1887, in "The Nude in the Era of the New Movement in American Art: Thomas Eakins, Kenyon Cox, and Augustus Saint Gaudens" (Ph.D. dissertation, Princeton University, 2000), 101–23. Comstock confiscated 117 photographs of works of art —mostly French nudes—in 1887. A variety of New York artists spoke to the press in Knoedler's defense, including Augustus Saint-Gaudens, John La Farge, and William Merritt Chase, who argued that Comstock had no art background and thus no right to judge art as decent or indecent.
107. Braun, *Picturing Time*, 249.
108. These sales arrangements are described in "Wonders of the Camera," *New York Times* (March 5, 1888).
109. Dr. Francis X. Dercum to George E. Nitzsche, May 10, 1929. University of Pennsylvania Archives.
110. Hendricks, *Eadweard Muybridge*, 171.
111. Solnit, *River of Shadows*, 39.
112. Solnit, *River of Shadows*, 139.

113. Solnit, *River of Shadows,* 144.

114. Hendricks, *Eadweard Muybridge,* 167.

115. H. L. Bell, Sr., to George E. Nitzsche, December 7, 1923, University of Pennsylvania Archives; quoted in Mileaf, "Poses for the Camera," n. 23.

116. Margaret McHenry, *Thomas Eakins Who Painted* (privately printed for the author, 1946), 75.

117. Parry III, "Thomas Eakins's 'Naked Series,'" 74–75.

118. Coates is thoroughly discussed in Doreen Bolger, "'Kindly Relations': Edward Hornor Coates and Swimming," in *Thomas Eakins and the Swimming Picture,* ed. Doreen Bolger and Sarah Cash (exh. cat., Amon Carter Museum, Fort Worth, 1996), 36–48.

119. Lubin, *Picturing a Nation,* 225.

120. Lubin, *Picturing a Nation,* 258.

121. Kathleen A. Foster, *Thomas Eakins Rediscovered* (New Haven: Yale University Press, 1997), 179.

122. Waugh, *Hard to Imagine,* 48.

123. Elizabeth Johns, "An Avowal of Artistic Community: Nudity and Fantasy in Thomas Eakins's Photographs," in *Eakins and the Photograph,* ed. Danly and Leibold, 67.

124. Weinberg, *Male Desire,* 19.

125. Mileaf, "Poses for the Camera," 31.

CHAPTER FIVE

Scandalous Exposures

1. "Prof. Eakins Resigns," *Philadelphia Press* (February 15, 1886), 4.

2. "The End of Eakins," *Philadelphia Evening Item* (February 15, 1886), 1.

3. Kathleen A. Foster and Cheryl Leibold chronicle the events of this difficult time with enormous clarity and skill in *Writing About Eakins: The Manuscripts in Charles Bregler's Thomas Eakins Collection* (Philadelphia: University of Pennsylvania Press, 1989).

4. TE to Edward H. Coates, February 1886, Archives of the Pennsylvania Academy of the Fine Arts.

5. TE to Edward H. Coates, n.d. (ca. March 10, 1886), quoted in Foster and Leibold, *Writing About Eakins,* 216–18. Eakins' polite letter to Emily Sartain on March 7, 1886, is also preserved in the Pennsylvania Academy Archives.

6. "Indignant Art Students," *Philadelphia Evening Bulletin* (February 16, 1886), 6.

7. "The Eakins Affair," *Philadelphia Evening Item* (February 18, 1886), 1.

8. "Forming a Students' League," *Philadelphia Press* (February 19, 1886), 2.

9. "The Academy Life School," *Philadelphia Evening Bulletin* (February 19, 1886), 4.

10. "Eakins Defended," *Philadelphia Evening Item* (February 22, 1886), 1.

11. The depth of resentment on the part of all these writers suggests that Alice Barber may be the woman in Eakins' arms in the manner of *The Rape of the Sabines.*

12. TE to Edward Hornor Coates, February 15, 1886, quoted in Foster and Leibold, *Writing About Eakins,* 214.

13. TE to John V. Sears, Philadelphia Sketch Club, March 13, 1886, Philadelphia Sketch Club Collection.

14. TE to Emily Sartain, March 25, 1886, Pennsylvania Academy of the Fine Arts Archives.

15. William J. Crowell to TE, March 24, 1886, Charles Bregler's Thomas Eakins Collection at the Pennsylvania Academy of the Fine Arts; quoted in Foster and Leibold, *Writing About Eakins,* 174. Benjamin Eakins' affidavit is lost.

16. Marc Simpson distinguishes between local newspaper accounts of the insurrection at PAFA ("revolt against the generosity of the Academy was deemed rude or foolish") and the national art press, which was "more inclined to favor the students and their enterprise, as well as to downplay the accusations against Eakins." Marc Simpson, "The 1880s," in *Thomas Eakins,* ed. Darrel Sewell (Philadelphia: Philadelphia Museum of Art, 2001), 115.

17. Quoted in Foster and Leibold, *Writing About Eakins,* 215–16.

18. Sarah Burns discusses negative reaction to *The Gross Clinic* in light of contemporary concerns about grave robbing and the ugly horrors of Civil War–era surgery and research involving vivisection. It should be pointed out that there is no evidence that Eakins ever dissected anything alive, or saw a living animal dissected. Sarah Burns, *Painting the Dark Side: Art and the Gothic Imagination in Nineteenth-Century America* (Berkeley: University of California Press, 2004), 188–220.

19. Anatomy was not the only subject that required cadavers. Suzanne M. Shultz writes that "Samuel David Gross, M.D., taught operative surgery on cadavers." Suzanne M. Shultz, *Body Snatching: The Robbing of Graves for the Education of Physicians in Early Nineteenth Century America* (Jefferson, N.C.: McFarland, 1991), 19.

20. Shultz, *Body Snatching,* 20.

21. A. M. Lassek, *Human Dissection: Its Drama and Struggle* (Springfield, Ill.: C. C. Thomas, 1958), 222, quoted in Shultz, *Body Snatching,* 55.

22. W. S. Forbes, M.D., "History of the First Anatomy-Act of Pennsylvania," *Philadelphia*

Medical Journal (November 26, 1898), 1131.

23. William Williams Keen, "Personal Recollections," typed manuscript, undated, Archives of the College of Physicians of Philadelphia, 132.
24. Forbes, "History of the First Anatomy-Act," 1131.
25. Forbes, "History of the First Anatomy-Act," 1133.
26. Shultz, *Body Snatching*, 85.
27. Forbes, "History of the First Anatomy-Act," 1133.
28. Forbes, "History of the First Anatomy-Act," 1134.
29. Forbes directed that the revised Anatomy Act add the requirement that the coroner actually deliver the bodies, rather than just collecting them. Forbes, "History of the First Anatomy-Act," 1134.
30. "More Ghouls Caught," *Philadelphia Press* (December 6, 1882), 1.
31. "More Ghouls Caught," 1.
32. "More Ghouls Caught," 1.
33. "More Ghouls Caught," 2.
34. "More Ghouls Caught," 1.
35. "The Ghouls Denounced," *Philadelphia Press* (December 8, 1882), 1–2.
36. "More Ghouls Caught," 2.
37. Many of the students at Jefferson in these years were Southerners, seeking education as close to home as they could find it. Alan C. Braddock, "Displacing Orientalism: Thomas Eakins and Ethnographic Modernity" (Ph.D. dissertation, University of Delaware, 2002), 397–99. Cecil Helman's account of medical education in apartheid South Africa provides a poignant footnote to this racial hatred in the nineteenth century. She writes of her own medical education in twentieth-century South Africa: "The bodies on the slabs are black, or brown or a grayish-pink. There is no *apartheid* among the dead in our dissecting room but, clustered at one end, the coloured students—barred from ever touching naked white flesh—are permitted only to dissect the bodies of their own kind." Cecil Helman, *The Body of Frankenstein's Monster: Essays in Myth and Medicine* (New York: W. W. Norton, 1991), 115.
38. "The Ghouls Denounced," 2.
39. "McNamee Confesses," *Philadelphia Press* (December 14, 1882), 1.
40. Suzanne M. Shultz writes that the problem of African-American grave robbing was written about as early as the eighteenth century in America. In the pre–Civil War period, "the black population was aware of the grave robbing and cadaver business but was powerless to do anything about it. The most they could hope for if they wished to remain in their graves was to die during the summer when classes were not in session and bodies decomposed rapidly. Shultz, *Body Snatching*, 39.
41. A Listener, "Light out of Darkness," *Philadelphia Inquirer* (December 12, 1882), 3.
42. "The Ghouls Committed," *Philadelphia Press* (December 16, 1882), 1.
43. "Dr. Forbes' Defense," *Philadelphia Inquirer* (March 16, 1883), 2.
44. "The Acquittal of Dr. Forbes," *Philadelphia Inquirer* (March 19, 1883), 2.
45. Forbes included the text of both acts in his "History of the First Anatomy-Act."
46. Julie S. Berkowitz, *Adorn the Halls: History of the Art Collection at Thomas Jefferson University* (Philadelphia: Thomas Jefferson University, 1999), 242.
47. Foster and Leibold, *Writing About Eakins*, 119.
48. TE to Frances Crowell, April 1890, Charles Bregler's Thomas Eakins Collection at the Pennsylvania Academy of the Fine Arts.
49. These charges were mentioned in a letter from Susan to Fanny, complaining of Thomas Eakins' treatment by the family and denying the charges. Foster and Leibold, *Writing About Eakins*, 292–98.
50. Quoted in Foster and Leibold, *Writing About Eakins*, 114.
51. Jennifer Doyle, "Sex, Scandal, and Thomas Eakins's *The Gross Clinic*," *Representations* 68 (Fall 1999), 9–10.
52. My sense here that the meaning of the phrase is hard to gauge first was put forth by Kathleen A. Foster. She writes, "it is possible [Wilde] was simply invoked as the premier of criminally decadent artists." Foster and Leibold, *Writing About Eakins*, 116.
53. Eve Kosofsky Sedgwick, *Epistemology of the Closet* (Berkeley: University of California Press, 1990), 94–95.
54. Mary Warner Blanchard, *Oscar Wilde's America: Counterculture in the Gilded Age* (New Haven: Yale University Press, 1998), 1.
55. For a fascinating account of Wilde's tour, see Blanchard, *Oscar Wilde's America*, 1–43.
56. On March 3, 1895, the day after Wilde filed suit against the marquess, the *Philadelphia Record* carried a review of Wilde's *Importance of Being Earnest* staged at the St. James Theater in London. The reviewer concluded, "Mr. Wilde, appearing at the end, bowed his acknowledgment of a reception which must at all events have gone to increase in his eyes the importance of being Oscar, said nothing, and offended no one." Anonymous, untitled, *Philadelphia Record* (March 3, 1895), 4.
57. "Oscar Wilde Libelled," *Philadelphia Evening Bulletin* (March 2, 1895), 6.
58. Merlin Holland, *The Real Trial of Oscar*

Wilde (New York: HarperCollins/Fourth Estate, 2003), xxvi.

59. "Wilde Scored," *Philadelphia Evening Bulletin* (April 4, 1895), 1.
60. "Oscar Wilde on the Stand," *Philadelphia Press* (April 4, 1895), 1.
61. "Terrible Ordeal for Oscar Wilde," *Philadelphia Inquirer* (April 4, 1895), 2.
62. Holland, *The Real Trial*, 138.
63. For a full transcript of the trial, see Holland, *The Real Trial*. The cross-examination of Wood is recorded on pp. 115–19.
64. "Oscar Wilde's Case Closed," *Philadelphia Times* (April 5, 1895), 1.
65. "Oscar Wilde in a Cell," *Philadelphia Record* (April 6, 1895), 2. For a full account of these events, see Holland, *The Real Trial*.
66. Untitled editorial, *Philadelphia Evening Bulletin* (April 5, 1895), 4.
67. *Philadelphia Times* (April 6, 1895), 4. Throughout coverage of the trial, Wilde was referred to as "the aesthete" and the "Apostle of Aestheticism."
68. "A Blow to Erotics," *Philadelphia Evening Bulletin* (April 8, 1895), 4.
69. Moses Harman, "Heywood Again Under Arrest," *Kansas Liberal* (June 8, 1883), 3; quoted in Jesse F. Battan, "The Word Made Flesh: Language, Authority, and Sexual Desire in Late Nineteenth-Century America," in *American Sexual Politics: Sex, Gender, and Race Since the Civil War*, ed. John C. Fout and Maura Shaw Tantillo (Chicago: University of Chicago Press, 1993), 105–6.
70. Battan also notes that "the goal of Victorian prudery was to use language to properly socialize desire." Battan, "The Word Made Flesh," 105, 121.
71. Kirby Farrell, "Wilde on Trial: Psychic Injury, Exhibitionism, and the Law," in *Processes of Institutionalisation: Case Studies in Law, Prison, and Censorship*, ed. Uwe Böker and Julie A. Hibbard (Essen: Die Blaue Eule, 2001), 63.
72. Farrell, "Wilde on Trial," 63–64.
73. Blanchard, *Oscar Wilde's America*, xii.
74. Holland, *The Real Trial*, xxxiii–xxxiv.
75. James M. Saslow, *Pictures and Passions: A History of Homosexuality in the Visual Arts* (New York: Viking, 1999), 202.
76. Quoted in Holland, *The Real Trial*, 221.
77. Quoted in Holland, *The Real Trial*, 223.
78. Quoted in Holland, *The Real Trial*, 80–81.
79. TE to Jacob Mendez DaCosta, January 9, 1893, transcribed copy, Lloyd Goodrich and Edith Havens Goodrich Archive, Philadelphia Museum of Art.
80. Berkowitz, *Adorn the Halls*, 244.

CONCLUSION
Thomas Eakins' Family Values

Epigraph: Walter Isaacson, *Benjamin Franklin: An American Life* (New York: Simon and Schuster, 2003), 149.

1. J. Eliot Woodbridge, *Cowperthwaite: Seven Generations from Hugh Born in 1648* (Princeton, N.J.: privately printed, 1983), 21.
2. For example, in 1850, he was awarded the contract to produce diplomas for the University of Pennsylvania Medical College. Elizabeth Lamotte Cates Milroy, "Thomas Eakins' Artistic Training, 1860–1870" (Ph.D. dissertation, University of Pennsylvania, 1986), 35.
3. Milroy, "Thomas Eakins' Artistic Training," 37.
4. Kathleen A. Foster, *Thomas Eakins Rediscovered* (New Haven: Yale University Press, 1997), 12.
5. Goodrich writes: "It is said that [Benjamin] told his son before they parted: 'You learn to paint the best you can, Tom; you'll never have to earn your own living.'" Lloyd Goodrich, *Thomas Eakins* (Cambridge: Harvard University Press, 1982), 1:15. Subsequent scholars, including Kathleen A. Foster and Elizabeth Milroy, have noted the subtle pressures Benjamin placed on his son to succeed financially as a painter. Nonetheless, Benjamin did effectively support his son financially through most of his career.
6. Collection of the Joseph Hirshhorn Museum and Sculpture Garden.
7. Michael Fried also describes the tenderness of this image. Michael Fried, *Realism, Writing, Disfiguration: On Thomas Eakins and Stephen Crane* (Chicago: University of Chicago Press, 1987), 39–40.
8. TE to Benjamin Eakins, October 13, 1866, Charles Bregler's Thomas Eakins Collection at the Pennsylvania Academy of the Fine Arts.
9. TE to Eliza Cowperthwaite, July 17, 1867, Charles Bregler's Thomas Eakins Collection at the Pennsylvania Academy of the Fine Arts.
10. TE to Mrs. Benson, February 12, 1897, Lloyd Goodrich and Edith Havens Goodrich Archive, Philadelphia Museum of Art.
11. "The Society of American Artists," *Art Interchange* 2, no. 6 (March 19, 1879), 42.
12. Samuel D. Gross, "The Live Physician. Charge to the Graduates of the Forty-Third Annual Commencement of the Jefferson Medical College of Philadelphia" (Philadelphia, 1868), 15, Jefferson Medical College Archives.
13. James McNeill Whistler, *Notes, Harmonies, Nocturnes* (exh. cat., London, 1884).
14. Fairman Rogers, "The Schools of the Pennsylvania Academy of the Fine Arts," *Penn Monthly* 22 (June 1881), 453.
15. Alan C. Braddock, "Displacing Orientalism: Thomas Eakins and Ethnographic

Modernity" (Ph.D. dissertation, University of Delaware, 2002), 403.

16. "Eakins Defended. Mr. H. T. Cresson Answers Mr. Bement's Remarks in 'The Item' About the Artist," *Philadelphia Evening Item* (February 22, 1886), 1.

17. Caroline Eakins' death certificate lists her as dying of "exhaustion from mania" on June 4, 1872. She was buried at Woodlands Cemetery on June 7, 1872. Philadelphia City Archives, Record Series 76:21, Death Register, 1860–1903.

18. Woodbridge, *Cowperthwaite: Seven Generations*, 21.

19. Margaret McHenry, *Thomas Eakins Who Painted* (privately printed for the author, 1946), 4.

20. Isaacson, *Benjamin Franklin*, 93.

21. Charles Coleman Sellers, *Mr. Peale's Museum: Charles Willson Peale and the First Popular Museum of Natural Science and Art* (New York: W. W. Norton, 1980), 3.

22. Scholars in the past have noted Eakins' Quaker heritage, and sometimes used it to explain aspects of the artist's life. Bryson Burroughs described Eakins' "Quaker-like ... plainness, reserve and integrity" in 1937. Elizabeth Johns supposed it might have been the reason he didn't fight in the Civil War. William Inness Homer has gone the farthest, discussing "secular" Quakerism as an "important source for Eakins' thinking" in several respects. Bryson Burroughs, "An Estimate of Thomas Eakins," *Magazine of Art* (July 1937); Elizabeth Johns, *Thomas Eakins: The Heroism of Modern Life* (Princeton: Princeton University Press, 1983), 11; and William Inness Homer, *Thomas Eakins: His Life and Art* (New York: Abbeville, 1992), 219–21. An excellent new study of Quakerism and the arts is Emma Jones Lapsansky and Anne A. Verplanck, eds., *Quaker Aesthetics: Reflections on a Quaker Ethic in American Design and Consumption* (Philadelphia: University of Pennsylvania Press, 2003).

23. William Wade Hinshaw, *Encyclopedia of American Quaker Geneaology* (Ann Arbor: Edwards Brothers, 1938), 210.

24. This quote is found in a letter from Evan H. Turner, director of the Philadelphia Museum of Art, to Seymour Adelman, in which he quotes a letter he had just found in the Cathedral Archives of SS Peter and Paul, dated April 10, 1948, from Cardinal Dougherty, in which he added: "Whether or not he was an atheist I have not heard. He seemed to be an amiable character." Thomas Eakins Research Archive, Philadelphia Museum of Art.

25. TE to Fanny Eakins, April 1, 1869, Archives of American Art.

26. Hugh Barbour and J. William Frost, *The Quakers* (New York: Greenwood, 1988), 174.

27. "Well suited to Quaker professions of simplicity, row homes on Arch, Vine and Mount Vernon Streets combined quality, comfort, and practicality." Philip S. Benjamin, *The Philadelphia Quakers in the Industrial Age, 1865–1920* (Philadelphia: Temple University Press, 1976), 31.

28. Joseph E. Haines, *A History of Friends' Central School* (Overbrook, Pa.: Magee, 1938), 55.

29. Homer, *Thomas Eakins*, 220.

30. Lloyd Goodrich, transcript of an interview with David Wilson Jordan, May 2, 1930, Lloyd Goodrich and Edith Havens Goodrich Archive, Philadelphia Museum of Art.

31. Walter Joseph Homan, *Children and Quakerism* (Berkeley, Calif.: Gillick, 1939), 9.

32. Biographical files for these doctors are located in the College of Physicians of Philadelphia.

33. Leonard S. Kenworthy, *Quaker Education: A Source Book* (Kennett Square, Pa.: Quaker Publications, 1987), 4.

34. Clara Marshall, *The Woman's Medical College of Pennsylvania: An Historical Outline* (Philadelphia: P. Blakiston, 1897), 10; Steven J. Peitzman, *A New and Untried Course: Woman's Medical College and Medical College of Pennsylvania, 1850–1998* (New Brunswick, N.J.: Rutgers University Press, 2000), 5, 89.

35. Henry Ossawa Tanner, "The Story of an Artist's Life," *The World's Work* 18, no. 2 (June 1909), 11665.

36. Lloyd Goodrich, transcript of an interview with Mrs. Mary Hallock Greenewalt, May 19 and May 20 [no year given], Lloyd Goodrich and Edith Havens Goodrich Archive, Philadelphia Museum of Art. David Lubin agrees with this assessment of Eakins' humanist (and more specifically feminist) contributions in paint when he praises *Edith Mahon* (1904) as a "stunning late portrait" which "draws on a variety of traditional artistic discourses of defeat and disjunction and in so doing appears to deliver an intense psychological study of female subjectivity" that is a "powerful analogue to the fiction of the period by writers such as Kate Chopin, Charlotte Perkins Gilman, and Edith Wharton." David Lubin, "Projecting an Image: The Contested Cultural Identity of Thomas Eakins," *Art Bulletin* 84, no. 3 (September 2002), 512.

37. William C. Brownell, "The Art Schools of Philadelphia," *Scribner's Monthly* 18, no. 5 (September 1879), 742.

38. Leslie Miller to Lloyd Goodrich, April 23, 1930, Lloyd Goodrich and Edith Havens Goodrich Archive, Philadelphia Museum of Art.

39. Miller to Goodrich, April 23, 1930.
40. Miller to Goodrich, April 23, 1930.
41. McHenry, *Thomas Eakins Who Painted*, 51.
42. Goodrich, interview with Jordan.
43. Howard H. Brinton, "Quaker Education in Theory and Practice," *Pendle Hill Pamphlet*, no. 9 (undated), 42–43.
44. A fascinating corollary for Eakins is Alfred Kinsey, who stood at the center of his own peculiar and loyal scientific tribe in the twentieth century.
45. "Fine Arts—The Society of American Artists," *New York Daily Graphic* (March 8, 1879), 38.
46. Jeanette Toohey, "Susan Macdowell Eakins: A Modest Reappraisal," in *Susan Macdowell Eakins, 1851–1938* (exh. cat., Woodmere Art Museum, 2001), 4.
47. David Sellin, "Eakins and the Macdowells and the Academy," in *Thomas Eakins, Susan Macdowell Eakins, Elizabeth Macdowell Kenton: An Exhibition of Paintings, Photographs, and Artifacts* (exh. cat., North Cross School, Roanoke, Va., 1977), 16.
48. Toohey, "Susan Macdowell Eakins," 4–5.
49. Louise Lippincott, "Thomas Eakins and the Academy," in *In This Academy: The Pennsylvania Academy of the Fine Arts, 1805–1976* (exh. cat., Pennsylvania Academy of the Fine Arts, 1976), 170.
50. Eakins referred to "both of our studios" in TE to Frances Crowell, April (?), 1890, Charles Bregler's Thomas Eakins Collection at the Pennsylvania Academy of the Fine Arts.
51. The Pennsylvania Academy of the Fine Arts gives this painting's date as 1872, but in Toohey, "Susan Macdowell Eakins" (p. 6), it is dated to the first half of the 1880s, which probably makes more sense.
52. Charles Bregler, "Thomas Eakins as a Teacher—Second Article," *Arts* 18, no. 1 (October 1931), 42.
53. Goodrich, *Thomas Eakins*, 2:109.
54. Goodrich, *Thomas Eakins*, 2:98.
55. Published in Benjamin Franklin, *Writings* (New York: Library of America, 1987), 302–3.

INDEX

Page numbers in *italics* refer to illustrations